Measuring Medical Professionalism

MEASURING MEDICAL PROFESSIONALISM

David Thomas Stern, Editor

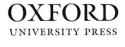

OXFORD
UNIVERSITY PRESS

2006

OXFORD
UNIVERSITY PRESS

Oxford University Press, Inc., publishes works that further
Oxford University's objective of excellence
in research, scholarship, and education.

Oxford   New York
Auckland   Cape Town   Dar es Salaam   Hong Kong   Karachi
Kuala Lumpur   Madrid   Melbourne   Mexico City   Nairobi
New Delhi   Shanghai   Taipei   Toronto

With offices in
Argentina   Austria   Brazil   Chile   Czech Republic   France   Greece
Guatemala   Hungary   Italy   Japan   Poland   Portugal   Singapore
South Korea   Switzerland   Thailand   Turkey   Ukraine   Vietnam

Published by Oxford University Press, Inc.
198 Madison Avenue, New York, New York 10016

www.oup.com

Oxford is a registered trademark of Oxford University Press

Library of Congress Cataloging-in-Publication Data

Measuring medical professionalism / David Thomas Stern, editor.
    p. ; cm.
Includes bibliographical references and index.
ISBN-13: 978-0-19-517226-3
ISBN-10: 0-19-517226-4
1. Medicine—Ability testing. 2. Physicians—Rating of. 3. Physicians—Professional
ethics. 4. Clinical competence—Evaluation. 5. Medical care—Quality control—
Measurement. I. Stern, David Thomas. [DNLM: 1. Physician's Role. 2. Evaluation
Studies. 3. Professional Competence—standards. 4. Professional Practice—standards.
W 21 M484 2005]
R837.A2M43 2005
610.69—dc22   2005007759

9 8 7 6 5 4 3 2 1
Printed in the United States of America
on acid-free paper

Foreword

Jordan Cohen

When I was dean of the medical school at SUNY Stony Brook, we had a vice president for buildings and grounds who had spent most of his earlier career in the military. He had a tough job supervising a large group of mainly unskilled laborers, but the physical condition of the campus under his watch was the best I've ever seen. The grass was always well kempt, graffiti was scrubbed clean as soon as it appeared, broken windows were replaced almost immediately, and dormitory floors were spotless. I asked him once how he managed to maintain such high standards among his workers. His answer taught me one of the most valuable lessons I've ever learned about the importance of evaluation. His secret, he said, was contained in a simple principle: "They don't respect what you *expect*; they respect what you *inspect*." He made it a point to rigorously evaluate the outcomes of the work his employees performed against the high standards he established. It didn't take long for the appearance of the whole campus to reflect the wisdom of this assessment-driven, outcomes-oriented approach to superior performance.

This book attempts to apply that principle to a task far more important than maintaining an immaculate university campus. Ensuring that students of medicine at all levels not only acquire but consistently demonstrate the attributes of medical professionalism is arguably the most important task facing medical educators here at the beginning of the twenty-first century. As noted in detail in chapter 2, many previous attempts have been made to define professionalism, and despite some differences in emphasis and scope, little substantive disagreement exists about the qualities of mind and standards of behavior that constitute this quintessential feature of the complete physician. Thus, we have a good understanding of what to *expect* in this arena. We have much less understanding, however, of how to *inspect* for its presence. And that is why the present volume is so welcomed. What it adds is a much-needed examination of the methods available to assess whether an individual actually manifests the attributes of professionalism.

Why is it so important to ensure that physicians not only understand the core values of professionalism but also conduct themselves in accordance with its precepts in their everyday professional dealings, especially with their patients? Another way of posing that question is to ask, Why is it important to maintain the medical profession's implicit contract with society? For it is professionalism that is the medium though which individual physicians fulfill the lofty expectations that society has of medicine. If norms of physician behavior fall short of the responsibilities called for by medical professionalism, both presumed signatories to the social contract—the profession and the public—are destined to suffer irreparable harm.

For the medical profession, what's at stake is a set of very special privileges that we too often take for granted. Those privileges include (1) the ability to self-regulate, to set our own standards (e.g., medical school admission criteria, licensure requirements, qualifications for board certification, credentials needed for hospital privileges, accreditation standards for medical schools, hospitals, residency programs, and continuing medical education providers); (2) a degree of autonomy in our interactions with patients that is virtually unheard of in any other sector of society; (3) a level of public esteem that surpasses virtually all other lines of work; and (4) an enviable measure of security as evidenced by unparalleled opportunities for well-compensated employment. These exceptional privileges are not birthrights to which doctors are entitled just because they have an MD degree; they are tenuous accommodations granted by society, in return for which society has legitimate expectations. Failing to deliver on those expectations, that is, falling short on the responsibilities of professionalism, will surely result in a withdrawal of the tremendous advantages that now accompany our profession's status.

But as high as the stakes are for the profession, they are much higher still for the public. What medical professionalism affords the public (and individual patients) is of profound and inestimable value, albeit not widely acknowledged. Having a physician imbued with professionalism offers patients by far the best hope for experiencing a beneficial outcome when encountering our increasingly sophisticated and inherently risky health care system. Nothing can substitute for having a trustworthy physician to safeguard a patient's interest: not laws, not regulations, not a patient's bill of rights, not watchdog federal agencies, not fine print in an insurance contract. Nothing. And it is professionalism that is the foundation of trust— trust between the medical profession and society, and trust between doctor and patient. Only by adhering to the fundamental precepts of professionalism can physicians establish the requisite trust that both sustains medicine as a moral enterprise and assures patients that their interests are always of paramount concern.

Why is the task of inculcating and sustaining professionalism such a challenge? Why have medical educators been urged so strongly in recent years to address professionalism in their curricula and to mount effective evaluations of their students' professional attributes? Why must we worry about whether students are being well armed to withstand the threats to professionalism? The answer to these questions is rooted both in certain timeless realities and in the peculiarities of this moment in medicine's history. Among the timeless challenges to sustaining professionalism's behavioral norms, the most basic is human nature itself. All of us have been hard-wired by eons of evolution to look out first for number one. Self-protection is the hallmark of survival. Self-interest, the antithesis of professionalism, is a powerful instinct to overcome. Compounding the innate tendency to serve one's own interests are the innumerable opportunities that physicians have—and always have had—to yield to temptation. Operating in the unwitnessed privacy of the examining room and with the presumed authority of their exclusive knowledge, physicians have always been in a virtually unique position to exploit routine encounters to extract private gain. Few have the inherent conflicts of interest that physicians are forced to contend with on a daily basis. Yet another abiding challenge to professionalism is pressure from physician peers. When many of one's colleagues are seen to abrogate their professional responsibilities, as appears regrettably to be an increasing problem in the present era, the difficulty of sustaining one's commitment to professionalism is understandably intensified.

As if these classic challenges to professionalism were not enough to worry about, we have the added burden of living at a time when medicine finds itself inundated by a wave of commercialism. Whether by intent or otherwise, our country has chosen to rely on the commercial marketplace in an effort to control the escalating costs of health care. As a consequence, medicine is increasingly being viewed by policy makers and others as no different from any other commercial entity. In their view, medicine is just another business. Witness the terminology that has crept into common usage: doctors are commonly referred to as providers; patients, as consumers; health care services, as commodities. As a salient reminder of the fundamental difference between commercialism and professionalism, consider their starkly contrasting mottos. Commercialism's is *caveat emptor*, buyer beware. Medicine's is *primum non nocere*, first do no harm.

The health care system has learned some very important lessons from the world of commerce, and these lessons must be acknowledged. For example, over the past few decades medicine has become more attentive to wasteful effort and expenditures, to sound back-office business procedures, and to the need to systematize routine care. The danger posed by commercialism lies not in medicine's adopting its business-like processes but in medicine's adopting its core ideology. Self-interest, the dominant paradigm of the marketplace, is the very antithesis of the self-sacrifice called for by medicine's commitment to the primacy of our patients' interests. And that is where professionalism enters the picture. For it is the mandates of professionalism that serve to keep self-interest in check; professionalism is the bulwark that prevents physicians' unavoidable conflicts of interest from corrupting the patient–physician relationship and dissipating trust. The last thing most people want is to be distrustful of their physician's motives.

For this reason, measuring medical professionalism in students at all levels should be a top priority of medical educators. We still have much to learn about how to make such measurements as reliable as those we depend upon to evaluate other aspects of physician performance. But the techniques are improving steadily, and those who digest this book will be in the best position to lead this critical field forward.

Acknowledgments

For at least a thousand years, physicians have worked to maintain the highest standards of behavior for this profession. In the last 20 years, medical educators have ventured into the area of assessing professional behavior with the intent of ensuring that physicians exhibit the excellence, humanism, accountability, and altruism that are expected of today's doctors. This exploration has not been a solitary one, but rather a group effort, with a vigorous, open dialogue in the community of medical educators. This book marks a point in time where we can now begin to assert that measuring professional behavior is possible. While there is still a great deal of work to be done, the ideas in this book form the foundation of what is likely to be a more comprehensive assessment of professionalism in physicians for the future.

The ideas in this book derive not only from the authors' individual work but also from the discussions we have had together at meetings and conferences over the years. The Association of American Medical Colleges has dedicated time to research professionalism at meetings for many years, and our dialogue at these meetings has rapidly moved the field forward. Since 1988, the Arnold P. Gold Foundation has created a home and a meeting place for those of us dedicated to this work. Not only was this book outlined at one of their "Barriers to Humanism in Medicine" symposia, but the foundation also followed up with additional support for the research and development of the text. The Gold Foundation (particularly Sandra and Arnold Gold) have provided us with a greater sense of community and purpose and have helped us all work together towards the ultimate goal of ensuring humanistic medical care.

My own work as editor has been supported not only by the Gold Foundation, but also by the University of Michigan, the VA Ann Arbor Healthcare System, and the Institute on Medicine as a Profession at Columbia University. I am grateful for the mentoring, critical feedback, and advice of Jim Woolliscroft, Carl Schneider, David Rothman, and M. Roy Schwarz, who have guided me through various parts of this process. My wife, Deb, has provided limitless enthusiasm and support for my work and my writing, and my boys remind me every day that we are doing this for more than academic reasons.

There is no reason that a group of researchers who focus on professionalism necessarily have to demonstrate the best of professional behaviors themselves. But they do. These authors are more than expert researchers or physicians, they demonstrate the highest degree of collegiality, intellectual integrity, compassion, and teamwork—they practice what they preach. This book is a testament to their diligent and energetic efforts as a team.

Contents

Contributors

Louise Arnold, PhD
Associate Dean and Professor
School of Medicine
University of Missouri, Kansas City

DeWitt C. Baldwin, Jr., MD
Scholar-In-Residence
Accreditation Council for Graduate Medical Education

Jordan J. Cohen, MD
President
Association of American Medical Colleges

Steven R. Daugherty, MD
Assistant Professor
Department of Psychology
Rush Medical College

Kelly Fryer-Edwards, PhD
Assistant Professor
Department of Medical History and Ethics
University of Washington School of Medicine

Shiphra Ginsburg, MD, MEd, FRCOC
Assistant Professor of Medicine
Mount Sinai Hospital
University of Toronto

Fred Hafferty, MD
Professor, Department of Behavioral Sciences
University of Minnesota Medical School, Duluth

Mohammadreza Hojat, PhD
Director, Jefferson Longitudinal Study
Research Professor, Psychiatry and Human Behavior
Center for Research in Medical Education and Health Care

Audiey Kao, MD, PhD
Vice President, Ethics Standards
American Medical Association

Debra Klamen, MD
Associate Dean for Education and Curriculum
Professor and Chair, Department of Medical Education
Southern Illinois University School of Medicine

David C. Leach, MD
Executive Director
ACGME

Lorelei Lingard, PhD
Associate Professor, Department of Paediatrics and Wilson Centre for
    Research in Education
University of Toronto
BMO Financial Group Professor in Health Professions Education Research

Helen Loeser, MD, MSc
Associate Dean, Curricular Affairs
School of Medicine
University of California, San Francisco

Deirdre C. Lynch, PhD
Research and Evaluation Specialist
Research Department
ACGME

John J. Norcini, PhD
President and CEO
Foundation for the Advancement of International Medical Education
    and Research
FAIMER®

Maxine A. Papadakis, MD
Professor of Clinical Medicine
Associate Dean for Student Affairs
School of Medicine
University of California, San Francisco

Linda E. Pinsky, MD
Associate Professor of Medicine
Adjunct Assistant Professor of Medical Education
Division of General Internal Medicine
University of Washington School of Medicine

Lynne Robins, PhD
Director, Teaching Scholars Program
Department of Medical Education and Biomedical Informatics
University of Washington School of Medicine

Donnie J. Self, PhD
Professor of Humanities in Medicine
Texas A and M College of Medicine

David Thomas Stern, MD, PhD
Associate Professor of Internal Medicine and Medical Education
Research Associate Professor, Center for Human Growth & Development
Director, Michigan Global REACH
Director, Minority Health and Health Disparities International Research
    Training Program
University of Michigan Medical School
VA Ann Arbor Healthcare System

Patricia M. Surdyk, PhD
Executive Director
Institutional Review Committee
ACGME

Jon Veloski, MS
Director of Medical Education Research
Center for Research in Medical Education and Health Care

Reed Williams, PhD
Professor and Vice Chair for Educational Affairs
Department of Surgery
Southern Illinois University School of Medicine

Norma Elizabeth Wagoner, PhD
Dean of Students and Deputy Dean for Education Strategy
University of Chicago Pritzker School of Medicine
Professor, Department of Organismal Biology and Anatomy
Division of the Biological Sciences and The College
The University of Chicago

Measuring Medical Professionalism

I

A Framework for Measuring Professionalism

David Thomas Stern

> A pious man stands in a long line at the gates of heaven, wait-
> ing for his audience with St. Peter. After an hour, a man in a
> white coat and stethoscope walks up to the front of the line,
> past St. Peter, and right into heaven. The pious man, upset
> about the break in protocol, asked St. Peter, "Why did that
> doctor skip the line and go right in?" "Oh him?" said St. Peter,
> "That's God—he just thinks he's a doctor."

Doctors are human. We make mistakes of knowledge, technique, and judgment. What characterizes physicians is not infallibility, but a personal and professional obligation to strive for excellence, humanism, accountability, and altruism. For medical educators, these principles of professionalism have special meaning. Excellence implies not only excellent knowledge and skills, but also a commitment to exceed ordinary standards. Humanism represents the principles of respect, compassion, empathy, honor, and integrity. Accountability reflects the action of doctors responding to the needs of patients, health care systems, communities, and the profession itself. Altruism demands that the best interests of patients, not self-interest, guide physicians (see chapter 2 for a full description of these and related terms). This book is about how to measure these principles of professionalism.

Who Cares About Measuring Professionalism?

Our patients and the public care about professionalism because of not only the sensational stories highlighted in the press but also what they hear from friends and what they experience themselves. As an extreme example, Michael Swango is a physician now serving consecutive life sentences in prison for murdering patients. The shocking story of how he made it through medical school, residency training, and practice without being stopped makes people wonder if physicians are fulfilling their professional responsibility to protect the public (Stewart 1999). Harold Shipman murdered at least 15 patients in the United Kingdom, and possibly as many as 250 (O'Neill 2000). Extreme cases such as these have helped to mobilize the U.S. public to support creation of a National Practitioner Data Bank. In the United Kingdom, it led the General Medical Council to overhaul methods to ensure the competency and oversight of physicians.

Patients and the public care about professionalism not only because of these egregious cases of unprofessional, immoral, or illegal behavior, but also because of personal experiences with physicians. No physician is immune from the cocktail party conversation with a friend about the poor quality care received by another doctor. Those conversations are rarely about technical incompetence—patients see our medical education system as teaching knowledge and skills quite well—but more commonly about a physician who was rude, insensitive, impatient, or inattentive.

The profession itself cares about professionalism not only because we feel responsible for these egregious cases, but also because we want to promote routine professional behavior among health care providers. Those of us in academic medicine spend inordinate amounts of time working to dismiss the rare student whom we believe should not practice medicine for reasons of professionalism. Hospital credentialing committees and state medical boards are similarly challenged by physicians with repeated episodes of inappropriate professional behavior who must have their licenses revoked to protect the public. But more often, we see lapses in professional judgment and poorly managed conflicts of interest every day. Medical students lie about participation in conferences; residents treat other doctors rudely; practicing physicians accept money for patient research enrollment (New York Times 1999; Relman and Lundberg 1998; Stern 1998; Kassirer 1995).

What Can Be Done About Professionalism?

The consistent response of teachers, medical boards, and medical professional organizations has been to encourage the measurement of professionalism (Association of American Medical Colleges 1998; Accreditation Council for Graduate Medical Education 2004; Institute for International Medical Education 2000). The ability to accurately measure professionalism will allow us to detect and dismiss those students or physicians with extremes of deviant behavior. Measuring professionalism will allow us to provide formative feedback to physicians across the educational continuum. Measures of professionalism can be used to reward those physicians who are most altruistic, humanistic, and compassionate. Measuring professionalism as an outcome of medical education parallels the trend in medicine to measure outcomes of patient care as an indicator of health care quality (Committee on Quality of Health in America 2000). Measuring professionalism will allow educators to detect changes in professionalism as a result of educational interventions.

This emphasis on outcomes makes educational sense. Even outstanding curricula, abundant resources, and well-trained teachers do not guarantee that students will learn. Teachers must set expectations, design experiences, and assess learners. Assessments tell teachers whether expectations are clear and whether students learn from their experiences. Assessments also motivate students to learn what is important. While some medical assessments have career-changing consequences (e.g., licensing examinations), others provide an opportunity for highly motivated medical students to work diligently to improve their competence (e.g., informal mid-clerkship feedback).

The greatest challenge to measuring professionalism has been the absence of a convincing set of tools with which to measure professional behaviors. This is a particularly vexing problem for admissions committees, clerkship directors, medical school deans, residency program directors, hospital credentialing committees, and state medical boards. Aside from routine end-of-month clerkship and rotation evaluations (usually containing only one or two items related to professionalism), and the occasional peer evaluation form, physicians have a limited set of methods available with which to provide feedback on professionalism. While educators have made great strides over the past 50 years in assessing knowledge, and over at least the past 20 years in assessing skills, the assessment of behaviors and professionalism has lagged.

Our failure to measure professionalism sends a conflicting message to both students and practicing physicians. While we profess and encourage professionalism, we do little to ensure its presence (Stern 1998). Our medical students attend closely to abilities in

knowledge and skills not only because they are important for medical competence but also because they are perceived as "counting"
for something in the educational process. Students who aren't
graded on professional behaviors infer that instructors don't care
about professionalism and that professionalism is therefore unimportant (Eisner 1985). Practicing physicians are no different. Without accurate feedback on professionalism, continuing medical education for physicians focuses on enhancing clinical expertise rather
than on professionalism.

Why Is It So Difficult to Measure Professionalism?

The first problem in measuring professionalism is finding the opportunities to observe professional behaviors. Most faculty are well
aware that they observe students only on their best behavior and that
they have limited opportunities to see students in realistic settings.
Most practicing physicians observe each others' behaviors only in the
hallways and conference rooms—rarely with patients. The solution
to this problem is to expand the number of observers and the settings in which they observe. In this book, we present methods of assessment for faculty, nurses, peers, and patients as a means for ex-
tending the sample of observed behaviors across individuals and
settings.

The second problem is finding a way to describe those observations. Description "should enable readers to get a feel for the place
or process and, where possible and appropriate, for the experience
of those who occupy the situation" (Eisner 1991, p. 89). We provide
examples of recently developed methods for describing even subtle
professional behaviors: a clerkship evaluation form designed to capture comments about a medical student talking with the family of a
recently deceased patient; a standardized patient rating form that allows the description of a student's ability to use understandable language; a peer rating form useful for identifying a colleague whose
patient data you would accept in the face of contradictory reports.

The next problem is determining whether those observations
are representative. Teachers tend to assume that if people behave
badly in one situation, they will behave badly in all situations. This
is what psychologists call "attribution error" (Sabini et al. 2001). People rarely behave identically even in identical situations. It is even
less likely that people will behave identically far in the future or un-

der different circumstances (i.e., late at night, after a stressful day, or in the face of personal problems). For this reason, I, along with others, have advocated the use of "lapses in professionalism" rather than "unprofessional behavior" when discussing inappropriate behaviors (Ginsburg et al. 2000). This rhetorical stance avoids the immutable label of "unprofessional" when talking about a single event and helps prevent unnecessary overgeneralization.

Yet, we must often make conditional judgments based on limited observations. To avoid overgeneralization and attribution bias, two approaches are necessary. First, the more frequently we observe an individual student or physician in varied settings, the more confidence we can have in the summative judgment. Measuring professional behaviors in multiple ways is therefore a requirement of high-quality assessment. This kind of triangulation is a fundamental element of validation in qualitative inquiries of all kinds (Denzin and Lincoln 1998). Second, having multiple observers in each setting allows for a "consensual validation" in which independent experts reach the same conclusions, increasing the likelihood that an assessment is accurate and appropriate (Eisner 1991, p. 112).

Once you have adequately observed and described an individual's behavior, there is still the problem of deciding if it was a positive professional behavior or a lapse. Can we say of professionalism only what Justice Stewart said of obscenity—that I "know it when I see it?" (*Jacobellis v. Ohio* 1964). Perhaps, but perhaps that isn't so bad. This nihilistic approach to assessment contains within it a pearl of wisdom. Most people who evaluate students, residents, and practicing physicians have developed a detailed and nuanced perception of how doctors should behave. Eliot Eisner has described this as *connoisseurship*, "the ability to make fine-grained discriminations among complex and subtle qualities" (Eisner 1991). Just as the oenophile distinguishes between wines made with cabernet or merlot grapes, experienced teachers can detect and discriminate between students who are responsible and thorough and those who are not.

Yet being a connoisseur does not guarantee that you can accurately describe what you perceive. A connoisseur does not necessarily possess the ability to describe and compare differences among students. If connoisseurship is the observation or input, *critique* is the public report, or output (Eisner 1991). It is this public report that is necessary for educational assessment. Assessment is a complex, multistage task that involves observation, description, and the determination of value. This book provides readers with these tools for the critique of professionalism.

Characteristics of an Effective Assessment

An ideal evaluation of a student's professionalism, then, might be to have a team of assessment experts eavesdrop on every conversation of every individual throughout the day. While researchers do this (Stern 1996a, 1996b, 1998), it is obviously not practical for large-scale assessment. Instead, researchers have developed methods for sampling behavior, with varying degrees of reliability, validity, and proximity to reality. These sampling methods range from self-administered psychometric surveys, to standardized patient encounters, to faculty and peer evaluation forms, to the analysis of reflective portfolios and essays. Educators have not identified any one of these methods as the gold standard of assessment for professionalism; however, their utility can be weighed by a set of criteria that any measurement tool should meet.

First, evaluation should occur in as realistic a context as possible. It is unrealistic, for example, to expect an overworked intern's noontime written description of how he would behave toward an irritated nurse at 2 A.M. to bear much resemblance to his actual behavior. Context is particularly relevant for professionalism because professional behavior is heavily influenced by forces of social desirability (the desire to provide answers that make the person appear to behave appropriately, even when in reality the individual would not behave this way), personal values, and organizational hierarchy. Imagine a faculty member asking a student, "How much time should you spend talking with this patient and his family?" The student is likely to respond to this question with a socially desirable answer, "As much time as the patient needs without interfering with my other patient care responsibilities." Of course, the amount of time a student actually spends with a patient will as likely depend on a myriad of other circumstances, including the student's interest in the patient, fatigue, conflicting seminars, and getting home. The closer to the context of real experience, the more valid the evaluation of professionalism is likely to be.

Next, an ideal evaluation must include a situation that involves conflict. As with moral reasoning (Oser 1986), professionalism is best evaluated when values conflict with one another (Stern 1996; Coulehan and Williams 2003). An evaluation that invites a student to choose between being honest and dishonest in the abstract offers no challenge—the student will always choose honesty. But professional challenges rarely appear as simple choices between right and wrong; they are more often choices among equally worthy values—such as responsibility to patients versus respect for teachers and the hospital hierarchy. For example, what will a student do when she is not sure her resident has obtained appropriately informed consent for a patient prior to surgery? Observing a student's response to this conflict provides a demonstration of the student's level of professionalism (Ginsburg et al. 2003).

Perhaps unique to the assessment of professionalism is the philosophy that the "correct" resolution of a dilemma is not the only measure of professionalism. As we explain in chapter 2, professionalism is demonstrated through an aspiration to and wise application of principles. This does not necessarily mean that the professional must act perfectly in every situation. To insist on such stringency would mean that even a single mistake would permanently label an individual "unprofessional" (Ginsburg et al. 2000). Physicians demonstrate professionalism by resolving a dilemma wisely. The reasoning behind the resolution of a dilemma is critical, even when someone makes a mistake. Evaluating reasoning strategies is a particular challenge addressed in several chapters of this book (see chapters 5, 11, and 12).

Context, conflict, and resolution are foundational criteria for measuring the quality of professionalism evaluation instruments (Ginsburg et al. 2000). In addition, two elements of the evaluation setting influence the observations of assessed behavior. The first is transparency. A few methods to assess professionalism involve various degrees of nondisclosure and entrapment (e.g., secret standardized patients). Such evaluations will likely lead those being evaluated refusing to participate, resisting this surreptitious behavior in other ways, or increasing institutional mistrust. Educators must remember that individuals being measured should be included and informed as assessment is designed and implemented and should be encouraged to provide feedback. This allows assessors to apply measurement tools fairly and ultimately makes for higher quality assessment.

The second aspect of setting is symmetry, the idea that all levels in the organizational hierarchy are evaluated using the same methods. In many modern business settings, all employees are subject to "360" evaluations, in which supervisors, peers, and subordinates all provide performance feedback to the individual at the center of the "360-degree circle." Every employee from the CEO to the mailroom participates. In medical education, we expect our entering students to behave as professionals and to adopt the expected norms of the profession, including self-evaluation and continued quality improvement. With this backdrop, it should be no surprise that when faculty propose professionalism assessments for students, one of the students' first reactions will be to ask about the professionalism assessments in place for faculty. Particularly for such personal and sensitive domains as compassion, responsibility, and respect, students are likely to ask if the evaluators themselves have been, or are undergoing, similar assessments. This concern from students is reasonable, and educators designing systems should be prepared to answer questions about symmetry. In an ideal health care system, all participants would engage in regular assessment and feedback for knowledge, skills, and professional behaviors—starting with the leadership and moving down to the entering medical students. However, the resistance of faculty and practicing physicians, and the dependent position of students within the educational hierarchy, means that evaluation often starts at the lowest educational level. Regardless of the sequence, symmetry demands that evaluation occur across all levels, with each institution defining the pathway to implementation that is most feasible within its culture.

Assessment for What Purpose?

Before designing a system to assess professionalism, one must be very clear about the purpose of assessment. For example, assessments of professionalism could be used to select among applicants, to remove those unfit for practice, to provide anonymous feedback, or to determine if an educational program is effective in teaching professionalism. The choice of outcome is intimately linked to the assessment method. For example, if the purpose is purely formative (to be used only for feedback and improvement), the individuals being assessed are potentially more likely to behave naturally, knowing that the assessment doesn't really "count." If the assessment is summative (to be used for promotion, graduation, or another high-stakes event), performance is more likely to be biased toward social desirability. An example of this, developed in more detail in later chapters, is the use of peer assessment. Peer assessment seems to work well when used to identify those who excel in professional behavior and may merit an award. But when used as a component of grades, peer assessment has higher stakes and students either don't participate or conspire against the system to provide only excellent assessments of peers (Arnold et al. 2004). If an educator begins by collecting information for formative assessment and subsequently tries to use that information for a summative purpose, students will likely treat the formative assessment as summative, and the quality of the data collected will deteriorate under the influence of social norms.

For these reasons, evaluators must decide the purpose of evaluation prior to developing an evaluation system. One could use the same system (involving evaluators, data management, oversight, recording, and feedback) for multiple measures, but those measures should fall within either formative or summative assessment. Educators planning both formative and summative assessments should use separate and independent systems.

Designing Assessments of Professionalism

The following steps should guide the assessment of professionalism:

1. Develop an institutional plan for assessing professionalism. Approaches developed in isolation by one group or department will lead to challenges of symmetry.
2. Discuss and agree upon the meaning of professionalism as applied to your organization using a wide range of participants, including those being evaluated and those affected by the professional behaviors of those being evaluated (e.g., other health care professionals, patients).
3. Select a set of behaviors on which to focus.
4. Decide whether the purpose of the evaluation is formative or summative. If some evaluations are formative and others are summative, separate administrative systems are likely to be needed.
5. Identify a set of instruments to measure behaviors:
   a. Consider context, conflict, and resolution.
   b. Consider transparency and symmetry.
   c. Use multiple raters and multiple types of measurement to enhance validity.
6. Train evaluators to improve both their connoisseurship and their criticism of professional behaviors.

7. Implement and evaluate the success of the program (from the perspectives of both evaluators and of those being evaluated), with an eye toward making further modifications.

The chapters that follow offer insight into these stages. Chapter 2 provides a historical background of professionalism, explores definitions suggested by others, and identifies a clear definition of professionalism for use in assessment. This chapter provides material that faculty can use as part of a conversation at individual institutions to discuss professionalism at the local level.

The next set of chapters (3–12) provide detailed information on instruments to evaluate professional behaviors. Each describes the history of the measurement tool, its reliability and validity and its use in medical settings and offers practical suggestions for implementation. Chapters 13 and 14 discuss the challenges of applying these evaluation tools to admissions and accreditation—two critical assessment points in the transition from student to professional physician. Together, these chapters should prepare educators to develop a system for assessing professionalism that reflects its importance in medicine. In the final chapter, Fred Hafferty identifies some of the most important issues in professionalism across measurement tools and provides new challenges for physicians, educators, and professional organizations.

Chapters 2–14 stand alone as a resource for individuals searching for the best evidence and advice about implementing professionalism assessments. Ultimately, the outcomes of interest for this book are whether the reader finds it useful, whether it serves the purpose of enhancing professional behaviors of students and physicians, and whether enhanced professionalism improves the quality of care for patients.

References

Accreditation Council for Graduate Medical Education. Outcomes Project. Available at: http://www.acgme.org/outcome/. Accessed September 24, 2004.

Arnold L, Shue C, Kritt B, Stern D. Medical students' views on peer assessment of professionalism. J Gen Intern Med 2005; in press.

Association of American Medical Colleges. Learning Objectives for Medical Student Education: The MSOP Report. Association of American Medical Colleges, Washington, DC, 1998.

Committee on Quality of Health in America. To Err Is Human: Building a Safer Health System. Kohn LT, Corrigan JM, Donaldson MS, Eds. National Academies Press, Washington, DC, 2000.

Coulehan J, Williams P. Conflicting professional values in medical education. Cambridge Quarterly of Healthcare Ethics 2003;12:7–20.

Denzin NK, Lincoln YS. The Landscape of Qualitative Research: Theories and Issues. Sage Publications, Thousand Oaks, CA, 1998.

Eisner E. The Educational Imagination. 2nd ed. Macmillan, New York, 1985.

Eisner E. The Enlightened Eye: Qualitative Inquiry and the Enhancement of Educational Practice. Macmillan, New York, 1991.

Ginsburg S, Regehr G, Hatala R, McNaughton N, Frohna A, Hodges B, Lingard L, Stern DT. Context conflict, and resolution: a new conceptual framework for evaluating professionalism. Academic Medicine 2000; 75(10):S6–S11.

Ginsburg S, Regehr G, Lingard L. The disavowed curriculum: understanding student's reasoning in professionally challenging situations. J Gen Intern Med 2003;18:1015–1022.

Institute for International Medical Education, Core Committee. Global minimum essential requirement in medical education. Medical Teacher 2002;24:130–135.

Jacobellis v. Ohio, 378 U.S. 184, 197, 1964 (Stewart, J., concurring).

Kassirer JP. Managed care and the morality of the marketplace. N Engl J Med 1995;333:50–52.

New York Times. Patients for hire, doctors for sale. New York Times, May 22, 1999;A12.

O'Neill B. Doctor as murderer. Death certification needs tightening up, but it still might not have stopped Shipman. BMJ 2000;320:329–330.

Oser FK. Moral education and values education: the discourse perspective. In: Handbook of Research on Teaching (Wittrock MC, ed.). New York, Macmillan, 1986;917–941.

Relman AS, Lundberg GD. Business and professionalism in medicine at the American Medical Association. JAMA 1998;279:169–170.

Sabini J, Siemmann M, Stein J. The really fundamental attribution error in social psychological research. Psychoanalytic Inquiry 2001;12:1–15.

Stern D. Hanging Out: Teaching Values in Medical Education. PhD Dissertation. Stanford University, Stanford, CA, 1996a.

Stern D. Values on call: a method for assessing the teaching of professionalism. Academic Medicine 1996b;71(10 suppl):S37–S39.

Stern D. Practicing what we preach? An analysis of the curriculum of values in medical education. American Journal of Medicine 1998;104(6):569–575.

Stewart JB. Blind Eye: How the Medical Establishment Let a Doctor Get Away With Murder. Simon and Schuster, New York, 1999.

2

What Is Medical Professionalism?

Louise Arnold and David Thomas Stern

With the rising interest in professionalism in medicine has come a plethora of definitions for the concept of professionalism. They range from the simplest straightforward statement to treatises covering several pages (ABIM et al. 2002; Cruess et al. 2000a; Accreditation Council for Graduate Medical Education 1999; Medical School Objectives Project Writing Group 1999). Medical educators, teachers, and students struggle with the meaning of the concept. Not infrequently, they paraphrase Justice Potter Stewart's definition of obscenity (Jacobellis v. Ohio 1964) and claim they may not be able to define professionalism intelligibly but "know it when they see it." Although individual observers may have the luxury of such a stance, when groups must agree on acceptable professional behaviors, they must all refer to the same overall concept and component dimensions. This chapter seeks to articulate a definition of professionalism.

The need for an explicit definition of professionalism is most pressing in the arena of assessment since measurement must be psychometrically and consequentially sound. These requirements demand a definition of professionalism that is clear, complete, and concise. The definition must circumscribe the parameters of professionalism and specify the content—the domains and dimensions that professionalism includes and excludes. It must also logically lead to transparent operational methods to observe professional behaviors. This chapter therefore offers a definition for the purpose of assessment that can serve as a referent for subsequent chapters. To achieve a psychometrically and consequentially sound definition of professionalism, we first outline the domains of professionalism and then sharpen our focus by exploring the issue of how professionalism can be viewed across the continuum of a medical career.

Historical Roots

Despite radically different cultural and healing traditions, physicians around the globe subscribe to professional values. Accordingly, one approach to developing a definition of professionalism is to look for universal values among physicians. In 1999, a conference was held in Beijing, China, to compare the foundations of professionalism and ethics between two independent and distinct traditions—the Western Hippocratic approach and the Eastern Confucian approach. At the conclusion of this meeting, Tom Murray of the Hastings Center for Healthcare Ethics remarked on the similarities, not the differences:

> [E]very culture knows illness; and every culture makes provision for caring for people who are ill. Disease and early death disrupt the lives of individuals and families, cause physical suffering as well as great emotional pain and loss. Disease makes medicine necessary. The specific values served by medicine and the virtues cultivated in doctors flow from our shared experiences of illness, love, compassion, and caring for those in need. Given our shared humanity, our common experiences of illness, the immense value we place on enduring human relationships, it is no surprise that we come to similar conclusions about values in medicine and virtues in physicians. (Murray 2000, p. 545)

The core values of professionalism, therefore, derive from the universality of disease and begin with caring or compassion. Caring over time creates the value of responsibility. The shared responsibility for care engenders trust and respect by both physician and patient. The maintenance of trust demands integrity and confidentiality. The humanistic values we consider core to the practice of medicine are thus biologically grounded in the nature of disease and the natural emotional connections between individuals. This universal humanistic core can be found in all definitions of professionalism in medicine and constitutes the foundation upon which the practice of medicine is built.

Beyond the humanistic core, the historical development of other values, including service, maintenance of competence, autonomy, and self-regulation, is more complex. These values are those of a "profession," which have been conjoined with humanism to create the more recent connotation of "professionalism." Physicians in Hellenic Greece were expected to subscribe to the Hippocratic oath, vowing a commitment not only to compassionate care but also to service (Cruess et al. 1997). In medieval England, along with the emergence of the learned professions came the notion of the elite professional with obligations to society (and to individual patients; Kimball 2000). Judge Louis Brandeis (1912) defined a profession as providing service to society with the following elements: First, a profession is an occupation for which the necessary preliminary training is intellectual in character, involving knowledge and to some extent learning, as distinguished from mere skill. Second, it is an occupation that is pursued largely for others and not merely for oneself. Third, it is an occupation in which the amount of financial return is not the accepted measure of success.

Abraham Flexner, leader of modern U.S. medical education reform in the early twentieth century, further expanded the definition of a professional beyond humanism and service by including both elements of excellence and self-regulation:

> [P]rofessions involve essentially intellectual operations with large individual responsibility; they derive their raw material from science and learning; this material they work up to a practical and definite end; they possess an educationally communicable technique; they tend to self-organization; [and] they are becoming increasingly altruistic in motivation. (Flexner 1915)

These developments reflect the increasing emphasis on the rise of scientific medicine of the early 1900s (Ludmerer 1985). "[M]edicine

. . . ha[d] for the first time become a science in the sense given to that term in modern usage. Previously . . . it was described in the ancient documents largely as an 'art and mystery'" (Anonymous 1910). With science as a foundation of proven medical treatment, expertise became a fundamental responsibility of the good physician, above and beyond compassionate and committed care.

The elements of self-regulation have their origins in the occupational guilds (Starr 1982) but were legally established as state medical boards were created in the early 1900s. The American Medical Association's Committee on Medical Education, Abraham Flexner, the university medical schools, and others contributed to the development of these boards in order to codify the self-regulating nature of the medical profession (Ludmerer 1985), since who, other than physicians, would be competent to judge the qualifications and continued competence of physicians? While state medical boards today contain lay members, they continue to be organized and guided by physicians as a professional right and obligation.

Although humanism and definitions of the "professional" have long histories, the word "professionalism" as currently used is a recent phenomenon in medicine. As late as the 1970s, the literature in medical education did not specifically refer to professionalism (Arnold 2002). There was interest in physician and student characteristics now labeled as professional, but they were treated as a residual category referring to qualities that were not cognitive. The 1980s witnessed a shift in the conceptualization of noncognitive attributes of physicians when the American Board of Internal Medicine (ABIM 1983) laid out the dimensions of humanism, consisting of respect, compassion, and integrity. In the 1990s, the ABIM turned to using the word "professionalism" and explicitly delineated its elements, including not only humanism but also altruism, duty and service, accountability, and excellence (ABIM 1994).

By the end of the 1990s and early into the 2000s, more than 60 medical schools reported that they had specified criteria for evaluating students' professionalism and had implemented a rigorous process of evaluating students' professionalism (Swick et al. 1999; Kao and Lim 2003). Increasing numbers of specialty and professional societies have joined the ABIM in defining professionalism (Adams et al. 1998; ABIM et al. 2002; Medical School Objectives Project Writing Group 1999; Association of American Medical Colleges 2004; Accreditation Council for Graduate Medical Education, 1994).

The challenge of these recent descriptions of professionalism is that they could be construed, albeit mistakenly, as subsuming all competencies of a physician—an approach that would make definition and measurement of professionalism unreasonable.

A Definition Guiding Assessment of Professionalism

The efforts to define professionalism by physicians and medical educators along with social scientists and ethicists suggest the following definition for assessment of professionalism (see figure 2-1):

> *Professionalism* is demonstrated through a foundation of clinical competence, communication skills, and ethical and legal understanding, upon which is built the aspiration to and wise application of the principles of professionalism: excellence, humanism, accountability, and altruism.

This definition points to several fundamental elements of knowledge and skills that are necessary but not sufficient for professionalism—clinical competence, ethical understanding, and communication

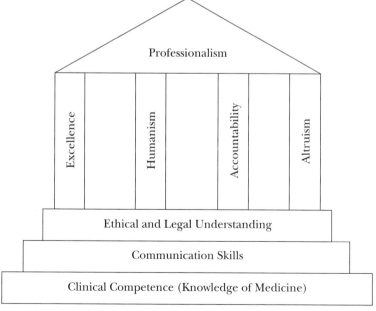

Figure 2-1   A definition of professionalism.

skills. It indicates the domains of direct interest for assessment by recognizing that knowledge, attitudes or aspirations, and skills underpin the application of the principles of professionalism. The definition introduces the idea of professionalism as virtue toward which physicians continually strive and thereby offers a bridge to medical ethics. It refers to those additional necessary and sufficient elements of professionalism—excellence, humanism, accountability, and altruism—as aspirational principles but avoids arguments of which precise terms should be used for each principle and highlights the application of those principles in observable behaviors. The wise application of those principles implies that these values may conflict at times, and those who can wisely resolve those conflicts may be identified as "professional."

Included in our definition of professionalism is the foundational understanding of ethics as applied to medicine. While the study of ethics can also be construed to include other domains of professional behavior (Christakis and Feudtner 1993), we include here a more limited definition (Brody 2003) in which ethics is viewed as a discipline focused on issues in the classic domains of beneficence, nonmaleficence, justice, and autonomy (Pellegrino and Thomasma 1981). A deep understanding of those principles, and the common situations in which they apply to medical care, forms the core of this element.

Communication skills are also included as part of the foundation for professionalism, since communication is the means through which professional behavior is enacted (Stern 2002). It is necessary but insufficient for professionalism and variably included in definitions of professionalism for that reason. More commonly, communication skills are included as a separate domain (Medical School Objectives Writing Group 1999; Accreditation Council for Graduate Medical Education 1999; Institute for International Medical Education 2002), in part because the methods used to evaluate communication skills have recently been much improved (see chapter 4). Communication skills include the ability to communicate not only with individual patients but also with their families, across cultural gaps, with members of the health care team, and with the public.

Principles of Professionalism

Although technical knowledge, skills, ethics, and communication are foundational to professionalism, principles, as statements of values, are central to the definition of professionalism and distinguish professionalism from the concept of clinical competence. ABIM's Project Professionalism identified key principles of excellence, accountability, duty, altruism, respect, and other humanistic qualities such as compassion and empathy, as well as honor and integrity (ABIM 1994). They may be usefully categorized under four headings and briefly defined as follows. Excellence begins with commitment to competence, understanding of ethical principles and values, knowledge of legal boundaries, and communication skills. However, its unique element involves a commitment to exceed ordinary standards. Accountability entails fulfilling the implied contract governing the patient-physician relationship as well as the profession's relationship to society. It includes self-regulation, standard setting, management of conflicts of interest, duty or the free acceptance of service, and responsibility. Altruism demands that the best interests of patients, not self-interest, guide physicians. Respect, compassion, and empathy, plus honor and integrity, comprise humanism.

Despite concern that we cannot all agree on what constitutes professional behavior, most professional organizations do subscribe to these principles (although they may disagree over details). Some organizations or authors would add a principle here and there, vary the emphasis given to a particular principle, or define a principle somewhat differently (Arnold 2002). For example, self-regulation appears on the list of only some writers' principles (Cruess et al. 1997, 1999, 2000a, 2000b). Responsibility figures in the definition of professionalism applied to medical students (Gibson et al. 2000; Phelan et al. 1993; Papadakis et al. 1999) but is more implied in the definitions for graduate medical education and practicing physicians. Altruism is the salient principle for the ABIM (1994); empathy as part of humanism is central to another author (Hafferty 2001), and autonomy is critical for still others (Cruess et al. 1997, 2000b). At times, differences in defining a principle lead to overlaps between them. For example, humanism involves integrity in an early ABIM formulation, but in Project Professionalism integrity is separate from humanistic qualities (compare ABIM 1983, 1994). Altruism, compassion, and empathy are sometimes used interchangeably (McGaghie 2002). The boundary between ethics and professionalism itself can be blurred (Brody 2003). No one of these definitions from different organizations and authors is superior to another. However, there is sufficient agreement about the principles of professionalism to serve as an organizing concept for the measurement of dimensions deemed important by all.

Since the principles of professionalism are central, a closer albeit brief substantive examination is appropriate to convey the rich-
ness of the phenomena each embodies and to articulate the definitions of each as further guides to the assessment of professionalism.

Excellence

The notion of excellence begins with a commitment to competence
in technical knowledge and skills, ethical and legal understanding,
and communication skills. However, commitment to meeting minimal standards is not adequate for the quintessence of excellence is
a continual conscientious effort to exceed ordinary expectations
(ABIM 1994). It therefore embraces the concept of lifelong learning, itself a multifaceted concept. According to Hojat et al. (2003b),
lifelong learning is a set of self-initiated activities and information-
seeking skills that are activated in individuals with a sustained motivation to learn and the ability to recognize their own learning needs.

Another expression of excellence is dedication to the continuous improvement of the quality of care by reducing medical error,
increasing patient safety, minimizing overuse of health care resources, and maximizing health outcomes (ABIM et al. 2002). To
improve quality of care, physicians in collaboration with other health
professionals must generate better measures of quality of care and
use these measures in routine evaluation of the performance of all
participants, organizations, and systems responsible for health care
delivery (ABIM et al. 2002). Further, physicians must help create,
support, and maintain mechanisms to encourage continuous improvement of quality of care.

A further aspect of excellence involves the promotion of scientific knowledge and technology (ABIM et al. 2002). According to the
ABIM charter, physicians must uphold scientific standards, promote
research, and produce new knowledge based on scientific evidence
and physician experience. Moreover, physicians have the duty to
safeguard and maintain the integrity of their medical knowledge and
technology and to assure the integrity of the use of that knowledge
and technology.

Humanism

Humanism denotes a sincere concern for and interest in humanity,
a vital principle to guide a profession rooted in the interaction be-

tween people in need of assistance and people offering it. The following quote speaks to the rationale for this principle:

> The practice of medicine is that it is an intensely personal matter. . . . The treatment of a disease may be entirely impersonal; the care of a patient must be entirely personal. The significance of the intimate personal relationship between physician and patient cannot be too strongly emphasized, for in an extraordinarily large number of cases both diagnosis and treatment are directly dependent on it. . . . One of the essential qualities of the clinician is interest in humanity, for the secret of the care of the patient is in caring for the patient. (Peabody 1927, p. 877)

Humanism has been articulated to include respect, compassion, and empathy, plus honor and integrity (ABIM 1992). In fact, it has been widely defined in terms of these components that are to guide physicians' relationships in the professional setting (Arnold 2002). Discussion of each of these components is therefore warranted.

Respect refers to regard for another person with esteem, deference, and dignity. Applied to medicine, respect is the "personal commitment to honor other [peoples'] choices and rights regarding themselves and their medical care" (ABIM 1992, p. 2). Respect includes a sensitivity and responsiveness to a person's culture, age, gender, and disabilities (Accreditation Council for Graduate Medical Education, 1999). It presents physicians with a special challenge since signs of respect may vary across cultures. Nevertheless, it has been called the essence of humanism (ABIM 1994), since it signals recognition of the worth of the individual human being and his or her belief and value system (Abbot 1983). Respect is due patients and requires confidentiality, privacy, and informed consent. It also is accorded to colleagues in the medical as well as other health care professions, learners, institutions, systems, and processes (Association of American Medical Colleges and the National Board of Medical Examiners 2002).

Empathy and compassion have been variously defined. Cognitive in nature, empathy is the ability to understand another person's perspectives, inner experiences, and feelings without intensive emotional involvement (Hojat et al. 2003a; Marcus 1999). To be understood is a basic human need and the backbone of patient-physician relationships. But empathy is not just an ability to understand another person, that is, to stand in the patient's shoes, and to view the world from a patient's perspective without losing sight of one's personal role and responsibility. Empathy is more than understanding. It is multidimensional and includes the capacity to communicate that understanding (Hojat et al. 2002; Feighny et al. 1998). Some authors add an emotional dimension to empathy that points to the capacity to enter into or join the experiences and feelings of another person (Hojat et al. 2002; Halpern 2003). But that capacity is conceptually more relevant to sympathy, which in turn could interfere with a necessary objectivity in medical care (Hojat et al. 2002).

A factor analysis of empathy among physicians confirmed its multidimensional character with perspective taking, the core ingredient of empathy. Such items as "an important component of the relationship with my patients is my understanding of the emotional status of the patients and their families" and "I try to understand what is going on in my patients' minds by paying attention to their non-verbal cues and body language" convey the meaning of the dimension of perspective taking. Other items, reversed scored, such as "It is difficult for me to view things from my patients' perspective" or "I try not to pay attention to my patients' emotions in interviewing and history taking" indicated additional dimensions of empathy such as standing in the patient's shoes and conveying empathy, respectively (Hojat et al. 2002).

Closely aligned with empathy, compassion is the feeling or emotion when a person is moved by the suffering or distress of another and by the desire to relieve it (Oxford English Dictionary 1989). It refers to an individual's inner resources—his or her affective assets, awareness of others, and accumulated wisdom derived from life experiences (McGaghie et al. 2002). In medicine, it involves an appreciation that illness engenders special needs for comfort and help but without excessive emotional involvement that could undermine professional responsibility for the patient (ABIM 1992), as well as the expression of that appreciation through appropriate sensitive communication and actions. Compassion also extends to peers, co-workers, and self (Association of American Medical Colleges and the National Board of Medical Examiners 2002).

Honor and integrity refer to "being fair and truthful, keeping one's word, meeting commitments, and being straightforward" (ABIM 1994, p. 6). These qualities pertain to relationships with patients, colleagues, other health care professionals, and learners. They apply to a variety of activities, including patient care, academic assignments, scholarly work, and research. Behavioral examples of these qualities include admitting errors, addressing errors of others, and crediting the work of others appropriately. In contrast, negative examples of behavior relevant to this principle include stealing, cheating on examinations, misrepresenting data, falsifying documents, and impersonating others (Association of American Medical Colleges and the National Board of Medical Examiners 2002).

Accountability

Accountability refers to the "procedures and processes by which one party justifies and takes responsibility for its activities" (Emmanuel and Emmanuel 1996, p. 229). It can involve 11 different parties that could be held accountable or hold others accountable (Emmanuel and Emmanuel 1996). The multiplicity of accountability levels include responsibility to patients for fulfilling the implied contract governing the patient-physician relationship, to colleagues, to the profession for adhering to medicine's time-honored precepts, and to society for addressing the health needs of the public.

Responsibility represents the most personal behavioral application of accountability. In a conservative definition, one is responsible "to" [patients, families, society] and accountable "for" [quality of care, upholding principles, reporting conflicts of interest]. Responsibility involves availability when "on call," acceptance of inconvenience to meet patients' needs, and endurance of unavoidable risks to oneself when a patient's welfare is at stake. It also connotes advocacy for individual patients so they may receive the best possible care (see discussion of public service, below). It involves an obligation to collaborate with other health professionals, to provide leadership when appropriate, and to defer to the leadership of others when indicated (Medical School Objectives Writing Group 1999).

Central to our definition of accountability are self-regulating activities for which physicians can be held accountable, and range from their professional competence and legal and ethical conduct to financial performance (ABIM 1994; ABIM et al. 2002; Medical School Objectives Project Writing Group 1999; Emmanuel and Emmanuel 1996). Standard setting for current and future members of the profession, engagement in internal scrutiny and acceptance of external scrutiny, and remediation and discipline of members who fail to meet those standards are also relevant to accountability (ABIM et al. 2002).

Physicians have both individual and collective obligations to participate in these processes.

Realizing that conflicts of interest are inevitable in the practice
of medicine, they are taking an increasingly central role as evidence
for the maintenance of professionalism (ABIM et al. 2002). The growing number of financial arrangements with insurance and pharma-
ceutical companies, efforts to attend to cost, and joint affiliations of
doctors with laboratory and evaluation facilities warrants this attention. While complete avoidance of such conflicts is rarely possible,
most organizations recommend disclosure and external monitoring
of such relationships to ensure that the perceptions of patients and
peers are not adversely influenced (Coyle 2002).

Public service, involving the free acceptance of duty to serve patients and the public, connotes advocacy for individual patients so
they may receive the best possible care, for access to health care for
everyone but especially for traditionally underserved populations,
and for social justice (ABIM 1994; ABIM et al. 2002). In addition, it
encompasses the use of systematic approaches to promoting, maintaining, and improving the health of individuals and populations
through counseling individual patients and their families and
through public education and action (Medical School Objectives
Project Writing Group 1999). In one sense, it merges with the definition of responsibility as applied to communities, rather than just
individuals (ABIM et al. 2002).

The Unique Place of Altruism

Altruism is clearly included in most definitions of professionalism,
and yet it remains a challenge to categorize. It could be included in
the domain of excellence (demanding the best for patients), accountability (avoiding self-interest), or humanism (selfless behavior).
In medicine, altruism demands that patients' best interests, rather
than the interests of physicians, guide behavior (ABIM 1994). The
Medical School Objectives Project Writing Group (1999) points to
potential threats to physicians' altruism inherent in various financial
and organizational arrangements for the practice of medicine and
calls for physicians "to advocate the interests of one's patients over
ones' own interest" (p. 5). More wide-ranging literature on altruism,
of interest to theologians, philosophers, social scientists, and biolo-
gists, presents varied views on the concept of altruism. For example,
operational definitions include emergency helping behavior, proso-

cial behavior, positive societal behavior, charity, social responsibility, and volunteerism (Kilpatrick and McCullough 2004).

The literature does agree that altruism is expressed in specific situations as behavior designed to benefit another person. Whether that action must also involve risk to the actor's well-being, some sacrifice on the part of the actor, or renunciation of self care in order to qualify as altruistic are questions unsettled in the literature. The essence of altruism remains, however, as actions aimed at increasing the welfare of others, particularly those in need (Piliavin and Charng 1990; Batson 2002). It is grounded in compassion with a deep sense of connection to others (McGaghie et al. 2002).

Although the concept of professionalism and the meaning attached to the principles that lie at its heart are rich and varied, sufficient agreement is apparent in the literature that a core definition of professionalism is available to guide the assessment of learners' and practitioners' professionalism.

Professionalism Across the Continuum of a Medical Career

Should these principles of professionalism be expected and evaluated equally across the continuum of a medical career? Are the dilemmas a medical student faces relevant to a practicing physician and vice versa? Are the values of a professional so clear that they can be expected beginning on the first day of medical school? One view suggests that the principles of professionalism are stage specific, dependent upon context. The other asserts that the principles apply throughout a career.

Studies documenting the context dependency of professional behavior (Hartshorne and May 1928–1930; Carlo et al. 1991; Rezler et al. 1992; Marcus 1999; Simmons et al. 1992; Wolf et al. 1989; Testerman et al. 1996; Satterwhite et al. 1998; Garfinkel 1997), the perspectives and practices of medical educators (Novack et al. 1999; Feighny et al. 1998; Swick et al. 1999; Kao and Lim 2003; Gibson et al. 2000; Phelan et al. 1993; Papadakis et al. 1999), and the views of learners (Christakis and Feudtner 1993; Ginsburg et al. 2002; Arnold et al. 1998; Brownell et al. 2001) generate the contention that the relevance of the various principles of professionalism changes during a medical career as a result of role responsibilities. Thus, educational activities and assessment should highlight those principles related to the daily work of medical students, residents, or physicians in practice. In short, what a physician needs to know and do and what therefore should be assessed depend on career stage. Resident physicians, for example, would recommend that because principles of professionalism related to societal issues are not intimately germane to their patient care tasks while principles related to caring for individual patients are, assessment of their professionalism should be directed to their commitment to excellence and their respect and compassion for patients (Brownell et al. 2001).

At the same time, evidence also exists for the alternative proposition that the principles of professionalism apply throughout a physician's career. Basic research on the development of moral behavior as well as studies of learners in medical education (Burton 1963; Nelsen et al. 1969; Clark et al. 1987; Rushton 1980; Rogers and Coutts 2000; Stewart 1999; Papadakis et al. 2004) suggests that the specificity of professional behavior according to context is an overstatement. In addition, professional organizations have delineated a comprehensive set of principles that apply equally to medical students, residents, and/or physicians in practice (Medical School Objectives Writing Group 1999, Accreditation Council for Graduate Medical Education 2004; ABIM 1994; Arnold 2002). Moreover, effective pedagogy that enables learners to anticipate and practice their future in safe surroundings also supports the notion that the principles of professionalism are relevant to all stages of a medical career. Similarly, developmental relationships among the principles of professionalism (Clark et al. 1987; Damon 2001; Eisenberg et al. 1991; Christakis and Feudtner 1993; Arnold 2002; Castellani and Wear 2000; Ginsburg et al. 2000; Shaffer 1993; Rushton 1980) argue for an assessment approach that examines learners' progress toward acquiring, embracing, and demonstrating the principles of professionalism throughout their career. Finally, the dynamic nature of human development, including the active participation of learners and the cyclical progression of learning, renders the decision to postpone assessment of some principles of professionalism until a later career phase and the selection of those principles less than straightforward (Archer 1989; Weidman et al. 2001; Clark et al. 1987; Santrock 2001; Merz 1961; Stockmeyer and Williams 1988; Papalia et al. 2001; Francis et al. 2001; Branch 2000; Self and Baldwin 1998; Satterwhite et al. 1998; Rennie and Crosby 2002). On what grounds, then, can a choice be made between equally worthy stances?

An approach that merges the two propositions offers a way forward: Assess each principle of professionalism at each stage of a medical career, but contextualize the principles, set stage-specific achievement levels, and approach assessment of professionalism from a developmental perspective. In contextualizing the principles, the assessment of each principle and the indicators that measure the achievement of learners and practitioners with respect to these principles should be tied to daily role responsibilities. For example, assessing medical students' accountability might well be operationalized as the timely completion of assignments in basic science in small groups or in following through with patient care tasks on clerkships. Measurements of residents' accountability might include the timeliness with which they complete patient care notes, while assessment of practitioners' accountability could include participation in peer review committees examining quality of patient care provided by colleagues. Another way to tailor the principles of professionalism to the role of student, resident, and practitioner involves Miller's pyramid of learning—the familiar "know, can, do" schema (Miller 1990; see figure 2-2). The pyramid provides for teaching and assessing knowledge, then competence or the capacity to apply, and finally actual performance in practice. By adapting the pyramid to professionalism, learners would be expected to reach stage-specific achievement in knowledge, competence, and performance depending upon the principle at hand. In fact, several studies of the longitudinal as-

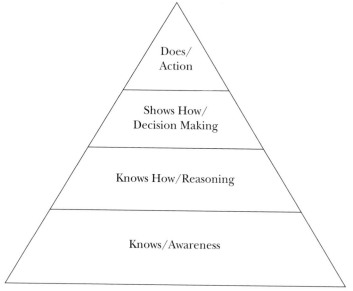

Figure 2-2   Combined Miller–Rest model for professionalism assessment.

sessment of the ethical development of medical students (Roberts et al. 1997) and residents (Larkin 1999) adopted this approach. Initially, only learners' ethical knowledge was tested. The following year their knowledge of ethics and competence in applying ethical principles to simulated scenarios were examined. In the final year, learners' ethical knowledge, competence, and performance in actual clinical settings were assessed. This scheme can be applied more generally with the construction of a matrix, to indicate levels of assessment by career stage.

Developmental models might also promote assessment of professionalism according to career stage. Extension of Rest and Narvaez's adaptation of the stages of moral development to professional development is a case in point (Rest and Narvaez 1994; Baldwin and Bunch 2000). Depending upon the principle of professionalism at hand and a physician's career stage, assessment of professionalism would be progressively and cumulatively directed toward the following developmental stages. The first stages are awareness or the ability to identify the principles of professionalism in clinical and professional situations and the ability to reason through these principles. Later stages encompass the ability to prioritize these principles relative to other values and finally possession of the character and skills to act, based on these principles. Figure 2-2 illustrates this approach (Stern 2002). It suggests, for example, that students would first be assessed for their ability to recognize that there are conflicts between professionalism principles in simulated or real clinical scenarios and then for their ability to reason and reach a choice from among competing principles in these scenarios. Assessment for the behavior they demonstrate or take when faced with conflicting principles in real time would complete this approach.

Other developmental models that specify the depth with which a student, resident, or physician has incorporated the principles of professionalism into his or her professional identity may also be helpful. Forsythe et al. (2002) have adopted Kegan's (1982) schema on the development of the self to understanding the development of a professional identity among army cadets. They argue that the developmental level stage of a cadet has a great deal to do with how he or she relates to the ideals or content of professionalism. Cadets at a relatively early stage (stage 2) see professional values and standards as rules to be followed to achieve something personally important or to avoid negative consequences. Their perspective is self-focused. In the transition to stage 3, cadets shift their focus to understanding themselves as part of a profession, not in terms of their own individual interests. Thus, cadets at stage 3 internalize their profession's values and understand them not just as rules to be followed but also as internal qualities expected of all members of their profession. Their identity at stage 3 is a shared identity, however, and includes all the expectations of the profession. These cadets have not yet achieved a mature autonomous identity and have difficulty resolving competing expectations that are part of professional practice. The transition to stage 4 involves a change in understanding the self as a member of a profession to being a professional. Stage 4 officers own the profession's values, can assess them, and are able to reconcile clashes between personal and professional values.

In this description of the development of the professional self lies a key to understanding how learners in medicine may experience and deal with the conflicts they encounter between equally worthy principles of medicine. That issue, of how learners resolve these conflicts, should be as much a part of assessing professionalism as are the matters of whether, how often, and how far learners have lapsed from the principles of professionalism. An array of reflective techniques can assist in assessing how and why learners resolve conflicts among professional principles.

A developmental view of professionalism has important and beneficial consequences for assessing it. It does not cast professionalism as a series of innate traits or attributes. Rather, it casts professionalism as a continual striving toward principles, toward virtues. It takes account of growth spurts observed in physicians' professionalism as they live out their careers, of transitions and plateaus in their growth, and even of regression. The developmental view highlights the need for formative, longitudinal assessment of learners' professionalism, for the use of qualitative methods involving self assessment and reflection, and for setting stage-specific cut points for acceptable and unacceptable behavior, depending, perhaps, upon the principle of professionalism involved.

Summary

For the purposes of assessment, *professionalism* is demonstrated through a foundation of clinical competence, communication skills, and ethical and legal understanding, upon which is built the aspiration to and wise application of the principles of professionalism:

excellence, humanism, accountability, and altruism. These elements cannot be measured with a single tool or a single item but demand the use of multiple observations, using multiple methods, over time. Each principle of professionalism is broad and contains the domains of knowledge, skills, and behaviors. The foundational knowledge and skills of professionalism could be taught and measured at an early stage and provide the focus of the early chapters in this book. While the measurement of general medical competence is not included, chapters 3–5 provide guidance for the measurement of ethical and legal knowledge, communication skills, and moral reasoning skills.

The measurement of professional behavior is substantially more complex and is the focus of chapters 6–12. Each chapter provides a means through which one or more principles of professionalism could be measured. It is not expected that any one of these methods will suffice; rather, the comprehensive assessment of professionalism in an individual or group may require the use of multiple choices from among these selected methods. Similar among them, however, is that each method provides a description of how to measure behaviors in the context of practice, in a manner that could be adopted to reflect the developmental perspective and yet maintain an aspirational view to the ideal medical professional.

From a practical perspective, the definition of professionalism provided here should be considered a starting point for an organizational response to the definition and assessment of professionalism. In order for assessment to have meaning, the group participating in the evaluation must agree on the definitions of terms and the principles underlying assessment. Moreover, the definition of professionalism that an organization crafts must also reflect the denotation and connotations that accumulating scholarship on professionalism attributes to the concept. Our recommendation is to use this book as an organizational guide to the principles of professionalism to be assessed at your institution.

References

Abbot LC. A Study of Humanism in Family Physicians. J Fam Pract. 1983; 16:1141–1146.

ABIM. Subcommittee on Evaluation of Humanistic Qualities in the Internist. Evaluation of Humanistic Qualities in the Internist. Ann Intern Med. 1983;99:720–724.

ABIM. Guide to Awareness and Evaluation of Humanistic Qualities in the Internist. Philadelphia, PA: American Board of Internal Medicine, 1992.

ABIM. Project Professionalism. Philadelphia, PA: American Board of Internal Medicine, 1994.

ABIM. American College of Physicians–American Society of Internal Medicine Foundation, European Federation of Internal Medicine. Medical Professionalism in the New Millennium: A Physician Charter. Ann Intern Med. 2002;136:243–246.

ACGME Outcome Project. Enhancing Residency Education Through Outcomes Assessment; General Competencies. Version 1.2. Chicago, IL: Accreditation Council for Graduate Medical Education, 1999. Available at: http://www.acgme.org/outcome/comp/compFull.asp. Accessed March 22, 2004.

Adams J, Schmidt T, Sanders A, Larkin GL, Knopp R. Professionalism in Emergency Medicine. Acad Emerg Med. 1998;5:1193–1199.

Anonymous. The Making of Doctors. New York Times, June 12, 1910;12.

Archer SL. The Status of Identity: Reflections on the Need for Intervention. J Adolesc. 1989;12:345–359.

Arnold EL, Blank LL, Race KEH, Cipparrone N. Can Professionalism Be Measured? The Development of a Scale for Use in the Medical Education Environment. Acad Med. 1998;73:1119–1121.

Arnold L. Assessing Professional Behavior: Yesterday, Today, and Tomorrow. Acad Med. 2002;77:502–515.

Association of American Medical Colleges and the National Board of Medical Examiners. Embedding Professionalism in Medical Education: Assessment as a Tool for Implementation. Baltimore, MD, May 15–17, 2002 (Invitational Conference).

Association of American Medical Colleges Group on Educational Affairs. Professionalism Project Website. Available at: www.acgme.org/outcome/comp/compFull.asp. Accessed on March 22, 2004.

Baldwin DC Jr., Bunch WH. Moral Reasoning, Professionalism, and the Teaching of Ethics of Orthopedic Surgeons. Clin Orthoped Rel Res. 2000;378:97–103.

Batson CE, Bolen MH, Cross JA, Neuringer-Benefiel HE. Where Is Altruism in the Altruistic Personality? Journal of Personality and Social Psychology. 1986;50(1);212–220.

Branch WT. Supporting the Moral Development of Medical Students. J Gen Intern Med. 2000;15:503–508.

Brandeis LD. Business—A Profession. Address Delivered at Brown University Commencement Day. October 1912.

Brody H. Professionalism, Ethics, or Both? Does it Matter? Med Hum Rep. 2003;24:1–4.

Brownell AKW, Cote L. Senior Residents' Views on the Meaning of Professionalism and How They Learn About It. Acad Med. 2001;76:734–737.

Burton R. Generality of Honesty Reconsidered. Psychol Rev. 1963;70:481–499.

Carlo G, Eisenberg N, Troyer D, Switzer G, Speer AL. The Altruistic Personality: In What Contexts Is It Apparent? J Pers Soc Psychol. 1991;61:450–458.

Castellani B, Wear D. Physician Views on Practicing Professionalism in the Corporate Age. Qual Health Res. 2000;10:490–506.

Christakis DA, Feudtner C. Ethics in a Short White Coat: The Ethical Dilemmas That Medical Students Confront. Acad Med. 1993;68:249–254.

Clark MS, Powell MC, Ovellette R, Milberg S. Recipient's Mood, Relationship Type, and Helping. J Pers Soc Psychol. 1987;43:94–103.

Coyle SL. Physician–Industry Relations. Part 1: Individual Physicians. Ann Intern Med. 2002;136(5):396–402.

Cruess RL, Cruess SR. Teaching Medicine as a Profession in the Service of Healing. Acad Med. 1997;72:941–952.

Cruess RL, Cruess SR, Johnston SE. Renewing Professionalism: An Opportunity for Medicine. Acad Med. 1999;74:878–884.

Cruess RL, Cruess SR, Johnston SE. Professionalism and Medicine's Social Contract. J Bone Joint Surg Am. 2000a;82(8):1189–1194.

Cruess RL, Cruess SR, Johnston SE. Professionalism: An Ideal to Be Sustained. Lancet. 2000b;356:156–159.

Damon W. The Moral Child. New York: Free Press, 1988. In: Santrock JW. Adolescence. 8th ed. Boston: McGraw Hill, 2001; 405.

Eisenberg N, Miller PA, Shell R, McNalley S, Shea C. Prosocial Development in Adolescence: A Longitudinal Study. Dev Psychol. 1991;27:849–857.

Emmanuel EJ, Emmanuel LL. What Is Accountability in Health Care? Ann Intern Med. 1996;124:229–239.

Feighny KM, Arnold L, Monaco M, Munro JS, Earl B. In Pursuit of Empathy and Its Relation to Physician Communication Skills: Multidimensional Empathy Training for Medical Students. Ann Behav Sci Med Educ. 1998;5:13–21.

Flexner A. Is Social Work a Profession? School and Society. June 26, 1915;26(1):904.

Forsythe GB, Snook S, Lewis P, Bartone P. Making Sense of Officership: Developing a Professional Identity for 21st Century Army Officers. In: Snider D, Watkins G, eds. The Future of the Army Profession. New York: McGraw Hill, 2002;357–378.

Francis J, Fraser G, Marcia JE. Cognitive and Experimental Factors in Moratorium-Achievement (MAMA) Cycles. Unpublished manuscript, Department of Psychology, Simon Fraser University, Burnaby, British Columbia, 1989. In: Santrock JW. Adolescence. 8th ed. Boston: McGraw Hill, 2001;310.

Garfinkel PE, Bagby RM, Waring EM, Dorian B. Boundary Violations and Personality Traits Among Psychiatrists. Can J Psychiatry. 1997;42:758–763.

Gibson DD, Coldwell LL, Kiewit SF. Creating a Culture of Professionalism: An Integrated Approach. Acad Med. 2000;75:509.

Ginsburg S, Hatala R, McNaughton N, Frohna A, Hodges B, Lingard L, Stern D. Context, Conflict, and Resolution: A New Conceptual Framework for Evaluating Professionalism. Acad Med. 2000;75:S6–S11.

Ginsburg S, Regehr G, Stern D, Lingard L. The Anatomy of the Professional Lapse: Bridging the Gap Between Traditional Frameworks and Students' Perceptions. Acad Med. 2002;77:516–522.

Hafferty FW. Keynote Address. Overcoming the Barriers to Sustaining Humanism in Medicine: Influencing the Culture Through a Humanism Honor Society. Invitational Conference of the Arnold P. Gold Foundation. Secaucus, NJ, March 2001.

Halpern J. What Is Clinical Empathy? J Gen Intern Med. 2003;18:670.

Hartshorne H, May MS. Studies in the Nature of Character. Vol. 1. Studies in Deceit. New York: Macmillan, 1928–1930; 411.

Hojat M, Gonnella JS, Nasca TJ, Mangione S, Magee M. Physician Empathy in Medical Education and Practices: Experience With the Jefferson Scale of Physician Empathy. Semin Integrative Med. 2003a;1:25–41.

Hojat M, Gonnella JS, Nasca TJ, Mangione S, Vergare M, Magee M. Physician Empathy: Definition, Components, Measurement, and Relationship to Gender and Specialty. Am J Psychiatry. 2002;159:1563–1569.

Hojat M, Nasca TJ, Erdmann JB, Frisby AJ, Veloski JJ, Gonnella JS. An Operational Measure of Physician Lifelong Learning: Its Development, Components and Preliminary Psychometric Data. Med Teacher. 2003b;25(4): 433–437.

Institute for International Medical Education, Core Committee. Global minimum essential requirements in medical education. Med Teacher. 2002;24(2):130–135.

Jacobellis v. Ohio, 378 U.S. 184, 197, 1964 (Stewart J, concurring).

Kao A, Lim M, Sperick J, Barzansky B. Teaching and Evaluating Students' Professionalism in US Medical Schools, 2002–2003. JAMA. 2003;290: 1151–1152.

Kegan R. The Evolving Self: Problem and Process in Human Development. Cambridge, MA: Harvard University Press, 1982.

Kilpatrick SD, McCullough ME. An Annotated Bibliography of Research on Personality and Individual Differences in Altruism. Available at: http://www.unlimitedloveinstitute.org/publications/pdf/annotated/Annotated_Bibliography.pdf. Accessed March 29, 2004.

Kimball HR. Medical Professionalism: At a Crossroads? 11th Annual Coggeshall Memorial Lecture, University of Chicago, April 2000.

Larkin GL. Evaluating Professionalism in Emergency Medicine: Clinical Ethical Competence. Acad Emerg Med. 1999;6:302–311.

Ludmerer KM. Learning to Heal. New York: Basic Books Inc., 1985.

Marcus ER. Empathy, Humanism, and the Professionalization Process of Medical Education. Acad Med. 1999;74:1211–1215.

McGaghie WC, Mytko JJ, Brown WN, Cameron JR. Altruism and Compassion in the Health Professions: A Search for Clarity and Precision. Med Teacher. 2002;24:374–378.

Medical School Objectives Project Writing Group. Learning Objectives for Medical Student Education—Guidelines for Medical Schools: Report I of the Medical School Objectives Project. Acad Med. 1999;74:13–18.

Merz L. The Graduate School as a Socializing Agency: A Pilot Study of Sociological Aspects of Graduate Training in the Physical Sciences. Ithaca, NY: Cornell University, 1961.

Miller GE. The Assessment of Clinical Skills/Competence/Performance. Acad Med. 1990;65:S63–S67.

Murray TH. Closing Reflections. Chinese-American Conference on Medical Ethics in Practice, Teaching, and Research: May 1999, Beijing. Hastings Center Rep. July 2000;30(4):S45.

Nelsen EA, Grinder RE, Mutterer ML. Sources of Variance in Behavioral Measures of Honesty in Temptation Situations: Methodological Analyses. Dev Psychol. 1969;1:265–279.

Novack DH, Epstein RM, Paulsen RH. Toward Creating Physician-Healers: Fostering Medical Students' Self-Awareness, Personal Growth, and Well Being. Acad Med. 1999;74:516–520.

Oxford English Dictionary, 2nd edition. Oxford: Oxford University Press, 1989. Available at: http://www.oed.com. Accessed June 20, 2005.

Papadakis MA, Hodgson CS, Teherani A, Kohatsu ND. Unprofessional Behavior in Medical School Is Associated With Subsequent Disciplinary Action by a State Medical Board. Acad Med. 2004;79:244–249.

Papadakis MA, Osborn EHS, Cooke M, Healy K. A Strategy for the Detection and Evaluation of Unprofessional Behavior in Medical Students. Acad Med. 1999;74:980–990.

Papalia DE et al. Human Development. 8th ed. Boston: McGraw Hill, 2001; 507.

Peabody FW. The Care of the Patient. JAMA 1927;88:877–882.

Pellegrino ED, Thomasma DC. A Philosophical Basis of Medical Practice: Toward a Philosophy and Ethic of the Healing Professions. New York: Oxford University Press, January 1981.

Phelan S, Obenshain SS, Galey WR. Evaluation of the Non-cognitive Professional Traits of Medical Students. Acad Med. 1993;68:799–803.

Piliavin JA, Charng HW. Altruism: A Review of Recent Theory and Research. Annu Rev Sociol. 1990;16:27–65.

Rennie SC, Crosby JR. Students' Perceptions of Whistle Blowing: Implications for Self-Regulation. A Questionnaire and Focus Group Survey. Med Educ. 2002;36:173–179.

Rest JR, Narvaez D. Moral Development in the Professions: Psychology and Applied Ethics. Hillsdale, NJ: Lawrence Erlbaum Associates, 1994.

Rezler AG, Schwartz RL, Obenshain SS, Lambert P, Gibson JM, Bennahum DA. Assessment of Ethical Decisions and Values. Med Educ. 1992;26:7–16.

Roberts LW and the Subcommittee on Professional Attitudes and Values, Student Progress Assessment. Sequential Assessment of Medical Student Competence With Respect to Professional Attitudes, Values, and Ethics. Acad Med. 1997;72:428–429.

Rogers JC, Coutts L. Do Students' Attitudes During Preclinical Years Predict Their Humanism as Clerkship Students? Acad Med. 2000;75: S74–S77.

Rushton JP. Altruism, Socialization, and Society. Englewood Cliffs, NJ: Prentice-Hall, 1980; 55–57, 66, 71–72.

Santrock JW. Adolescence. 8th ed. Boston: McGraw Hill, 2001; 310, 395–396, 400–401, 404–406.

Satterwhite WM, Satterwhite MA, Enarson CE. Medical Students' Perceptions of Unethical Conduct at One Medical School. Acad Med. 1998;73: 529–531.

Self DJ, Baldwin DC Jr. Does Medical Education Inhibit the Development of Moral Reasoning in Medical Students? A Cross-sectional Study. Acad Med. 1998;73:S91–S93.

Shaffer DR. Developmental Psychology Childhood and Adolescence. 3rd ed. Pacific Grove, CA: Brooks Cole Publishing, 1993; 541–544.

Simmons JMP, Robie PW, Kendrick SB, Schumacher S, Roberge LP. Residents' Use of Humanistic Skills and Content of Resident Discussions in a Support Group. Am J Med Sci. 1992;303:227–232.

Starr P. The Social Transformation of American Medicine. New York: Basic Books, 1982.

Stern DT. Behavior-Based Methods for Assessing Professionalism. Invited Plenary Lecture, GSA/GSA-MAS/OSR Plenary Session, AAMC National Meeting, San Francisco, CA, November 10, 2002.

Stewart JB. Blind Eye: How the Medical Establishment Let a Doctor Get Away With Murder. New York: Simon and Schuster, 1999.

Stockmeyer J, Williams RH. Life Trek: The Odyssey of Adult Development. Atlanta, GA: Humanics New Age, 1988; 9–73.

Swick HM, Szenas P, Danoff D, Whitcomb ME. Teaching Professionalism in Undergraduate Medical Education. JAMA. 1999;282:830–832.

Testerman JK, Morton KR, Loo LK, Worthley JS, Lamberton HH. The Natural History of Cynicism in Physicians. Acad Med. 1996;71:S43–S45.

Weidman JC, Twale DJ, Stein EL. Socialization of Graduate and Professional Students in Higher Education: A Perilous Passage? ASHE-Eric Higher Educ Rep. 2001;28(3):1–112.

Wolf TM, Balson PM, Faucett JM, Randall HM. A Retrospective Study of Attitude Change During Medical Education. Med Educ. 1989;23:19–23.

3

Ethics, Law, and Professionalism:
What Physicians Need to Know

Audiey Kao

- A governor and state legislature intervene and order rein-
  sertion of a feeding tube of a woman in a persistent vegeta-
  tive state
- A physician informs his patient that a medical error has occurred, despite having serious concerns about the malpractice implications of such a disclosure
- A federal law setting national standards designed to protect
  the privacy of personal health care information is passed by
  the U.S. Congress
- A patient is asked if she has any further questions about
  the risks of the surgery before signing the consent form

The practice of medicine requires physicians to properly balance ethical principles with legal requirements and liabilities. In some cases,
a physician's ethical duty and legal responsibility are concordant, and
thus, the appropriate course of action is relatively clear and straightforward. For example, a physician needs to provide a patient with all
relevant information before soliciting consent for treatment. The

doctrine of informed consent is supported by the ethical principle of patient autonomy as well as by the legal concept of bodily integrity.

In other situations, however, the application of ethical principles in medical practice can conflict with statutory requirements or legal liability. For example, a physician who cares for suspected illegal immigrants struggles with whether to report his patients' residency status information to authorities as required under state law; or a physician must decide whether to continue aggressive medical treatment because the perceived liability risk of withdrawing life-sustaining care is seen as higher than the liability risk of continuing treatment. It is during these circumstances of discordance between ethics and law (or the legal consequences of certain physicians' decisions and conduct) that the principles of professionalism properly applied can aid in resolving challenging situations in medical practice. Wise resolutions of these situations provide examples of behavior that characterize the ideal professional.

In this chapter, we consider some common situations in which ethics, law, and professionalism interact in medicine. Many of these situations are those that physicians should be able to manage comfortably, while there are some that pose challenges. Any comprehensive assessment of professionalism should necessarily engage medical students and physicians in how they would handle straightforward cases as well as some challenging dilemmas.

Common Interactions of Ethics, Law, and Professionalism

Securing Informed Consent

Ethical Principle
Informed consent is the formal means for honoring the principle of respect for patient autonomy. Originally codified in the Nuremberg Code and subsequently in the Declaration of Helsinki, the duty to respect an individual's informed choice has since extended from human subjects research protections to all aspects of medicine (Faden and Beauchamp 1986). To comply with informed consent, a physician must provide the patient with all relevant information about the risks and benefits of the recommended intervention, including the risks and benefits of no intervention. Provided with this information, patients can choose what course to take as long as they are competent to make the decision and that the decision is a voluntary one,

that is, not coerced. It is important to keep in mind that this approach allows a patient to makes a choice the physician considers "unwise."

Physicians engaged in clinical research need to consider expectations patients have of them as clinicians and as researchers, and potential financial conflicts of interests of research. As more physicians, especially those in community practice, become more involved in clinical research, we must be mindful of the potentially conflicting roles of investigator and clinician and the potential for physicians to unduly influence patients' decisions to participate in trials that may or may not have any direct therapeutic benefit for them. According to the American Medical Association Code of Medical Ethics,

> When a physician has treated or continues to treat a patient who is eligible to enroll as a subject in a clinical trial that the physician is conducting, the informed consent process must differentiate between the physician's roles as clinician and investigator. This is best achieved when someone other than the treating physician obtains the participant's informed consent to participate in the trial. (American Medical Association 2002, p. 83)

In addition, physicians are often paid for recruiting research subjects and for participating in the implementation of the clinical trial. In such instances, the "nature and source of funding and financial incentives offered to the investigators must be disclosed to a potential participant as part of the informed consent process." The rate of financial compensation should not "vary according to the volume of subjects enrolled by the physician" (American Medical Association 2002, p. 83).

Legal Standard
In 1914, the New York Supreme Court firmly established the legal basis for patient autonomy under the constitutional right to bodily integrity. Based on a case in which a surgeon removed a tumor from an anesthetized patient without the patient's consent, Justice Benjamin Cardozo wrote in his decision: "It is trespass. Every human being of adult years and sound mind has a right to determine what shall be done with his own body; and a surgeon who performs an operation without his patient's consent commits an assault" (*Schloendorff v. Society of New York Hospital* 1914, p. 130).

Professionalism Challenge
There are few disputes from an ethical or legal perspective about the importance of securing informed consent as part of good medical practice and clinical research. Nevertheless, there may be some gray areas concerning the type and amount of information needed to inform the patient sufficiently before seeking consent. In the era of managed care, physician reimbursement methods and financial incentives have been increasingly recognized by the courts as relevant information to the informed consent process (Miller and Sage 1999). Legal decisions raise many unresolved practical considerations, including the form of disclosure, means of enforcing disclosure, and the potential impact of disclosure on patient trust. At the minimum, physicians should be prepared to answer questions about financial incentives if patients inquire.

Protecting Patient Confidentiality

Ethical Principle
Keeping in confidence the personal information that patients disclose lies at the heart of ethical medical practice and derives from the principle of nonmaleficence (or do no harm) and from the principle that demands respect for patient autonomy. When patient confidentiality is not protected, patients may be less likely to reveal personally sensitive medical information to their physicians. Yet, confidentiality is generally not viewed as an absolute rule and can be breached for ethically justifiable reasons such as the duty to prevent significant harm to identifiable third parties (e.g., cases of communicable diseases such as tuberculosis and HIV). *Tarasoff v. Regents of University of California* (1976) is a landmark case that explored the obligation of physicians to break confidentiality. In *Tarasoff*, a psychologist failed to warn a woman or her family when his patient threatened to murder the woman (which he subsequently did). The court found that the psychologist had an obligation to warn the potential victim even though it meant breaching confidentiality. In such cases, the ethical justification and legal requirements for breaching confidentiality are concordant.

Legal Standard
The right to privacy provides a legal foundation for patient confidentiality (Krulwich and McDonald 2000). While the word "privacy" does not appear in the U.S. Constitution, an individual's guaranteed right to privacy has been drawn from various Amendments, includ-

ing the Fifth and Ninth. In *Griswold v. Connecticut* (1965), a physician was charged with aiding and abetting "the use of a drug, medicinal article, or instrument for the purpose of preventing conception," a crime under Connecticut law, by providing contraceptives to unmarried people. The Supreme Court reversed the physician's conviction, and Justice Douglas, writing for the Court, concluded that "specific guarantees in the Bill of Rights have penumbras, formed by emanations from those guarantees that helped give them life and substance. Various guarantees create zones of privacy" (p. 484). The constitutional right to privacy acknowledged in *Griswold* ultimately found its most significant articulation in *Roe v. Wade* (1973).

The legal doctrine of privacy as it applies to patient confidentiality was made more uniform across states with passage of the federal Health Insurance Portability and Accountability Act (HIPAA) legislation. As a consequence of HIPAA, national standards govern the access, dissemination, and use of personally identifiable health information for purposes of patient care, business functions such as billing and marketing, and public health research.

Professionalism Challenge

In certain situations, physicians may have difficulty justifying a legal requirement to report patient information to third parties. This often occurs when a physician believes the legal duty to report will not reduce potential harm to others but, in fact, may increase potential harm to others, for example, Proposition 501 in California, which requires physicians to report the residency status of illegal immigrants. Such examples of physicians serving as "agents of the state" highlight the role of physicians as "double agents." In these circumstances, a physician has obligations to patients but also may have responsibilities to third parties including insurers, government agencies, and the courts. In resolving these double-agency conflicts with patient confidentiality, a physician should initially inform patients of reporting requirements to third parties. Under circumstances where a breach in confidentiality does not benefit identifiable third parties and actually harms the patient, the physician may be ethically justified in not obeying legal requirements for reporting.

Disclosing Difficult Information

Ethical Principle

The duty to disclose difficult information derives from respect for patient autonomy and is guided by the ethic of truth-telling (English

1994; Surbone 1997). Being honest with patients strengthens trust in the clinical relationship and gives them the knowledge necessary for "informed" consent. It is worth noting that disclosing difficult information such as "bad news" about a diagnosis and prognosis was not the accepted professional norm in the past. For example, in 1961 only 10% of surveyed physicians believed it was appropriate to tell a patient of a fatal cancer diagnosis; by 1979, 97% felt that such disclosure was appropriate (Novack et al. 1979). This physician attitude about not disclosing bad news was in part guided by a sense of paternalism and the principle of beneficence.

Legal Standard

Concerns about the legal consequences of disclosure can be operative in these situations. For example, in cases of disclosing medical errors to patients, physicians may be concerned that such disclosure will increase their legal liability to malpractice suits. Patients and physicians have different attitudes regarding such disclosure, as demonstrated by a study by Gallagher et al. (2003). Patients generally want to know about all harmful errors. They expect information about what happened, why the error occurred, how the error's consequences will be mitigated, and how recurrences will be prevented. Physicians agree that harmful errors should be disclosed, but they choose their words carefully and often avoid stating that an error occurred, why the error happened, or how occurrences would be prevented. Physicians in this study also worried that an apology would increase their malpractice risk.

Professionalism Challenge

Despite general consensus that physicians must be open and honest in disclosing difficult information to patients, circumstances may arise when the notion of "therapeutic privilege" is invoked. Therapeutic privilege is the permissibility of physicians to withhold information from a patient when it is believed that this information might harm the patient. An example of such a circumstance is a patient who has a psychiatric disorder such as hypochrondriasis. In various situations, the patient's physical symptoms are psychosomatic in nature. Disclosure of this diagnosis and recommending psychiatric treatment often can aggravate the situation. Therefore, a physician may choose to withhold this "bad news" while working toward establishing a relationship where recommendation for psychiatric treatment would be better received by the patient.

Some physicians are concerned that disclosure of difficult information such as the occurrence of a medical error may increase their legal liability. Some studies have suggested that disclosure of an error occurrence may actually reduce malpractice liability (Beckman et al. 1994; Kraman et al. 1999; Witman et al. 1996). Patients appreciate the physician's honesty and commitment to identify the factors that contributed to the error and "fixing" the problem for the future. Even if the evidence for reducing liability risk is not yet conclusive, it is important for physicians to learn how to better communicate difficult information to patients in ways that will reinforce trust and not undermine the therapeutic relationship.

Withholding or Withdrawing Care

Ethical Principle

As with informed consent, the operative ethical principle in decisions to withhold or withdraw care in competent patients is respect for individual autonomy and self-determination, as well as do no harm. In cases of withholding or withdrawing life-sustaining care as opposed to consent for routine medical tests or procedures, patients are often unable to make decisions for themselves due to incapacity created by the trauma, illness, or disease. In these cases, advance directives that establish a living will and designate a health care proxy can provide helpful guidance in addressing the situation. However, only one-fifth of patients have advance directives. This fact may in part be explained by the reality that such discussions often involve difficult and emotionally charged topics such as unfavorable prognoses and treatment failures, treatment choices and family responses to them, and the meaning of illness and the suffering it creates. Therefore, it is imperative that physicians have the communication skills to effectively engage patients in such "end-of-life" conversations so as to better understand and document patient wishes and preferences if such situations present themselves.

Legal Standard

While there is general uniformity of legal standards for informed consent, the legal standard that dictate the withholding or withdrawing of care are more variable across states, especially in the absence of a competent patient or advance directive. In landmark cases such as *Quinlan* (1976) and *Cruzan v. Director* (1997), the courts have recognized the right of patients and their proxies or surrogates to choose to withhold or withdraw life-sustaining treatment, including artificial nutrition and hydration. Yet in states such as New York with high legal standards about withholding or withdrawing care, the ability to use a "best interest" of the patient or "substituted judgment" standard (under which family members are permitted to make end-of-life decisions on behalf of the patient) is constrained.

Professionalism Challenge

In situations where there is disagreement among family members such as between a patient's spouse and parents, a physician's clinical determination that withdrawing care is appropriate may be undercut by concerns about legal liability or regulatory scrutiny. The wishes of a family member advocating a more aggressive medical approach may be given greater weight because the perceived legal risks of continuing treatment are less than those of stopping it. Under these circumstances, the ethic of "do no harm" or nonmaleficence must guide the decision to continue withholding or to withdraw care.

Measuring the Interactions of Ethics, Law, and Professionalism

An understanding of the principles of ethics and law related to medicine is a foundational component to any physician's overall professionalism. Physicians who practice compassionate and respectful care would be considered just as incompetent if they ignored these principles as if they practiced without an understanding of anatomy or pharmacology. Any comprehensive system to assess professionalism must therefore contain an element that measures the individual student's or physician's understanding of ethics and law.

Some would argue that the competent physician must not only have this understanding but also be able to demonstrate the ability to negotiate the dilemmas outlined in the preceding section. Ultimately, physicians demonstrate their abilities to negotiate ethical and professional dilemmas in practice, but the observation of these relatively infrequent events would be costly if performed in real time. In recent years, medical educators have developed assessment programs for just these purposes. Most assessments have been in the form of either multiple-choice question examinations or standardized patient scenarios, depicting students and physicians in scenarios that challenge their abilities to resolve ethical and professional dilemmas.

Written examinations (multiple-choice questions) are commonly used as a reliable method of assessing medical knowledge and understanding. These types of assessments have been developed for ethics, law, and professionalism, as well (Rezler et al. 1992; Mitchell et al. 1993). For example, Barry et al. (2000) have developed a six-item examination in medical professionalism covering the domains of conflicts of interest, confidentiality, physician impairment, sexual harassment, honesty, and acceptance of gifts. Two items from this examination follow:

> A pharmaceutical company approaches you about a clinical research project involving your office patients. Your patients with high blood pressure will be eligible to be treated with a new medication that has just been released by the FDA. The object of the study is to evaluate risks and benefits of this medication in an unselected office population. The pharmaceutical company will pay $250 per patient for the expenses generated by the study, and [the company will pay] one year's salary for a data manager and will supply the drug free of charge. Meetings to discuss the initiation of the study and follow-up results will be held in New Orleans and Honolulu. Your spouse will be invited as the company's guest to attend these meetings since they will take you away from home. Participating in the study would be considered appropriate professional behavior if:
> a. Your patients signed an informed consent
> b. Your patients sign an informed consent and your partners approve the study
> c. An oversight committee of the hospital where you have privileges or your regional medical society approves the study
> d. None of the above. (Barry et al. 2000, p. 141)

An established patient of yours presents with symptoms of depression. This is the second time in 3 months that the patient has visited you for these complaints. You wish to start treatment with antidepressant medication. As you are filling the prescription, the patient asks you not to document the diagnosis or medication in the chart. She is concerned that her employer will find out about her diagnosis and she could potentially lose her job like a co-worker did. She knows that her insurance company has access to her diagnosis. How do you proceed?
a. Inform the patient that you must document the diagnosis to provide any treatment.

    b. Agree to not document the diagnosis but prescribe the medication anyway.

    c. Agree to not document the diagnosis but refuse to provide the prescription.

    d. Terminate your relationship with the patient because she is inhibiting your ability to provide adequate care. (Barry et al. 2000, p. 142)

The reliability of multiple-choice examinations relates to the purpose of assessment, the number of domains being assessed, and the number of questions posed. Because case-based questions provide the most realistic item stems and because knowledge is often case specific (Case & Swanson 1996), a single domain should be sampled many times. In practical terms, for formative assessment a single domain could be assessed with only one or two cases. For high-stakes summative assessment, a domain such as patient confidentiality would be assessed with at least 7–10 cases. If the domain is considered more broadly to be "medical ethics," a sampling across multiple subdomains (e.g., confidentiality, end-of-life decisions) would produce a longer discipline-based assessment (for more details on multiple-choice examination item writing and exam blueprinting, see Case & Swanson 1996).

    The content and face validity of written examinations in ethics, law, and professionalism are usually excellent, since the cases are written by experts in the field and scoring algorithms are designed by these same individuals (Barry et al. 2000; Rezler et al. 1992; Mitchell et al. 1993). Written assessments can be used to evaluate not only "correct answers" but also the recognition of ethical dilemmas and aspects of the reasoning process (Smith et al. 2004; Hebert et al. 1992; Knabe et al. 1994; Myser et al. 1995; for a detailed description of tests of moral reasoning, see the Baldwin and Self chapter in this volume). Whether results of written examinations predict ethical behavior in real-world practice (predictive validity) remains unknown. No studies as yet have made a direct connection between knowledge of ethics, law, or professionalism and more ethical, legal, or professional practice. This lack of evidence does not imply that none exists; to the contrary, these principles are likely to be the foundation upon which ethical and professional behavior is based.

    An assessment method for ethics that moves closer to the real-world context is the objective structured clinical examination

(OSCE) using standardized patient (SP) and/or patient proxies, who are often portrayed by trained actors. These individuals are employed to simulate a potential clinical encounter between patient and clinician. These SP assessment methods are used to evaluate how a medical student or physician would decide and behave when presented with a hypothetical but real-world–based clinical scenario. Because of the same case specificity mentioned above for multiple-choice questions, many cases are necessary for high-stakes reliability (summative assessment). Fewer cases could be used if the purpose is for feedback alone. Methodological issues such as sources of measurement error and standard setting that may undermine the reliability and validity of SP as an assessment can be addressed with proper OSCE design (Norcini and Boulet 2003; details of simulations are presented in chapter 4).

A few sample cases from published materials on ethics OSCEs are outlined below:

- A generally healthy patient presents himself to the physician reporting that he had unprotected anal intercourse with a homosexual lover. Results of an HIV test are positive, and the patient does not want his wife to know of his HIV status (Singer et al. 1996).
- A patient is evaluated with suspected herpes encephalitis and a diagnostic lumbar puncture is indicated. Informed consent for the procedure is needed, but changes in his mental status raise the possibility of impaired decisional capacity (McClean and Card 2004).
- A 48-year-old woman is scheduled for elective angioplasty and wants to speak with her physician about completing an advanced directive (Gallagher et al. 1999).

The published data on OSCEs using SP as a performance-based assessment method for clinical ethics show relatively low test reliability (Singer et al. 1996). OSCEs with SPs that focus simply on generic skills to be measured, such as history taking or physical examination, are generally more reliable. On the other hand, a clinical case content that is richer and more nuanced, such as with ethics OSCEs, the high number of stations required to achieve high-stakes reliability would make maintaining such an evaluation regime cost prohibitive for most institutions. Therefore, "ethics" OSCEs with SPs should not typically be used as a method of summative evaluation and are better suited for formative assessment.

Practical Suggestions for the Assessment of Ethics,
Law, and Professionalism

Multiple-choice examinations are relatively simple to administer but
challenging to design. Writing good multiple-choice ethics items is
extremely challenging, as evidenced by the fact that the National
Board of Medical Examiners does not have a subject-based examination in ethics, despite vigorous efforts to write and include ethics
questions on all examinations (S. Case and K. Holtzman, personal
communication). While efforts continue to develop a bank of good
ethics-related questions, the lack of reliability for even short ethics
examinations should not discourage educators from using them for
the purposes of formative feedback and potentially to identify outliers in ethics knowledge (on either the high or the low end). Although the reliability of an examination may be low, performance
at the extremes can still be useful for evaluative purposes.

OSCE-type examinations are very useful for formative feedback
and provide students with the opportunity to experience ethical decision making in a controlled setting. Even without the evaluative
component, such experiences can be useful for desensitizing students to delicate and challenging situations before they are called
upon to make decisions and counsel patients in the clinical setting.
As a summative assessment tool, the ethics OSCE remains too expensive and has too low a reliability to advocate as a universal requirement. That said, for those institutions with well-established
OSCE programs, it makes sense to include some ethics-based cases
because of the opportunity they provide for student practice. Therefore, a comprehensive OSCE, and competency assessment in general, that covers domains of professionalism sends a powerful message to physicians and the public that our medical educational system
values ethical reasoning and communication skills on the same level
as scientific knowledge and technical abilities. Good doctoring requires it.

References

American Medical Association, Council on Ethical and Judicial Affairs. Man-
    aging conflicts of interest in the conduct of clinical trials. JAMA.
    2002;287:78–84.
Barry D, Cyran E, Anderson RJ. Common issues in medical professionalism:
    room to grow. Am J Med. 2000;108:136–142.

Beckman HB, Markakis KM, Suchman AL, Frankel RM. The doctor-patient relationship and malpractice: lessons from plaintiff depositions. Arch Intern Med. 1994;154:1365–1370.

Case SM, Swanson DB. Constructing Written Test Questions for the Basic and Clinical Sciences. Philadelphia: National Board of Medical Examiners, 1996.

Cruzan v. Director, 497 US 702, 1997.

English DC. Truth-telling. In: Bioethics: A Clinical Guide for Medical Students. New York: W.W. Norton and Company, 1994; 38–43.

Faden R, Beauchamp TL. A History and Theory of Informed Consent. New York: Oxford University Press, 1986.

Gallagher TH, Pantilat SZ, Lo B, Papadakis MA. Teaching medical students to discuss advance directives: a standardized patient curriculum. Teach Learn Med. 1999;11:142–147.

Gallagher TH, Waterman AD, Ebers AG, Fraser VJ, Levinson W. Patients' and physician's attitudes regarding the disclosure of medical errors. JAMA 2003;289:1001–1007.

Griswold v. Connecticut, 381 US 479, 85 SCt 1678, 14 LEd 2d 510, 1965.

Hebert PC, Meslin EM, Dunn EV. Measuring ethical sensitivity of medical students: a study at the University of Toronto. J Med Ethics. 1992;18:142–147.

Knabe BJ, Stearns JA, Glasser M. Medical students' understanding of ethical issues in the ambulatory settings. Fam Med. 1994;26:442–446.

Kraman, S, Hamm, G. Risk management: extreme honesty may be the best policy. Ann Int Med. 1999;131:963–967.

Krulwich AS, McDonald BL. Evolving constitutional privacy doctrines affecting healthcare enterprises. Food Drug Law J. 2000;55:491–516.

McClean KL, Card SE. Informed consent skills in internal medicine residency: how are residents taught, and what do they learn? Acad Med. 2004;79:128–133.

Miller TE, Sage WM. Disclosing physician financial incentives. JAMA. 1999;281:1424–1430.

Mitchell KR, Myser C, Kerridge IH. Assessing the clinical ethical competence of undergraduate medical students. J Med Ethics. 1993;19:230–236.

Myser C, Kerridge IH, Mitchell KR. Ethical reasoning and decision-making in the clinical setting: assessing the process. Med Educ. 1995;29:29–33.

Norcini J, Boulet J. Methodological issues in the use of standardized patients for assessment. Teach Learn Med. 2003;15:293–297.

Novack DM, Plumer R, Smith RL, Ochitill H, Morrow GR, Bennett JM. Changes in physicians' attitudes toward telling the cancer patient. JAMA. 1979;241:897–900.

Quinlan, 355 A2d 647, 1976.

Rezler AG, Schwartz RL, Obenshain SS, Lambert P, Gibson JM, Bennahum DA. Assessment of ethical decisions and values. Med Educ. 1992;26:7–16.

Roe v. Wade, 410 US 113, 93 SCt 705, 35 LEd 2d 147, 1973.

Schloendorff v. Society of New York Hospital, 211 NY 125, 1914.

Singer P, Robb A, Cohen R, Norman G, Turnbull J. Performance-based assessment of clinical ethics using an objective structured clinical examination. Acad Med. 1996;71:495–498.

Smith S, Fryer-Edwards K, Diekema DS, Braddock CH III. Finding effective strategies for teaching ethics: a comparison trial of two interventions. Acad Med. 2004;79:265–271.

Surbone A. Truth-telling, risk, and hope. Ann NY Acad Sci. 1997;809:72–79.

Tarasoff v. Regents of University of California, 17 Cal 3d 425, 551 P 2d 334, 131 Cal Rptr 14 (Cal), 1976.

Witman AB, Park DM, Hardin SB. How do patients want physicians to handle mistakes? Arch Intern Med. 1996;156:2565–2569.

4

Using Standardized Clinical Encounters to Assess Physician Communication

Debra Klamen and Reed Williams

Communication underlies all medical work; taking histories, educating patients, developing alliances, and managing illnesses. Core professional values of compassion, responsibility, and integrity are all demonstrated through communication. In an average day, physicians communicate hundreds of bits of information, with patients, patients' families, and professional colleagues in either oral or written form. Measuring communication skills, and the demonstration of professional behaviors through communication, is the focus of this chapter.

Communication Modalities

Communication can be broken down into four broad modalities, and each modality may be employed "intentionally" or "unintentionally."

The first element of communication is the ability to speak—to communicate verbally. Of course, mastery of the language being spoken is a necessary but not sufficient condition for a patient to understand what the physician intends. In a more subtle way, the language the physician chooses to use, such as the highly technical "your cardiac enzymes show that you have had a myocardial infarction" versus the lay terminology "your tests have come back showing you probably have had a heart attack," also affects the physician's ability to communicate effectively.

Speaking as a communication device is influenced by the speaker's tone (angry, hopeful, frightened), volume, and rate, as well. In the context of public speaking, communication specialists (Dexter 1992) report that the speaker's words account for 7% of the impact upon the listener, while tone accounts for 38%. (More about the other 55% later.)

Listening is, of course, as essential as speaking if true communication is to occur. Even the most eloquent language will fall on effectively deaf ears if the physician is speaking fluent Italian and discussing the merits of the use of the latest antipsychotic medication and its effect on the dopamine pathway, while the listener speaks only English and has a third-grade education. Part of effective communication is matching the speaking capability of the speaker to the listening capability of the listener. Other factors may interfere with the listener's ability to listen, thus cutting off all hope of effective communication. A noisy environment in which there are many distractions, competition for the listener's attention, and a general noise level in the stratosphere will suspend all useful communication. The emotional state of the listener is also important. It is well known that in the throes of being given bad news, most patients do not remember much, if anything, that they were told (Quill and Townsend 1991). Any emotional state that is significantly elevated or depressed will interfere with the listener's ability to listen and thus interfere with communication in general. Finally, the motivation of the listener to receive the information and respond is also an important factor.

Nonverbal communication provides critical clues to both the content and context of spoken language. Gestures, facial expressions, and body posture convey copious amounts of information, without a word being spoken. Body language accounts for fully 55% of the communicator's impact upon the listener, based on communications research on public speaking (Dexter 1992). Patients can infer whether their physicians are bored, distracted, or carefully listening by physicians' use (often unconscious and unintentional) of nonverbal communications. Intentional nonverbal communication can be used to the physician's advantage; leaning slightly toward the patient and paying attention to an open body posture conveys interest in what the patient has to say, silently. Likewise, the physician can garner a great deal of information about the patient by paying attention to these same nonverbal communications. A patient who denies the use of alcohol or drugs, but at the same time avoids looking at the physician, while crossing his arms and angling his body away, is conveying a very different answer by his body language.

Written communication is the fourth modality, a critical one to the success of patient care. Health care professionals of all types must be able to read each other's notes in a clinical chart, and the clarity with which the information is conveyed is important for patient outcomes. Medication errors lead to 7,000 deaths per year, and illegible handwriting is one of the most preventable sources (Institute of Medicine 2000). In one study, the error rate on handwritten prescriptions was 10.2% (Shah et al. 2001). As time to care for individual patients shortens, and the medical record becomes more stylized, the ability to maintain a clear record of hypotheses, management, and plans in the patient's chart becomes ever more important. Written communication is sometimes all that is available to maintain the continuity of care of the patient across time and location—across shifts, between visits, and among treatment sites.

The effects of communication may be intentional (purposeful) or unintentional. In both cases, the effects are equally powerful. Purposeful communication refers to the effectiveness of an individual in achieving intended outcomes when communicating with another person or persons. It is not easy to articulate the wide variety of behaviors that an effective communicator employs in achieving these goals, however. Doubtless, truly excellent communicators with an established track record of success are consciously aware of using their skills in all four basic communication arenas to achieve their goals. Likewise, a poor communicator who conveys unintended communications such as hostile tone of voice, tendency to clip off the end of other speakers' sentences, or repeated glancing at a watch leaves powerful (and negative) messages with the recipient of such behavior. Those who wish to measure communication skills must be aware of each of these four dimensions of communication, and the fact that they can be intended or not, and strive to capture elements of all in any evaluation of communication competence. Most assessment and training programs of physician communication have focused on communication with patients and families. An equally important but relatively uninvestigated realm of communication involves physician communication with other health professionals. The first part of this chapter deals with communication with patients and families. The second part deals with communication with other health professionals. The chapter ends with a section designed to help the reader understand the infrastructure and costs of designing and implementing a standardized clinical encounter program.

Communication With Patients and Families

Many authors have established descriptions of general routines used by physicians to communicate with patients. These routines are organized around the purpose of each element of the routine. Billings and Stoeckle (1999) discuss six broad tasks that characterize student encounters with patients: (1) beginning the interview and establishing a relationship with the patient, (2) eliciting from the patient information needed for diagnosis and management, (3) consultation with the student's preceptor (oral presentation of the case), (4) assessment and plan formulated in conjunction with the preceptor, (5) informing and counseling the patient (including the negotiation of a mutually agreeable plan and saying goodbye to the patient), and (6) the recording of the interview and discussion with the preceptor in written form. The Kalamazoo Consensus Statement (2001) notes seven essential elements of communication in medical encounters: (1) building the patient–physician relationship, (2) opening the discussion, (3) gathering information, (4) understanding the patient's perspective, (5) sharing information, (6) reaching agreement on problems and plans, and (7) providing closure. Greg Makoul developed a widely used framework to teach and evaluate communication skills entitled SEGUE, an acronym for Set the stage, Elicit information, Give information, Understand the patient's perspective, and End this visit (Makoul 2001). All of these frameworks, while varying slightly, have more in common than not, and all point to the essential general skills of physicians or physicians-in-training.

Additional communication skills elements, or variations from the above, may be needed depending on the specific purpose of the patient–physician communication. Potentially difficult encounters such as giving bad news, maintaining confidentiality, obtaining informed consent, and inquiring about sensitive areas of the patient's history all require a high degree of specific communication skills to be traversed successfully. These situations require a special combination of empathy and objectivity, which allows a somewhat formal, but comfortable and uncompromising, professional relationship to develop. Unfortunately, a recent survey found that communications (counseling, education) skills are the area least effectively used in meeting the health care needs of the U.S. population (McGlynn et al. 2003).

A number of other specific communication skills are needed. A physician may find herself needing the skills of persuasion, for example, as she tries to get a middle-aged woman to understand, and agree to, her first mammogram. This kind of work requires flexibility on the part of the physician, since each patient may require a different approach. Building trust and confidence is another specific communication skill, which is probably done on multiple levels, verbal and nonverbal, intentionally and not, that physicians need if they are to develop a working and therapeutic alliance with their patients. Checking facts and ensuring the reliability of information that is received are part of the general gathering of information but may come to the forefront of needed skills in patients who are being evasive or are hiding the truth for one reason or another. The ability of the physician to reassure and calm patients, while also remaining calm, is especially critical in situations that are potentially painful or life threatening, such as in situations in which bad news must be delivered. Indeed, knowing what to say or do in a wide variety of interactions with patients may mean the difference between effective and noneffective communication. Finally, conflict resolution skills are vital since patients and physicians will inevitably find themselves at odds in the course of their relationship, for example, when a patient is angry about waiting to be seen longer than the patient feels is appropriate. All of these skills make up the wide repertoire of abilities that a physician must be able to use in daily practice, and without which he or she cannot be considered fully competent (see table 4-1).

Assessment of Communication Skills Involving Physician Communication With Patients and Family Members

Physician communication skills directed toward patients and families have long been evaluated by faculty observation of trainees in real clinical settings, although this method is fraught with difficulty.

Table 4-1   Communication Competencies

Data collection
Delivering bad news
Inquiring about sensitive areas of the patient's history (e.g. sexual history)
Patient education/counseling
Interviewing process (general)
Establish a relationship with the patient
Opening the discussion
Close the encounter
Understanding patient's point of view
Persuading
Negotiating a mutually agreeable plan
Conflict resolution[a]
Building trust/confidence
Reassuring/calming Patients[a]
Checking facts/insuring reliability of information[a]
Checking patient understanding of information provided[a]
Obtaining informed consent[a]
Communicating with children[a,b]

---

[a]A communication area that has been underemphasized with respect to development of assessment methods and training programs. [b]Work with standardized patients who are minors is challenging secondary to legal and work issues with children.

A relatively large number (up to 30) of observations across different patient contexts and behaviors must be obtained in order to provide a stable estimate of communication and interpersonal competence (Carline et al. 1992; Wenrich et al. 1993; Tamblyn et al. 1994). Such large numbers of observations are needed because communication skills are situation and case specific. Live clinical events vary with the presenting condition, the patient, and the physician. Measuring communication skills in a reliable fashion with three rapidly changing sources of variation posed such a great challenge that researchers in the 1970s thought to minimize the variation from presenting conditions and from patients, in order to measure differences in individual physician performance (Barrows 1993).

Standardized patients are nonphysicians carefully trained to perform in multiple roles of patient, teacher, and evaluator while realistically replicating a patient encounter. They receive intensive instruction (often 15–25 hours per case) and use their own bodies as teaching material (Stillman and Swanson 1987). Once trained to enact a particular patient encounter, the SP can, with very high fidelity, play that part repeatedly over time and with different students. Thus, they can provide a controlled environment in which clinical situations and/or difficult patient communication scenarios can be experienced by learners. Issues such as setting variability and the need for patient confidentiality can be controlled or eliminated. Students, since they are all seeing the same "case," can be compared with their peers, as well as to a preestablished gold standard for the case. Standardized patients are often trained to evaluate the encounters and give detailed feedback to students.

The usual scenario of an SP interaction with a student for assessment purposes begins with the student introducing him or herself to the patient and beginning an interview, much as would occur in a real clinical setting. The student has been informed in advance as to the task of the particular case, for example, take a history and perform a physical examination, deliver bad news to the patient, or obtain informed consent. There is generally a time frame that may vary from 10 or 15 minutes for a simple task (obtaining an uncomplicated informed consent) to an hour or more (performing a complete history and physical examination.) Once the encounter has concluded, the SP may fill out paperwork evaluating the interaction with the student, and/or meet with the student "out of character" to discuss the student's performance and give feedback. Students may or may not have postencounter responsibilities, such as writing a progress note of the encounter, as well. Faculty may or may not observe the encounter as it occurs (usually through a video camera feed), or later using the tape that was created.

Standardized patients (SPs) have been used extensively in the training, formative feedback, and clinical skills evaluation of medical students, residents, and clinicians (Stillman et al. 1990). They have been studied extensively and shown to be reliable and valid (Colliver and Williams 1993).

Accuracy of Portrayal and Accuracy of Ratings

Several studies have examined the realism of SP performance and the accuracy of SP portrayal of case details. Realism has been best measured by establishing whether experienced physicians detected SPs when sent unannounced into their offices. Detection has run in the 10–20% range. However, in the one study where the reasons for detection were studied, the detection occurred in approximately one-third of the cases because the patient did not fit the physician's practice (Russell et al. 1991). Across the studies, SPs were more than 90%

accurate in portraying details of the case (Tamblyn et al. 1991a). Further their performances were stable across encounters and time.

SPs also appear to be very accurate raters, about as accurate as physicians in evaluating and rating the clinical performance of students. In one study, the average agreement in recording examinee performance was 82% (Tamblyn et al. 1991b). In one particularly interesting study, Pangaro et al. (1997) trained standardized examinees to perform at either the 40% or 80% level on the history and physical examination items of a checklist filled out by SPs to see how these examinees would be rated by the SPs who were unaware that the "trainees" they were examining were actually standardized themselves. The SPs rated the examinees trained to perform at the 80% correct rate as 77% correct, and the 40% correct group as 44% correct, providing a measure of the accuracy of the scoring process. The overall accuracy of the SPs in completing the checklists was 91%.

As might be expected, however, the number of items on which students are to be rated makes a difference in the accuracy of the SPs, with accuracy decreasing with increasing numbers of items (Vu et al. 1992). Of note is the fact that almost three-quarters of SP errors in recording were in the examinee's favor. Kopp and Johnson (1995) found agreements ranging from 78% to 97% when both SPs and faculty scored students' interpersonal skills. The differences were most often due to the SP giving credit on the checklist used when the faculty member did not. However, the two categories of raters (SPs and faculty) often do not rate the same facets of interpersonal and communication skills, even while viewing the same case. Cooper and Mira (1998) found that the communication skills emphasized by physician-teachers did not reflect the skills considered to be important by the SPs. Finlay et al. (1995) reported that although the SPs did produce a valid assessment of trainees' communication skills, they scored the trainees differently than did the clinicians; this is important to keep in mind when using SP raters instead of physician observers. Donnelly et al. (2000) noted that faculty proctor and SP global ratings of interpersonal skills were both reliable and valid, although the SPs tended to give slightly higher ratings than did the faculty proctors.

A group discussion of technical issues of SP application (Consensus Working Group 1993) concluded that SPs have an edge over outside observers in evaluating communication skills. Boulet et al. (1998) examined the high-stakes examination used to measure the clinical skills of graduates of foreign medical schools. They found that the overall interpersonal scores were reliable, generalizable, and valid. Their conclusion was that well-trained SPs could be used to assess the interpersonal skills of physicians in a reliable manner.

SP examinations also appear to be quite reliable, especially in the case of pass–fail decisions. In one study, the pass–fail decision reliability was 0.84 (dependability index with cutoff), based on data collected for six classes (Barrows et al. 1991). A number of cases are needed to achieve this level of reliability, 15 in the study mentioned, but this is still far less than the number that would be required to reach a level of 0.80 for the generalizability coefficient (40 in this case). Reliability is minimally affected by having more than one SP simulate the same case, as demonstrated by several studies (Swanson and Norcini 1989; Colliver et al. 1990 1993a).

Validity

If the use of SPs in examination formats is valid, one would expect increasing competence on these exams with increasing levels of training. Indeed, this has been the case, with several studies demonstrating that examination performance is higher with increasing levels of training (Barnhart et al. 1992; Petrusa et al. 1987; Stillman et al. 1991b).

Cohen et al. (1996) studied the global ratings SPs assigned trainees while assessing interpersonal and communication skills, and how these ratings compared to the use of SP checklists for the same purpose. Global ratings by expert physician observers were found to be more efficient and reliable than the checklist. Regehr et al. (1998) found that global rating scales scored by experts showed higher interstation reliability, better construct validity, and better concurrent validity than did checklists. In addition, they found that the presence of checklists did not improve the reliability or validity of the global rating scale over that of the global rating scale alone. Regehr et al. (1999) noted that while checklist scores are highly content specific, global ratings scales capture and evaluate a broader set of skills. Checklists, however, still have advantages for training purposes because they point out specific performance deficiencies that can be used for purposes of continued professional development.

Additionally, the use of checklists by SPs to document questions asked by trainees has given some cause for concern (Williams et al. 1999). Students quickly learn that SPs are filling out checklists, and that there are certain questions that must be asked to get credit for the case. This can lead to a closed-ended, rapid-fire questioning style that is counter to what expert interviewers are likely to do and counter to what educators would like their students to demonstrate (Billings and Stoeckle 1999). Indeed, when this kind of checklist is used in an examination setting, Hodges et al. (1999) have shown that scores of expert interviewers are similar to those of novices. Since the real issue is whether the examinee has learned the critical case details from the patient so that a correct diagnosis may be reached, testing data collection by asking trainees to record their findings on a patient findings questionnaire (Williams et al. 1999) may allow students to interview in a style consistent with accepted interviewing practices, rather than adapting to perceived test demands. SPs would still be asked to fill out process ratings evaluating the examinee's ability to form an alliance or conduct the interview smoothly, global items that do show increasing scores with increasing expertise of the interviewer (Hodges et al. 1999).

Researchers have used SPs for the assessment of a variety of advanced communication skills, as well (Roberts et al. 1999; Smith et al. 1994; Greenberg et al. 1999; Serwint 2002; Amiel et al. 2000). In these studies, students generally performed well and agreed that these types of assessment were important. They also noted feeling more confident about their skills around issues such as delivering bad news after training sessions using SPs. Good levels of face and content validity, as well as interrater agreement, were generally achieved.

A major advantage to the use of SPs in the assessment of communication skills is that one can see not only what physicians are capable of, but also how they actually perform in practice settings. This is usually achieved through the use of unannounced SPs, who come to see the physician in the guise of a real patient that might be seen in everyday practice. A number of studies have shown that, when cases are well developed and SPs are properly trained, experienced physicians cannot detect the presence of unannounced SPs in their office practices (Burri et al. 1976; Owen and Winkler 1974; Norman et al. 1983, 1985). Unannounced SPs have been used particularly in two areas of clinician practice: first, to ascertain variations and quality of practice among physicians with respect to a certain chief complaint or disease entity, and second, to evaluate the impact of continuing medical education on physician behavior (Beullens et al. 1997).

Colliver and Williams (1993), in their review of the SP literature, raised a number of threats to the validity and reliability of these
examinations. First, the fact that several different SPs often play the
same case during the course of an examination for multiple students
raises the concern of the variance of scores that might be produced.
A number of investigators (Colliver et al. 1991c, 1998; De Champlain
et al. 1999a; Swartz et al. 1999) in multiple studies have shown that
only a small amount of variance in scores comes from having more
than one patient do the case. These wash out when looking at an
overall exam score, versus a case score.

Second, security leaks are a concern, since large SP examinations with many trainees being tested typically take place over days
to weeks, using the same cases (Colliver et al. 1991a, 1992; Stillman
et al. 1991a; De Champlain et al. 1999b, 2000; Cohen et al. 1993).
In a test coaching scenario (De Champlain et al. 1999b), scores for
the coached individuals were one to two points higher than for those
who went in "cold." Since this exam did not count, the coaching differences would be even higher in a high-stakes examination situation. Thus, in a high-stakes exam, examiners should freely substitute
many equivalent cases to minimize this effect.

Third, experts set unrealistically high absolute performance
standards. This is because clinicians lack an adequate database of
observing students in actual performance situations performing
the full range of the tasks in question. Because they lack a basis
for comparison, they set the levels too high. In addition, since very
little research has been done regarding the relationship between
actual clinical practices and measurable patient outcomes, it is difficult to know what skills must be performed in order for a student to be ruled "competent." More research in this area is clearly
needed.

Other investigators have looked at the effect of gender (both
SP and trainee), ethnicity, sequence of cases, or day of the examination on SP ratings. Gispert et al. (1999) found no significant differences or associations between these variables for SPs. Likewise,
Lloyd et al. (1990) found no order effects. Bienstock et al. (2000)
found no bias attributable to the perceived student ethnicity affecting the examination that was studied. Colliver et al. (1991b) did find
that women trainees scored higher in attributes of personal manner,
but that men and women were scored equally well in interpersonal
and communication skills, regardless of the gender of the SP. Likewise, Chambers et al. (2001) Rutala et al. (1991), and Colliver et al.

(1993b) found no significant interaction between SP gender and trainee gender and concluded that male and female trainees were assessed equally.

Communicating With Professional Colleagues

Virtually all of the research and development using standardized clinical encounters to teach and assess communications has focused on encounters between the physician and the patient. Little research, development, and training using standardized clinical encounters have focused on communicating with professional colleagues. The increasing emphasis on the importance of teamwork in health care settings and the focus on the effectiveness of health care systems rather than that of individual health care practitioners assure us that this area will be receiving more attention in the future, especially in light of reports of errors that occur when excellent team communication is not maintained.

Anesthesiologists have been on the forefront in designing team resource training for health care professionals using simulation (Gaba and DeAnda 1988, 1989; Gaba 1992; Gaba et al. 1995, 1998; Holzman et al. 1995; Howard et al. 1992). Recently, similar work has been done in emergency medicine (Small et al. 1999) and surgery (Helmreich et al. 1999). This work has led to the initial identification of a list of communication-related competencies critical to team effectiveness. We have summarized these competencies in table 4-2.

Helmreich and Merritt (1998) is a very good resource for those interested in assessment and training of team resource management effectiveness. The book provides a number of measurement instruments in the appendices that have been adapted for use in medicine. They describe others used in aviation that can easily be adapted for use in medical team simulation activities designed to assess communication competence in its broadest sense. Howard et al. (1992) provide an example instrument used in evaluating videotaped simulated encounters for anesthesia crisis resource management. This instrument provides details about anesthesia critical incidents and communication performance elements, as well, allowing others to use it as a basis for simulations and subsequent communication performance evaluation.

Table 4-2   Team Resource Management Competencies Involving
Communication

Communication
Communicate clearly and precisely; use commonly accepted terminology
Ensure reception of intended data and meaning
Foster open exchange of information
Cross-check information; use check-backs to verify information transfer
Systematically hand off responsibilities during team transitions
Communicate decisions and actions to team members
Related Competencies
Focus the team; mobilize resources
Call for help early
Establish role clarity
Establish shared situation awareness; request and share situation awareness updates
Ensure availability of up-to-date key information; call out critical information during emergent events; offer and seek information to support planning and decision making
Distribute the workload; assign tasks to those with the skills to complete them; ensure that responsibility is clear
Establish priorities; identify and focus staff attention on key goals
Acknowledge the contributions of team members to team goals
Demonstrate mutual respect in all communication
Address professional concerns directly
Resolve conflicts constructively
Engage team members in planning and decision-making processes
Advocate and assert a position or corrective action
Request and offer assistance for task overload
Defuse interpersonal conflict (e.g., by saving for postevent discussion)

Infrastructure for Standardized Clinical Encounters

The infrastructure needed for a successful program of standardized clinical encounters to occur includes five areas which must be addressed. First, the program must be staffed. For a program to become integrated into the curricula surrounding it and used by faculty involved in the process of working with students, it is desirable to have it directed by a physician with an excellent knowledge of the SP field, or an educator with an excellent track record of working with basic science and clinical faculty. Faculty busy with the day-to-day education (course or clinical work) of students will be more easily drawn into using standardized clinical encounters as part of their educational or assessment procedures if there is an outreach "expert" on hand to tell them about the process, sell them on its merits, and help them through the development and implementation phases. An SP trainer is essential, since the training process and its quality directly affect the reliability, accuracy, and fidelity (in cases where unannounced SPs are used) of the cases developed. A skilled trainer will also help faculty with the process of developing cases, since the trainer will see up front what elements of the history have been omitted or underdeveloped and be able to fill in these details sooner rather than later. Finally, a secretary, or someone responsible for the copying, filing, and organization of the innumerable pieces of paper, videotapes, and other data that are produced with even one standardized clinical encounter, is essential.

The second area is the development of the cases themselves. Usually, cases are written by faculty members with the help and guidance of the SP trainer (either in person or by providing the group with a template to use). Once the goals and objectives of the course or clerkship have been set, examples of ideas for cases naturally flow from them. For example, in a course on ethics, interviewing skills, and professional behavior, it seems natural that one might develop a standardized clinical encounter in which the student is asked to obtain informed consent. As another example, at the University of Illinois in Chicago, in preparation for a senior clinical competence examination, volunteer faculty were asked to agree upon a list of diagnoses and clinical skills that they considered most important from a long list of goals and objectives culled from the third-year clerkship lists. This list was then used to create a blueprint matrix of diagnoses and clinical tasks that was used as the substrate for each of the 12 cases developed. In addition, case revisions are needed as questions arise or diagnostic testing or treatment methods change— faculty time is needed for this, as well.

The third needed element of a standardized clinical encounter program is the production phase. Whether or not the encounters are used for training, formative feedback, or summative assessment, SPs will need to be trained. Typically, at least several hours of training are needed for each patient, and this number goes up depending on the complexity and length of the case to be portrayed. Standardized patients should be paid for training time, although the cost may be less than the hourly rate for the actual performances. For a medical school class, it is common that several actors portray each case, given fatigue and scheduling issues. This multiplies the number of patients that must be trained. Materials must be printed and readied for use during the encounters. These may include check-lists, other rating scales, patient-finding questionnaires, posten-counter multiple-choice or short-answer questions, or forms on which the SPs can write their comments. The use of computers for SPs and students to record their answers is also a possibility. However, if computers are to be used, different costs arise. Banks of computers are necessary if more than one student and SP are to be running at a time. Software designed for the management of such data input must be purchased and installed, as well as maintained. Finally, videotapes of the encounters should be made (for live review for quality assurance, or later review by students and faculty). The tapes themselves must be purchased, as well as the video equipment to make use of them. Other small but essential details should not be overlooked in this phase. If students are to be physically examining patients, the tools to do so must be supplied. These may include the soap to wash hands, tongue depressors, cotton swabs, disposable specula, and examining tables and drapes for the patient's comfort, among a host of others.

The implementation of the standardized clinical encounter brings with it another complete set of costs and details. These, however, may vary somewhat, depending on whether the encounters are conducted in a medical education setting or unannounced in a practicing physician's office. In a medical education setting, more often than not multiple students come through the site in a given time period, and multiple stations are required for students to rotate through. This kind of work requires the presence of multiple SPs, and rooms for them to be encountered. It is also helpful to hire an extra, trained SP to watch the cases as they progress on video; this helps with the maintenance of high levels of fidelity to the originally written cases. If physician examiners are to be present, listening to presentations by students after their meetings with the SPs, scoring written material immediately after they are produced by the students, or watching live encounters on videotape, they must be present for the duration of the training session or examination as well. Support staff need to be present because they perform several key roles. First, they provide the timing of the stations and facilitate the movement of students between them. Second, they collect and collate material produced by the students or SPs, either for immediate or later scoring. Finally, they maintain a watchful eye on the examinees, keeping talking and sharing of information between them to a minimum.

As might be surmised from the word "unannounced," such SPs require different environmental preparation for their encounters with physicians in actual practice. For example, if realism is to be ensured, a referral for the patient's visit must be made, and a patient record must be created. A means of recording the session must be included, such as having an audiotape recorder carried in the purse of a female SP. The development of these cases is critical, as well. Indeed, for these patients to remain undetected, their training if anything needs to be more rigorous, and the cases they portray even more detailed. Forms to be filled out after the encounter with the physician will still need to be provided, and analysis of these forms still needs to occur. In many of these cases, the patient carried a concealed audio recorder into the physician's office to provide a detailed record of the encounter. During the encounter itself, however, many of the issues as noted in the paragraph above simply are not relevant.

After the training sessions or examinations, the analysis and reporting of the data collected must be undertaken. If all materials were produced in hard copy form, these data must be entered for analysis. If the computer was used and appropriate software installed beforehand, this part of the infrastructure (the data entry) will not be needed, although inevitably the data require cleaning in some form. The statistical analysis of the large amounts of data that are produced must be undertaken, and a report generated. These reports can have several audiences. Given the nature of the standardized clinical encounters, they are a rich source of feedback to the students. Some form of data about their performance should be provided to them. The more specific the information provided, the better. The course directors will be interested in how the students performed, whether the objective was a training session (Did the students like it? Did the students learn it?) or a high-stakes examination (Did the students pass the test?). Finally, in aggregate form, the data can help curriculum developers see where the "holes" are in their curricula based on student performance, and plan appropriate changes. Depending on the types and number of the analyses and reports that are needed, one or more individuals working for days to weeks may be required.

The reported costs of implementing a SP examination vary widely, depending greatly on whether or not faculty time for the development and implementation of the examination is donated or must be paid. Reznick et al. (1993) reported a cost range of $496–870

(Canadian dollars). Similarly, Cusimano et al. (1994) reported that the costs of administering a SP examination could be reduced from $35 per student per station to $1 per student per station if all test developers, SPs, support staff, and examiners could donate their time. Frye et al. (1989) reported a cost of $32 per student, while Williams et al. (1987) reported a cost of $118 per student for the SP resources and another $125 per student for supplies. This group concluded that "startup costs are high until there is a large station bank and many trained SP are gathered."

Conclusion

In summary, standardized clinical encounters are highly reliable and valid when assessing the communication skills of medical students, residents, physicians out in practice, and groups of physicians working as a team. These encounters are uniquely designed to allow examinees to show what they know how to and will do in a clinical setting. These encounters can be designed to simulate a wide variety of experiences that a physician might encounter in all sorts of clinical experiences, and can occur either in a testing setting or out in general practice and unannounced. The practice opportunities afforded by using standardized clinical encounters to train students and physicians appear to have lasting effects on behavior, superior to didactic lectures or other non-interactive material. While the costs of setting up an infrastructure to create, implement, and analyze the results of standardized clinical encounters may be high, especially in situations where expert faculty are not volunteering their time, it appears that this methodology is worth the expense, since the benefits gained are so great. There remain many areas of investigation into the use of these encounters, among them the effects on patient care and outcomes of training physicians in communication skills with this methodology, and the fascinating and critical area of attempting to improve communication between and among professional colleagues.

References

Amiel GE, Ungar L, et al. Using an OSCE to assess primary care physicians' competence in breaking bad news. Acad Med 2000;75(5):560–561.

Barnhart AJ, Marcy ML, Colliver JA, Verhulst SJ. A comparison of second- and fourth-year medical students on a standardized-patient examination of clinical competence: a construct validity study. Paper presented at the American Educational Research Association annual meeting, April 10, 1992, San Francisco, California.

Barrows H. An overview of the uses of standardized patients for teaching and evaluating clinical skills. Acad Med 1993;68(6):443–453.

Barrows HS, Colliver JA, Vu NV, Travis TA, Distlehorst LD. The clinical practice examination: six years experience. Springfield, IL: Southern Illinois University School of Medicine, 1991.

Beullens J, Rethans JJ, et al. The use of standardized patients in research in general practice. Fam Pract 1997;14(1):58–62.

Bienstock JL, Tzou WS, Martin SA, Fox HE. Effect of student ethnicity on interpersonal skills and objective standardized clinical examination scores. Obstet Gynecol 2000;96(6):1011–1013.

Billings JA, Stoeckle JD. The clinical encounter. A guide to the medical interview and case presentation. 2nd ed. St. Louis: Mosby Press, 1999.

Boulet JR, Ben-David MF, Ziv A, Burdick WP, Curtis M, Peitzman S, Gary NE. High-stakes examinations: what do we know about measurement? Acad Med 1998;73(10):S94–S96.

Burri A, McCaughan K, Barrows H. The feasibility of using the simulated patient as a means to evaluate clinical competence of practicing physicians in a community. In: Proceedings of the 15th Annual Conference on Research in Medical Education, 1976;295–299. Washington, DC: Association of American Medical Colleges.

Carline JD, Paauw DS. Thiede KW, Ramsey PG. Factors affecting the reliability of ratings of students' clinical skills in a medicine clerkship. J Gen Int Med 1992;7:506–510.

Chambers KA, Boulet JR, Furman GE. Are interpersonal skills ratings influenced by gender in a clinical skills assessment using standardized patients? Adv Health Sci Educ Theory Pract 2001;6:231–241.

Cohen DS, Colliver JA, Marcy MS, Fried ED, Swartz MH. Psychometric properties of a standardized-patient checklist and rating-scale form used to assess interpersonal and communication skills. Acad Med 1996;71(1 suppl):S97–S89.

Cohen R, Rothman AI, Ross J, Poldre P. Impact of repeated use of objective structured clinical examination stations. Acad Med 1993;68:S73–S75.

Colliver JA, Barrows HS, Vu NV, Verhulst SJ, Mast TA, Travis TA. Test security in examinations that use standardized-patient cases at one medical school. Acad Med 1991a;66:279–282.

Colliver JA, Marcy ML, Travis TA, Robbs RS. The interaction of student gender and standardized-patient gender on a performance-based examination of clinical competence. Acad Med 1991b;66(9 suppl):S31–S33.

Colliver JA, Marcy ML, Vu NV, Steward DE, Robbs RS. The effect of using multiple standardized patients to rate interpersonal and communication skills on the same case on the intercase reliability of the ratings. Paper presented at the annual meeting of the American Educational Research Association, Division I, April 8, 1993a, Atlanta, GA.

Colliver JA, Morrison LJ, Markwell SJ, Verhulst SJ, Steward DE, Dawson-Saunders E, Barrows HS. Three studies of the effect of multiple standardized patients on intercase reliability of five standardized-patient examinations. Teach Learn Med 1990;2:237–245.

Colliver JA, Robbs RS, Vu NV. Effects of using two or more standardized patients to simulate the same case on case means and case failure rates. Acad Med 1991c;66:616–618.

Colliver JA, Swartz MH, Robbs RS, Lofquist M, Cohen D, Verhulst SJ. The effect of using multiple standardized patients on the inter-case reliability of a large-scale standardized-patient examination administered over an extended testing period. Acad Med 1998;73:S81–S83.

Colliver JA, Travis TA, Robbs RS, Barnhart AJ, Shirar LE, Vu NV. Test security in standardized-patient examinations: analysis with scores on working diagnosis and final diagnosis. Acad Med 1992;67:S7–S9.

Colliver JA, Vu NV, Marcy ML, Travis TA, Robbs RS. Effects of examinee gender, standardized-patient gender, and their interaction on standardized patients' ratings of examinees' interpersonal and communication skills. Acad Med 1993b;68(2):153–157.

Colliver JA, Williams RG. Technical issues: test application. Acad Med 1993; 68:454–460.

Consensus Working Group. Highlight of group discussion of technical issues of SP application. Acad Med 1993;68(6):461–463.

Cooper C and M Mira. Who should assess medical students' communication skills: their academic teachers or their patients? Med Educ 1998; 32(4):419–421.

Cusimano MD, Cohen R, Tucker W, Murnaghan J, Kodama R, Reznick R. A comparative analysis of the costs of administration of an OSCE. Acad Med 1994;69:571–576.

De Champlain AF, MacMillan MK, King AM, Klas DJ, Margolis MJ. Assessing the impacts of intra-site and inter-site checklist recording discrepancies on the reliability of scores obtained in a nationally administered standardized patient examination. Acad Med 1999a;74: S52–S54.

De Champlain AF, MacMillan MK, Margolis MJ, King AM, Klass DJ. Do discrepancies in standardized patients' checklist recording affect case and examination mastery-level decisions? Acad Med 1998;73:S75–S77.

De Champlain AF, MacMillan MK, Margolis MJ, Klass DJ, Lewis E, Ahearn S. Modeling the effects of a test security breach on a large-scale standardized patient examination with a sample of international medical graduates. Acad Med 2000;75:S109–S111.

De Champlain AF, MacMillan MK, Margolis MJ, Klass DJ, Nungester RJ, Schimpfiauser F, Zinnerstrom K. Modeling the effects of security breaches on students' performances on a large-scale standardized patient examination. Acad Med 1999b;74:S49–S51.

Dexter D. (Producer and Director). Speaking effectively to 1 or 1000. [videotape]. Carlsbad, CA: CRM Films, 1992.

Donnelly MB, Sloan D, Plymale M, Schwartz R. Assessment of residents' interpersonal skills by faculty proctors and standardized patients: a psychometric analysis. Acad Med 2000;75:S93–S95.

Finlay IG, Stott NC, Kinnersley P. The assessment of communication skills in palliative medicine: a comparison of the scores of examiners and simulated patients. Med Educ 1995;29(6):424–429.

Frye AW, Richards BF, Philp EB, Phil JR. Is it worth it? A look at the costs and benefits of an OSCE for second year medical students. Med Teacher 1989;11:291–293.

Gaba DM. Improving anesthesiologists' performance by simulating reality. Anesthesiology 1992;76:491–494.

Gaba DM, A DeAnda. A comprehensive anesthesia simulation environment: re-creating the operating room for research and training. Anesthesiology 1988;69:387–394.

Gaba DM, DeAnda A. The response of anesthesia trainees to simulated critical incidents. Anesth Analg 1989;68:444–451.

Gaba DM, Howard SK, Flanagan B, Smith BE, Fish KJ, Botney R. Assessment of clinical performance during simulated crises using both technical and behavioral ratings. Anesthesiology 1998;89:8–18.

Gaba DM, Howard SK, Small SD. Situation awareness in anesthesiology. Hum Factors 1995;37:20–31.

Gispert R, Rue M, Roma J, Martinez-Carretero JM. Gender, sequence of cases and day effects on clinical skills assessment with standardized patients. Med Educ 1999;33(7):499–503.

Greenberg LW, Ochsenschlager D, O'Donnell R, Mastruserio J, Cohen GJ. Communicating bad news: a pediatric department's evaluation of a simulated intervention. Pediatrics 1999;103(6 pt 1):1210–1217.

Helmreich RL, Merritt AC. Culture at work in aviation and medicine. Burlington, VT: Ashgate, 1998.

Helmreich RL, Merritt AC, Wilhelm JA. The evolution of crew resource management training in commercial aviation. Int J Aviat Psychol 1999; 9:19–32.

Hodges B, Regehr G, et al. OSCE checklists do not capture increasing levels of expertise. Acad Med 1999;74(10):1129–1134.

Holzman RS, Cooper JB, Gaba DM, Philip JH, Small SD, Feinstein D. Anesthesia crisis resource management: real-life simulation training in operating room crises. J Clin Anesth 1995;7:675–687.

Howard SK, Gaba DM, Fish KJ, Yang G, Sarnquist FH. Anesthesia crisis resource management training: teaching anesthesiologists to handle critical incidents. Aviat Space Environ Med 1992;63:763–770.

Institute of Medicine. To err is human: building a safer health system. Washington, DC: National Academy Press, 2000.

Kalamazoo Consensus Statement. Participants in the Bayer-Fetzer Conference on Physician-Patient Communication in Medical Education. Essential elements of communication in medical encounters. Acad Med 2001; 76:390–393.

Kopp KC, JA Johnson JA. Checklist agreement between standardized patients and faculty. J Dent Educ 1995;59(8):824–829.

Lloyd JS, Williams RG, Simonton DK, Sherman D. Order effects in standardized patient examinations. Acad Med 1990;65(9 suppl):S51–S52.

Makoul, Greg. The SEGUE Framework for teaching and assessing communication skills. Patient Educ Coun 2001;45:23–34.

McGlynn EA, Asch SM, Adams J, et al. The quality of health care delivered to adults in the United States. N Engl J Med 2003;348:2635–2645.

Norman GR, Neufeld VR, Walsh A, Woodward CA, McConvey GA. Measuring physicians' performance by using simulated patients. J Med Educ 1985;60:925–934.

Norman G, Stillman P and C Woodward C. Simulated patients in evaluation of medical education. In Proceedings of the 22nd annual conference on Research in Medical Education. Washington, DC: Association of American Medical Colleges, 1983;240–244.

Owen A, Winkler R. General practitioners and psychosocial problems: an evaluation using pseudopatients. Med J Austr 1974;2:393–398.

Pangaro LN, Worth-Dickstein H, Macmillan MK, Klass DJ, Shatzer JH. Performance of "standardized examinees" in a standardized-patient examination of clinical skills. Acad Med 1997;72(11):1008–1011.

Petrusa ER, et al. An objective measure of clinical performance. Am J Med 1987;83:34–42.

Quill TE, Townsend P. Bad news: delivery, dialogue and dilemmas. Arch Intern Med 1991;151:463–468.

Regehr G, Freeman R, et al. Assessing the generalizability of OSCE measures across content domains. Acad Med 1999;74(12):1320–1322.

Regehr G, MacRae H, et al. Comparing the psychometric properties of checklists and global rating scales for assessing performance on an OSCE-format examination. Acad Med 1998;73:993–997.

Reznick R, Smee S, Baumber JS, Cohen R, Rothman A, Blackmore D, Berard M. Guidelines for estimating the real cost of an objective structured clinical examination. Acad Med 1993;68:513–517.

Roberts LW, Mines J, Voss C, Koinis C, Mitchell S, Obenshain SS, McCarty T. Assessing medical students' competence in obtaining informed consent. Am J Surg 1999;178(4):251–255.

Russell NK, Boekeloo BO, Rafi IZ, Rabin DL. Using unannounced simulated patients to evaluate sexual risk assessment and risk reduction skills of practicing physicians. Acad Med 1991;66(9):S37–S39.

Rutala PJ, Witzke DB, Leko EO, Fulginiti JV. The influences of student and standardized patient genders on scoring in an objective structured clinical examination. Acad Med 1991;66(9 suppl):S28–S30.

Serwint JR. The use of standardized patients in pediatric residency training in palliative care: anatomy of a standardized patient case scenario. J Palliat Med. 2002;5:146–153.

Shah SN, Aslam M, Avery AJ. A Survey of prescription errors in general practice. Pharm J 2001;267:860–862.

Small SD, Wuerz RC, Simon R, Shapiro N, Conn A, Setnik G. Demonstration of high-fidelity simulation team training for emergency medicine. Acad Emerg Med 1999;6:312–323.

Smith SR, Balint JA, Krause KC, Moore-West M, Viles PH. Performance-based assessment of moral reasoning and ethical judgment among medical students. Acad Med 1994;69(5):381–386.

Stillman PL, Haley JL, Sutnick AI, et al. Is test security an issue in a multistation clinical assessment? A preliminary study. Acad Med 1991a;66:S25–S7.

Stillman PL, Regan MB, et al. Results of a survey on the use of standardized patients to teach and evaluate clinical skills. Acad Med 1990;65(5): 288–292.

Stillman PL, Swanson DB. Ensuring the clinical competence of medical school graduates through standardized patients. Arch Intern Med 1987; 147(6):1049–1052.

Stillman PL, Swanson DB, Regan MB, et al. Assessment of clinical skills of residents utilizing standardized patients: a follow-up study and recommendations for application. Ann Int Med 1991b;114:393–401.

Swanson DB, Norcini JJ. Factors influencing the reproducibility of tests using standardized patients. Teach Learn Med 1989;1:158–166.

Swartz MH, Colliver JA, Robbs RS, Cohen DS. Effect of multiple standardized patients on case and examination means and passing rates. Acad Med 1999;74:S131–S134.

Tamblyn R, Benaroya S, Snell L, McLeod P, Schnarch B, Abrahamowicz M. The feasibility and value of using patient satisfaction ratings to evaluate internal medicine residents. J Gen Int Med 1994;9:146–152.

Tamblyn RM, Klass JF, Schabl GK, Kopelow ML. The accuracy of standardized-patient presentations. Med Educ 1991a;25:100–109.

Tamblyn RM, Klass DJ, Schabl GK, Kopelow ML. Sources of unreliability and bias in standardized-patient rating. Teach Learn Med 1991b;3:74–85.

Vu NV, Marcy MM, Colliver JA, Verhulst SJ, Travis TA, Barrows HS. Standardized patients' accuracy in recording clinical performance checklist items. Med Educ 1992;26:99–104.

Wenrich MD, Carline JD, Giles LM, Ramsey PG. Ratings of the performances of practicing internists by hospital-based registered nurses. Acad Med 1993;68:680–687.

Williams RG, Barrows HS, Vu NV, Verhulst SJ, Colliver JA, Marcy M, Steward D. Direct, standardized assessment of clinical competence. Med Educ 1987;21:482–489.

Williams RG, McLaughlin MA, Eulenberg B, Hurm M, Nendaz MR. The Patient Findings Questionnaire: one solution to an important standardized patient examination problem. Acad Med 1999;74(10):1118–1124.

5

The Assessment of Moral Reasoning and Professionalism in Medical Education and Practice

DeWitt C. Baldwin, Jr., and Donnie J. Self

Moral Judgment and Professionalism

The recent interest in professionalism has been fueled by at least two major concerns. The first is an effort on the part of organized medicine to reclaim its traditional autonomy, in the face of the increasing incursions of market forces and commercialism. The second, and more relevant to the theme of this book, is to reaffirm the traditional goal of medical education—to educate and train physicians with high levels of competence, compassion, and moral integrity, who will be worthy of the ideals of the profession and the trust of society. It is in ensuring and assessing these qualities that the study of moral development and moral judgment in medical students and residents has become relevant to the assessment of professionalism.

While there are relatively few studies that can be viewed as directly linking moral reasoning with the specific attributes and qualities of professionalism, the fault may lie as much with the limited attention paid to this topic until recently, as with the difficulties in elaborating a theory of professionalism. Apart from early contribu-

tions to the literature on professionalization by some pioneering sociologists (Parsons 1957; Greenwood 1957; Caplow 1954; Freidson
1970, 1994), little effort has been devoted to this topic until quite
recently. With the definition of professionalism used in this book,
however, we believe that moral judgment must be viewed as an essential component of professional behavior. It is also a component
of the "wise application of the principles of professionalism" (see
chapter 2). This application implies not only the awareness of moral
issues but also the demonstration of appropriate moral actions in
the contexts of education and clinical care.

Moral Reasoning and Moral Development

Although moral development has been addressed from both secular
and religious viewpoints, intellectual thought in the field of the psychology of moral development has been dramatically influenced in
recent decades by Lawrence Kohlberg's work on cognitive moral development (Kohlberg 1969, 1976, 1981, 1984). Stimulated by the
thought of Jean Piaget (1932/1965) and John Dewey (1954),
Kohlberg's initial research aimed at determining how children respond to specific moral issues at different ages. These same subjects
were interviewed every 3 years over a 25-year period, resulting in the
formulation, substantiation, and popularization of his now widely
known stage theory of moral development.

Based on more than 30 years of quantitatively reproducible research, Kohlberg's theory posits three levels of moral development:
preconventional morality, conventional morality, and postconventional, or principled, morality. Each level consists of two stages. Stage
1, at the preconventional level, is an authority–punishment stage, in
which what is considered right is defined by authority figures and
one behaves morally in order to avoid censure and punishment.
Stage 2 is based on an egoistic, instrumental exchange, in which
one's own needs determine what is considered right, although this
is modified by a sense of fairness in terms of equal exchange between
parties in agreement. Basically, it is an "I'll scratch your back if you'll
scratch mine" approach to morality.

Stage 3 begins the second, conventional level of mutual interpersonal expectations, peer relationships, and interpersonal con-
formity, in which what is considered right is what is expected by people close and important to you. "Being good" is seen as important

in the roles one occupies. Stage 4 has a societal maintenance and conscience orientation in which one fulfills one's agreed upon duties and contributes to the welfare of the group, institution, or society. Right is defined in terms of that which maintains a smoothly running society and avoids a breakdown of the system. Most medical students appear to function at this level (Self and Baldwin 1994).

Stage 5 begins the third, postconventional or principled level of moral reasoning, in which one emphasizes individual rights such as life and liberty, while endorsing a social contract that protects the rights of all persons, with a contractual commitment freely entered upon to serve the greatest good for the greatest number. It is based upon a rational calculation of the welfare of all humankind. Last, Stage 6 is based on a commitment to universal ethical principles of justice, equality, autonomy, and respect for the dignity of all human beings as individual persons. Although laws and social agreements are usually valid because they are based on these principles, when laws violate these principles, one acts in accordance with the principles. Right is whatever is required by a personal commitment to these universal ethical principles of justice, equality, autonomy, and respect for the dignity of all persons.

According to Kohlberg's theory, people proceed through these stages as they mature. The sequence is invariant, although the rate and end stage reached vary with the individual (Colby and Kohlberg 1987). Attainment of lower stages is necessary for progression to higher stages. People generally function at one stage and only partially at the stage below and the stage above. Research has established that one is unable to exceed one's achieved stage, or to "fake" higher scores on the various tests of moral reasoning (McGeorge 1975), although one may function at a lower level under conditions of stress or impairment. Stage attainment has been shown to be correlated with age and education (Rest et al. 1978; Rest and Thoma 1985; Rest 1986). The voluminous empirical research supporting the theoretical foundations of cognitive moral development theory has been summarized by Rest and colleagues (Rest 1986; Rest and Narvaez 1994; Rest et al. 1999a).

It should be noted that Kohlberg's theory has been criticized as being too heavily based on a cognitive-developmental model and on a particular Rawlsian/Kantian concept of justice. Based on her work with women, Carol Gilligan (1982) has suggested alternatively that women tend to have a different orientation than do men on morally problematic issues, focusing less on the justice or fairness dimensions of a situation than on caring or relational considerations. While her claim that the measures of moral reasoning based on Kohlberg's justice-based theory ignore the relational orientation of women and supposedly disadvantage them on justice-based tests of moral reasoning, research to date on medical students has consistently found that women score significantly higher compared with men on most Kohlbergian measures of moral reasoning (Self and Baldwin 1998; Self et al. 1998a). In the few studies where both justice-based and caring-based choices were offered, results indicated that while men tended to be more justice oriented and women more care oriented, each gender showed ample awareness and consideration of both orientations (Self and Skeel 1992; Gilligan and Attanucci 1988; Self et al. 2003).

Another criticism has been that Kohlberg's theory offers too little understanding of how moral reasoning or judgment is related to moral action or behavior (Blasi 1980), although Kohlberg saw moral judgment as only one element in the psychology of morality. Rest (1984) offered a broad model of moral functioning that included four major components or processes: (1) moral or ethical sensitivity, (2) moral judgment or reasoning, (3) moral motivation, and (4) moral action. This model attempts to account for the many possible elements that enter into moral action. While it does not propose that these components necessarily function sequentially, it does recognize the complexity of the process. Perhaps more important, it opens the door to the possibility of educational interventions designed to remediate identifiable deficiencies, such as a lack of sensitivity as to what constitutes a moral dilemma, or a less highly developed stage of moral reasoning. Thus far, validated instruments for assessing ethical or moral sensitivity, moral reasoning, and moral motivation, including professional identity formation (role-concept), have been developed and are supported in empirical studies by Bebeau et al. (1985; Bebeau 1994b, 2002; Bebeau and Thoma 1994). The same cannot be said, as yet, for direct assessment of moral action, although it is possible that measures such as objective structured clinical examinations (OSCEs) could serve to test the integrated performance of both competence and character. The reader is referred to Bebeau (2002) for a more thorough discussion of these measures.

Moral Reasoning in Medical Education and Practice

The reader is again referred to Bebeau (2002) for a recent review of 33 studies, involving some 6,000 respondents from five professions: medicine, veterinary medicine, dentistry, nursing, and law. Except where noted, most of these studies used the Defining Issues Test (DIT) of Rest (1979) and were conducted with students or trainees in these professions. Bebeau (2002) summarizes the major research findings under the headings of four main questions. For the first question, "Does professional education promote moral judgment development?" she finds that the data strongly suggest a negative answer. At a time when normal advances in levels of moral reasoning should be expected, health profession education (including medical education) apparently does little to enhance postconventional thinking. The answer to her second question, "Does the addition of ethics instruction promote reasoning development?" however, suggests the opposite: that such interventions, when appropriately conducted, are generally accompanied by significant increases in moral reasoning or judgment. Similarly, in answer to her third question: "Are there differences in moral judgment development among subgroups within a profession?" what data there are reveal some measurable differences between subgroups, based on maturity, region, culture, and gender, all of which deserve further exploration. Her final question, "Is moral judgment linked to professional performance?" is answered again in the affirmative by the literature (see below), which provides some of the strongest arguments for using measures of moral reasoning and judgment in the assessment of professionalism.

Clinical Competence and Performance

Ultimately, objective measures of moral reasoning must be found to be empirically related to measurable dimensions of professional behavior and performance if they are to gain widespread acceptance. In 1994, Self and Baldwin conducted a thorough review of studies of moral reasoning in medicine and medical education. That review documented considerable empirical evidence of a significant relationship between levels of moral reasoning and measures of clinical excellence in medical students, residents, and practicing physicians, strongly supporting the notion that the assessment of moral reasoning should be regarded as important in the assessment and teaching of professionalism.

In a pioneering study, Sheehan et al. (1980) reported a highly significant relationship ($P < .0001$) between the clinical performance of 244 pediatrics residents as assessed by their supervisors using 18 criteria and their moral reasoning scores as measured by the percentage of principled responses on the Defining Issues Test (DIT; Rest 1979). Residents with high levels of moral reasoning were seldom assessed as having low, or poor, clinical performance, while those with low moral reasoning scores were essentially never found among the highly rated clinical performers. This suggests that high levels of moral reasoning may serve to ensure qualities associated with excellence in clinical performance, as well as to protect against less than optimal performance. These findings were later confirmed by Sheehan et al. (1985) in a study of 39 family practice residents who were evaluated as they interacted with each of two simulated patients. A correlation of 0.38 was found between faculty ratings of resident performance and levels of moral reasoning as reflected by another measure of moral reasoning, the Moral Judgment Interview (MJI) of Kohlberg (1984).

Following up on Sheehan's work, Baldwin et al. (1996a) studied levels of moral reasoning in practicing orthopedic surgeons whose malpractice claims data were available from another study. Those orthopedists in the low-claims group (<0.20 claims per year [CPY]) were found to have significantly ($P < .04$) higher levels of moral reasoning (mean principled moral reasoning [P] score of 43.8) compared with orthopedists in the high-claims group (>0.40 CPY; mean P score of 38.0). Furthermore, the scatter plot for all scores revealed that when the mean P score was >40, there were 25 orthopedists in the low-claims group, compared with only 6 in the high-claims group. Only one orthopedist with a P score >50 was in the high-claims group, supporting Sheehan's idea that there may be a protective element, or "floor effect," provided by higher levels of moral reasoning, in this case against malpractice claims. Further support for a significant relationship between moral reasoning and clinical performance has been reported in studies of both dental and nursing students (Bebeau 1988, 1993; Bebeau and Thoma 1994; Meetz et al. 1988; Duckett et al. 1992; Duckett and Ryden 1994). Of note is Adamson et al.'s (2000) report that orthopedists rated as having better rapport with their patients and who took more time with and explained more to them had fewer malpractice suits and lower claim payments.

Professional Attitudes and Decision Making

Cook (1978) reported finding a significant correlation ($P < .001$) between levels of moral reasoning and attitudes toward aggressive

treatment of critically ill patients. Residents with more principled responses on the DIT were more sensitive to negative family attitudes
toward prolonging treatment and less active in their treatment procedures. Later, Cook and other members of Sheehan's group reported that higher levels of moral reasoning were found to be significantly associated with greater sensitivity to patient attitudes and
to less aggressive treatment of critically ill infants (Candee et al.
1979). They also found a significant negative correlation between
levels of activism in treating infants with severe defects and levels of
moral reasoning, concluding that

> those subjects who were shown to reason in terms of universal
> ethical principles were most likely in particular cases to tailor
> their treatment of critical illness to both the explicit and im-
> plicit rights of patients. This was shown by correlations between
> DIT scores and the family attitude factor (explicit rights) and
> the salvageability factor (implicit rights). (Candee et al. 1979,
> p. 98)

A positive correlation (P < .02) has also been reported between levels of moral reasoning on the DIT and the "degree to which physicians tend to use a physician-based disclosure standard, the amount
of tolerance they had of disagreement between doctor and patient,
and the amount of information the physician presumed that the patient wanted" (Silver and Weiss 1992, p. 63). Taken together, these
findings suggest that the moral development of physicians is related
to qualities associated with good clinical performance, such as excellence, empathy, respect, tolerance, openness, and integrity, qualities usually associated with professionalism.

Assessment of Moral Reasoning During Medical Education

The work of Rest and others has shown that it is not developmentally too late for growth in moral reasoning to occur in subjects with
higher education and professional credentials (Rest 1988; Bebeau
1994a). Using both repeated-measure and cross-sectional designs,
however, a number of researchers have found that without specific
intervention, significant changes are unlikely to occur in postconventional moral thinking among subjects during their undergraduate or graduate medical education (Self and Baldwin 1998; Self and

Olivarez 1996; Self et al. 1996a; George 1997). For example, using the DIT and a cross-sectional design, Self and Baldwin (1998) found no change in the moral reasoning scores of 488 medical students from several sequential classes at one institution over the 4 years of their medical education, or in any combination of years. They have reported the same findings for students in veterinary medicine (Self et al. 1996b). In addition to the failure of an expected progression of moral reasoning during professional education, these and other studies have shown that there is a narrowing of the range of moral reasoning scores and of stage development from the first to the fourth year, suggesting a strong socializing effect of medical education and a tendency toward regression to the mean (Self and Olivarez 1996; Self et al. 1998a). The authors are currently engaged in a long-term follow-up of the subjects from their earlier studies, to determine the course of moral reasoning in physicians as they age and mature in practice (Self et al. unpublished manuscript).

More recently, Patenaude et al. (2003), using the original MJI of Kohlberg (1984), have found that entering medical students used more higher stage moral reasoning, involving law and order (stage 4) and social-contract/legalistic (stage 5) orientations, than did these same students at the end of their third year, when they used more lower level instrumental relativist (stage 2) and interpersonal concordance (stage 3) orientations. Such findings appear to confirm the medical student claims of "ethical erosion" reported by Feudtner et al. (1994), as well as suggesting that moral development is not just inhibited during medical education, but profoundly influenced by it.

Stern et al. (2005) have recently found an intriguing correlation between clerkship professionalism and student immunization and course evaluation form completion. This study appears to confirm an earlier report by Givner and Hynes (1983). Studying first-year medical students taking a course in medical humanities, they found that students who lived up to their commitments to complete both pre- and posttest DITs (fulfillers) had significantly higher moral reasoning scores than did those who failed to complete both tests (nonfulfillers).

Effect of Courses or Curriculum

It is important to note that course or curricular interventions may effectively serve to elevate the moral reasoning skills of medical students (Self et al. 1991, 1996a). Over nearly two decades, this group has tested a number of such interventions with successive classes of students at one school, mainly using the DIT as the instrument of assessment (Self et al. 1989, 1992, 1993b). In the first of these, the Sociomoral Reasoning Measure (SRM) was used to assess the relative effects of lecture and case-study discussions as alternative methods of implementing a medical ethics curriculum. The results showed a statistically significant increase in the level of moral reasoning of students exposed to the medical ethics course, regardless of the format. Self et al. (1992) also found a statistically significant increase in the level of moral reasoning of students exposed to a medical ethics course compared with an unexposed control group, using the DIT.

Self et al. (1993a) additionally evaluated the use of film discussions of morally problematic issues for teaching medical humanities. A control group of first-year medical students with no exposure to the films, a group of first-year medical students who participated in the weekly 1-hour film discussions during the fall quarter only, and a group of first-year medical students who participated in the film discussions during both the fall and winter quarters were pre- and posttested with the DIT. Significant differences in the moral reasoning scores were found for both the one-quarter and the two-quarter exposure groups compared with the control group. In an unreported pilot study also using the DIT, we found that first-year students who were exposed to a course sequence of one quarter of medical ethics, involving small-group, case-based discussion of morally problematic issues, followed by one quarter of medical humanities, which included lectures and class discussion of topics in history, literature and the law, showed a significant rise in their moral reasoning, whereas students assigned to the reverse sequence of courses failed to show any increase in their scores (Self and Baldwin 2004).

In a large study of first-year medical students ($n = 729$) who had been exposed to varying amounts of small-group, case-based discussion of morally problematic issues, Self et al. (1998b) found that those who had participated in 20 or more hours of such instruction showed significant increases in their levels of moral reasoning. Along the same lines, both Bebeau (1988) and Bebeau and Thoma (1994) found that a combination of 12 hours of dilemma discussion, plus focused writing assignments, produced similar results among dental students. Hartwell (1995) also has reported that the use of student-centered, small-group discussions of moral problems in law produced significant increases in moral reasoning scores, with effect sizes estimated at 0.77–0.97. Recently, a study of theological students also found statistically significant increases in moral reasoning, as demonstrated by higher P scores on the DIT, in students taught ethics exclusively in a small-group, case-based approach, compared with students who were exposed to lectures only, or lectures plus 7 hours of case-based discussion (Bunch 2005). Separately, Self and Olivarez (1996) have reported that gains in moral reasoning attained by medical students in the first year are maintained throughout the 4 years.

The conclusion of most scholars in the field, then, is that assessment of moral reasoning and the other components of moral development can be a useful component of the assessment of course or curricular interventions. Of major interest to educators, of course, should be the widespread reports of the effectiveness of the small-group, case-based discussion format for raising levels of moral reasoning. Unfortunately, many of the studies described above have involved the use of volunteers or convenience samples rather than required participation. In conducting future outcome studies of curricular or educational interventions (e.g., current courses in professionalism), we advise making the use of moral reasoning tests a required part of student evaluation.

Institutional Applications

Institutional Climate

While little definitive research has been reported on the specific effect of the environment or "moral climate" on the moral development of students and trainees in professional settings, the findings discussed above on the apparent failure of professional school curricula to produce the expected increases in levels of moral reasoning in their students and trainees strongly suggest that this should be an important concern for educators. Feudtner et al. (1994), for example, found that 62% of their third- and fourth-year medical students believed that they had suffered "erosion" of their ethical principles since entering medical school, while Patenaude et al. (2003) have reported disturbing evidence of specific regression in students' moral reasoning between the first and third year of medical school. They have further hypothesized that this may be due to the heavy emphasis in medical education on "technical rationality," described elsewhere by Schon (1983) as a mode of "instrumental problem-solving made rigorous by application of scientific theory and technique," which may encourage students to regard patients as a problems to be solved rather than persons to be understood. At another level, Baldwin et al. (1991, 1996b, 1998) have documented differences in the prevalence of unprofessional behaviors, such as cheating, substance abuse, and mistreatment between schools. With regard to residents, what has been reported is consistent with that found with medical students: there is a general failure of subjects to make age-expected gains in moral reasoning during the period of graduate medical education (George 1997).

While simply aggregating and comparing the scores of medical students and faculty on a standard test of moral reasoning such as the DIT might conceivably offer some indication of the moral "climate" or environment of an institution, and even provide a means of comparing multiple institutions, it seems evident that the development of more definitive measures are needed in this area. In our experience, however, faculty have been highly resistant to such efforts in the past, while, apart from the work of George (1997), there has been relatively little research on the moral reasoning of residents.

Admissions

Given the reports in the literature described briefly above, it would seem desirable to select students for professional training who are most likely to exhibit qualities that have been shown to be significantly related to high clinical performance and professional behavior. The idea of using moral reasoning assessment as a screening tool to exclude persons, however, was deplored by Kohlberg because he viewed moral reasoning as a developmental process and therefore amenable to educational intervention. In addition, the lack of definitive long-term studies of specific behavioral and performance outcomes should preclude its use for this purpose. However, given the current interest in the teaching of professionalism, it may be time to begin conducting studies of the use and effectiveness of such a criterion in the admission process. We have suggested such a plan, involving long-term study of the use of such an instrument by a number of institutions, not just in predicting outcomes but also in aiding faculty to identify students likely to be handicapped in their clinical decision making and performance (Self and Baldwin 2000).

We are aware of only one published report on the formal use of the DIT in the admissions process. Benor et al. (1984) employed the DIT to assess applicants to two medical schools in Israel, each with distinctly different selection criteria. One, a traditional school, based its selection process almost exclusively on competitive cognitive performance criteria, while the other, an innovative, community-based school, employed a complex process involving noncognitive criteria and personal interviews. Students admitted to the latter school were found to have significantly higher P scores (50.08) than those rejected at this same school, those admitted to the traditional school, and those rejected at the traditional school. There was a moderate but significant correlation between P scores and interview scores, suggesting that interviews did result in selecting students with higher levels of principled thinking. One of us (D.C.B.) has proposed using at least one vignette containing a morally problematic issue during the interview process to assess how applicants respond.

Instruments for Assessing Moral Reasoning

Multiple instruments are available for assessing the development of moral reasoning. Among them are the original MJI of Kohlberg (1984), the SRM of Gibbs and Widaman (1982), the DIT of Rest (1979), and the Moral Reasoning and Orientation Interview of Self and Skeel (1992; see table 5-1 for an overview of these instruments). Only the MJI, SRM, and DIT are widely used and are described below.

Moral Judgment Interview

The original MJI is generally considered to be the most accurate instrument for measuring moral development. It consists of a 45-minute, semistructured, oral, tape-recorded interview in which the subject is asked to resolve three hypothetical moral dilemmas. Each dilemma is followed by a set of open-ended probe questions designed to reveal the logic of the moral reasoning. The subject is asked to state what the person in the story *should* do, and not just what he or she *would* do in such situations. The interview is transcribed and assigned scores from a possible low score of 100 to a maximum high of 500, which are correlated with the stages in cognitive moral development theory. The actual scoring is highly complex, and special training is required. Both the data collection from one-on-one interviews and the scoring are very time consuming and labor inten-

Table 5-1   Dimensions in Moral Judgment Assessment

	MJI	SRM	DIT
I. Domain			
A. Moral justification	X	X	
B. Moral evaluation			X
II. Task			
A. Spontaneous production	X	X	
B. Recognition (comprehension or preference)			X
III. Level			
A. Competence (the best one can do)	X (oral)		
B. Performance (what one actually does)	X (written)	X	X
IV. Administration			
A. Individual: interview	45 min		
B. Group: pencil and paper		50 min	30 min
V. Scoring			
A. Individually rated	X	X	
B. Objectively scored			X
VI. Average time to rate by experienced rater	**30 min**	**15 min**	**5 min**

Table adapted from Mark Tappan, Colby College, Personal communication 2005.

sive, which results in the MJI being the most expensive of the assessment instruments available. Limited success has been achieved with a version of the MJI that uses written responses instead of oral tape-recorded ones. This allows the assessment to be group administered and eliminates the need for transcriptions, reducing cost. However, it still has to be individually hand scored, and the quality of material is decreased.

The Sociomoral Reasoning Measure

Developed at Ohio State University by Gibbs and Widaman (1982), the SRM is a paper-and-pencil version of the original oral MJI that attempts to simplify the collection and scoring of moral reasoning data. Less complicated to score than the MJI, it is also much less time consuming and less expensive. Since it can be administered to groups, the SRM permits larger sample sizes than the MJI. Like the MJI, the SRM assesses the spontaneous generation of moral reasoning and justification, rather than merely the recognition or preference of given moral reasons. Scores on the SRM range from a low of 100 to a high of 400 and are highly correlated with the stages found in Kohlberg's cognitive moral development theory. Unfortunately, the SRM only assesses stages 1 through 4, and not the postconventional or principled reasoning of stages 5 and 6, which can result in a ceiling effect with some groups.

The Defining Issues Test

The DIT was developed by James Rest (1979) at the University of Minnesota and can be both group administered and computer scored. As is the case with the MJI, the DIT presents hypothetical moral dilemmas for resolution. Rather than asking open-ended probe questions, however, multiple choices are presented to the subject from which he or she is to select the most important in resolving the dilemma. Six moral dilemmas are presented, each with 12 possible choices representing various stages in Kohlberg's theory. A score is expressed in terms of the percentage of choices from a given stage and is generally reported in terms of the number or percent of principled responses (P score) by the subject. Misleading nonsense phrases are included to rule out indiscriminate or inattentive answers.

While the MJI and SRM seek spontaneous generation of moral reasoning, the DIT offers various considerations that the subject chooses to justify his or her position. The four most salient considerations from the 12 offered for each dilemma on the DIT are rank ordered and weighted. The sum of the weighted ranks creates stages or levels of moral reasoning.

Because of its ease of administration, scoring, and cost, and because it can be used for larger groups of subjects, the DIT has been used in hundreds of studies of moral reasoning, resulting in a high level of validation and an extensive literature (Rest and Narvaez 1994; Rest et al. 1997, 1999a). It is the single most widely used instrument for assessing moral reasoning and is recommended for proposed studies in medical education because of its ease of administration, its low cost, and its simple scoring method. Recently, members of Rest's group have extensively revised the DIT, with new, updated, and more appropriate vignettes, as well as newer scoring mechanisms that are held to be more sensitive and accurate (Rest and Narvaez 1998; Rest et al. 1999b; Bebeau and Thoma 2003). The new DIT2 is now available from the Center for the Study of Ethical Development at the University of Minnesota and is considered preferable for use in studies involving medical students and residents.

Summary

High-quality instruments exist for the assessment of moral reasoning in medical students and residents. The available research suggests that such an assessment is strongly related to many, if not most, of the qualities and attributes ascribed to professionalism in the literature. For instance, Baldwin (2003) found that when health professionals were asked to designate which of 52 commonly accepted descriptors were characteristics of either morality or professionalism, 62% were found to apply to both categories. Thus, it would appear that for most people there is considerable overlap at least in their naturalistic understanding of these two concepts.

In conclusion, the assessment of moral reasoning would appear to be a useful component of any overall evaluation of professionalism in medical education and, especially, in the evaluation of courses and educational interventions designed to enhance professionalism. In addition, it should prove valuable in studies of groups and institutional climate.

References

Adamson TE, Bunch WH, Baldwin DC Jr, Oppenberg A. The virtuous orthopaedist has fewer malpractice suits. Clin Orthopaed Rel Res 2000;378:104–109.

Baldwin DC Jr. Toward a theory of professional development: framing humanism at the core of good doctoring and good pedagogy. In: Enhancing the Culture of Medical Education Conference Proceedings. New York: Arnold P. Gold Foundation, January 17–19, 2003.

Baldwin DC Jr, Adamson TE, Sheehan JT, Self DJ, Oppenberg AA. Moral reasoning and malpractice: a pilot study of orthopedic surgeons. Am J Orthoped 1996a;25(7):481–484.

Baldwin DC Jr, Daugherty SR, Rowley BD. Observations of unethical and unprofessional conduct in residency training. Acad Med 1998;73:1195–1200.

Baldwin DC Jr, Daugherty SR, Rowley BD, Schwarz MR. Cheating in medical school: a survey of 31 schools. Acad Med 1996b;71:267–273.

Baldwin DC Jr, Hughes PH, Conard S, Storr CL, Sheehan DV. Substance use among senior medical students: a survey of 23 medical schools. JAMA 1991;265:2074–2078.

Bebeau MJ. The impact of a curriculum in dental ethics on moral reasoning and student attitudes. J Dent Educ1988; 52(1):49.

Bebeau, MJ. Designing an outcome-based ethics curriculum for professional education: strategies and evidence of effectiveness. J Moral Educ 1993; 22(3):313–332.

Bebeau MJ. Can ethics be taught? A look at the evidence revisited. NY State Dent J 1994a;60(1):51–57.

Bebeau MJ. Influencing the moral dimensions of dental practice. In: Rest JR, Narváez D, eds. Moral Development in the Profession: Psychology and Applied Ethics (pp. 121–146). Hillsdale, NJ: Lawrence Erlbaum Associates, 1994b.

Bebeau MJ. The defining issues test and the four component model: contributions to professional education. J Moral Educ 2002;31:271–295.

Bebeau MJ, Rest JR, Yamoor CM. Measuring dental students' ethical sensitivity. J Dent Educ 1985;49:225–235.

Bebeau MJ, Thoma SJ. The impact of a dental ethics curriculum on moral reasoning. J Dent Educ 1994;58(9):684–692.

Bebeau MJ, Thoma SJ. Draft Guide for DIT-2. Minneapolis, MN: Center for the Study of Ethical Development, University of Minnesota, 2003.

Benor DE, Notzer N, Sheehan TJ, Norman GR. Moral reasoning as a criterion for admission to medical school. Med Educ 1984;18:423–428.

Blasi A. Bridging moral cognition and moral action: a critical review of the literature. Psychol Bull 1980;88:1–45.

Bunch WH. Changing moral reasoning in seminary students. J Moral Educ 2005 (in press).

Candee D, Sheehan TJ, Cook CD, Husted S. Moral reasoning and physicians' decisions in cases of critical care. Proc Res Med Educ Conf 1979;18:93–98.

Caplow T. The Sociology of Work. Minneapolis, MN: University of Minnesota Press, 1954.

Colby A, Kohlberg L. The Measurement of Moral Judgment. Vol. 1: Theoretical Foundations and Research Validation (pp. 1–117). New York: Cambridge University Press, 1987.

Cook CD. Influence of moral reasoning on attitude toward treatment of the critically ill. Proc Res Med Educ Conf 1978;17:442–443.

Dewey J. Moral Principles in Education. New York: Philosophical Library, 1954.

Duckett L, Rowan-Boyer M, Ryden MB, Crisham P, Savik K, Rest J. Challenging misperceptions about nurses' moral reasoning. Nursing Res 1992;41:323–331.

Duckett LJ, Ryden MB. Education for ethical nursing practice. In: Rest JR, Narvaez D, eds. Moral Development in the Professions: Psychology and Applied Ethics (pp. 51–70). Hillsdale, NJ: Lawrence Erlbaum Associates, 1994.

Feudtner C, Christakis DA, Christakis NA. Do clinical clerks suffer ethical erosion? Students' perception of their ethical environment and personal development. Acad Med 1994;69:680–689.

Freidson E. Profession of Medicine: A Study of the Sociology of Applied Knowledge. New York: Dodd, Mead and Company, 1970.

Freidson E. Professionalism Reborn: Theory, Prophecy and Policy. Chicago: University of Chicago Press, 1994.

George JH. Moral development during residency training. In: Scherpbier AJJA, Van Der Vleuten CPM, Rethans JJ, Van Der Steeg AFW, eds. Advances in Medical Education (pp. 747–748). Dordrecht: Kluwer, 1997.

Gilligan C. In a Different Voice: Psychological Theory and Women's Development. Cambridge, MA: Harvard University Press, 1982.

Gilligan C, Attanucci J. Two moral orientations: gender differences and similarities. Merrill-Palmer Q 1988;34:223–237.

Gibbs JC, Widaman KF. Social Intelligence: Measuring the Development of Sociomoral Reflection (pp. 192–210). Englewood Cliffs, NJ: Prentice-Hall, 1982.

Givner N, Hynes K. An investigation of change in medical students' thinking. Med Educ 1983;17:3–7.

Greenwood E. Attributes of a profession. Social Forces 1957;2:44–55.

Hartwell S. Promoting moral development through experiential teaching. Clin Law Rev 1995;1:505–539.

Kohlberg L. Stage and sequence: the cognitive-developmental approach to socialization. In: Goslin D, ed. Handbook of Socialization Theory and Research (pp. 347–480). Chicago: Rand McNally, 1969.

Kohlberg L. Moral stages and moralization: the cognitive developmental approach. In: Lickona T, ed. Moral Development and Behavior: Theory, Research, and Social Issues (pp. 31–53). New York: Holt, Rinehart and Winston, 1976.

Kohlberg L. Essays on Moral Development. Vol. 1: The Philosophy of Moral Development. San Francisco: Harper and Row, 1981.

Kohlberg L. Essays on Moral Development. Vol. 2: The Psychology of Moral Development. San Francisco: Harper and Row, 1984.

McGeorge C. The susceptibility to faking of the defining issues test of moral development. Dev Psychol 1975;11:108.

Meetz HK, Bebeau MJ, Thoma SJ. The validity and reliability of a clinical performance rating scale. J Dent Educ 1988;52:290–297.

Parsons T. The Professions and Social Structure. Social Forces 1957;17: 457–467.

Patenaude J, Niyonsenga T, Fafard D. Changes in the components of moral reasoning during students' medical education: a pilot study. Med Educ 2003;37:822–829.

Piaget J. The Moral Judgment of the Child. Gabain M, trans. New York: Free Press, 1965 (originally published 1932).

Rest JR. Development in Judging Moral Issues. Minneapolis: University of Minnesota Press, 1979.

Rest JR. The major components of morality. In: Kurtines W, Gewirtz J, eds. Morality, Moral Development and Moral Behavior (pp. 24–38). New York: Wiley, 1984.

Rest JR. Moral Development: Advances in Research and Theory. New York: Praeger, 1986.

Rest JR. Can ethics be taught in professional schools? The psychological research. In: Ethics: Easier Said Than Done 1988;1:22–26.

Rest JR, Davidson M, Robbins S. Age trends in judging moral issues: a review of cross-sectional, longitudinal, and sequential studies of the defining issues test. Child Dev 1978;49:263–279.

Rest JR, Narvaez D. Moral Development in the Professions: Psychology and Applied Ethics. Hillsdale, NJ: Lawrence Erlbaum, 1994.

Rest JR, Narvaez D. Guide for DIT-2. Minneapolis, MN: Center for the Study of Ethical Development, University of Minnesota, 1998.

Rest JR, Narvaez D, Bebeau MJ, Thoma SJ. Post Conventional Moral Thinking: A Neo-Kohlbergian Approach. Mahwah, NJ: Lawrence Erlbaum, 1999a.

Rest JR, Narvaez D, Thoma SJ, Bebeau MJ. DIT2: devising and testing a revised instrument of moral judgement. J Educ Psychol 1999b;91:644–659.

Rest JR, Thoma SJ. Relation of moral judgment development to formal education. Dev Psychol 1985;21:709–714.

Rest JR, Thoma S, Edwards L. Designing and validating a measure of moral judgement: stage preference and stage consistency approaches. J Educ Psychol 1997;89(1):5–28.

Schon D. The Reflective Practitioner. New York: Basic Books, 1983.

Self DJ, Baldwin DC Jr. Moral reasoning in medicine. In: Rest JR, Narvaez DF, eds. Moral Development in the Professions (pp. 147–162). Hillsdale, NJ: Lawrence Erlbaum, 1994.

Self DJ, Baldwin DC Jr. Does medical education inhibit the development of moral reasoning in medical students? A cross-sectional study. Acad Med 1998;73:S91–S93.

Self DJ, Baldwin DC Jr. Should moral reasoning serve as a criterion for student and resident selection? Clin Orthopaed Rel Res 2000;378:115–123.

Self DJ, Baldwin DC Jr. The effect of course order on the moral reasoning of medical students. Unpublished manuscript, 2004.

Self DJ, Baldwin DC Jr, Dickey NW. Long term follow-up of medical student moral reasoning skills. Unpublished manuscript, 2004.

Self DJ, Baldwin DC Jr, Olivarez M. Teaching medical ethics to first-year students by using film discussion to develop their moral reasoning. Acad Med 1993a;68(5):383–385.

Self DJ, Baldwin DC Jr, Wolinsky FD. Evaluation of teaching medical ethics by an assessment of moral reasoning. Med Educ 1992;26:178–184.

Self DJ, Baldwin DC Jr, Wolinsky FD. Further exploration of the relationship between medical education and moral development. Cambridge Q Healthcare Ethics 1996a;5:444–449.

Self DJ, Jecker NS, Baldwin DC Jr. The moral orientations of justice and caring among young physicians. Cambridge Q Healthcare Ethics 2003;12:54–60.

Self DJ, Olivarez M. Retention of moral reasoning skills over the four years of medical education. Teach Learn Med 1996;8(4):195–199.

Self DJ, Olivarez M, Baldwin DC Jr, Shadduck JA. Clarifying the relationship of veterinary medical education and moral development. J Am Vet Med Assoc 1996b;209(12):2002–2004.

Self DJ, Olivarez M, Baldwin DC Jr. Clarifying the relationship of medical education and moral development. Acad Med 1998a;73(5):72–75.

Self DJ, Olivarez M, Baldwin DC Jr. The amount of small-group case-study discussion required to improve moral reasoning skills of medical students. Acad Med 1998b;73(5):521–523.

Self DJ, Schrader DE, Baldwin DC Jr, Wolinsky FD. A pilot study of the relationship of medical education and moral development. Acad Med 1991;66(10):629.

Self DJ, Schrader DE, Baldwin DC Jr, Wolinsky FD. The moral development of medical students: a pilot study of the possible influence of medical education. Med Educ 1993b;27:26–34.

Self DJ, Skeel JD. Facilitating healthcare ethics research: assessment of moral reasoning and moral orientation from a single interview. Cambridge Q Healthcare Ethics 1992;4:371–376.

Self DJ, Wolinsky FD, Baldwin DC Jr. The effect of teaching medical ethics on medical students' moral reasoning. Acad Med 1989;64(12):755–759.

Sheehan TJ, Husted SDR, Candee D, Cook CD, Bargen M. Moral judgment as a predictor of clinical performance. Eval Health Prof 1980;3:393–404.

Sheehan TJ, Candee D, Willms J, Donnelly JC, Husted SR. Structural equation models of moral reasoning and physician performance. Eval Health Prof 1985;8:379–400.

Silver A, Weiss D. Paternalistic attitudes and moral reasoning among physicians at a large teaching hospital. Acad Med 1992;67:62–63.

Stern DT, Frohna AZ, Gruppen LD. The prediction of professional behaviour. Med Educ 2005;39:75–82.

6

Using Surveys to Assess Professionalism in Individuals and Institutions

DeWitt C. Baldwin, Jr., and Steven R. Daugherty

While surveys have been used by social scientists for more than 50 years in studies of medical education, these early efforts primarily followed the investigators' disciplinary interests in the process of socialization and professionalization among medical students. They were aimed at gathering extensive amounts of data on student demographics, background, characteristics, expectations, experiences, opinions, and career plans, as well as their values, attitudes, behavior, and self-image during exposure to the intense environmental influence of medical education. A classic example of this type of survey questionnaire can be found in Appendix D of Merton et al.'s *The Student-Physician* (1957). It was nearly 40 pages in length and consisted of 72 separate and exhaustive questions, each seeking numerous subsets of information. This survey was administered to successive classes of medical students at Cornell, Case Western Reserve, and the University of Pennsylvania during the 1950s, and the findings constitute a classic study of medical education.

In the years since, surveys have been used fairly extensively by institutions to assess changes in the medical student population and experience. A major example is the Annual Graduation Question-naire of the Association of American Medical Colleges (AAMC), which has been sent to all senior medical students in the United States since 1978. This survey provides a cross-sectional picture of student responses to a large number of prescribed questions. Such data are excellent for viewing trends and tracing patterns of response over time. In general, however, the data are presented primarily as averages or distributions and do not provide much information re-garding individual variation or elaboration as to incidence or cause. An example is given by the data reporting students' experiences of having been harassed or abused, which have been recorded since the early 1990s (Kassebaum and Cutler 1998).

Assessing Unprofessional Behaviors and Attitudes

Most surveys conducted during the 1980s were aimed at examining the prevalence of certain specific negative events and behaviors on the part of students, such as substance abuse and cheating, with the aim of mitigating or preventing such experiences and producing healthier and more ethical physicians. For example, McAuliffe et al. (1986), Clark et al. (1987), and Conard et al. (1988) all utilized sur-veys to establish prevalence rates for various forms of substance use and abuse among medical students in a number of medical schools, while a study by Sierles et al. (1980) reported alarmingly high rates of academic dishonesty among students at two medical schools. In a different mode, Rowley and Baldwin (1988) surveyed a national sam-ple of medical school administrators regarding school policies about substance use and abuse.

Baldwin et al. (1988, 1991a) provided early empirical data on students' experiences of perceived mistreatment and abuse at 1 and, later, 10 medical schools. They followed with evidence of similar events and behaviors among a large, national random sample of res-idents (Baldwin and Daugherty 1997). These studies were followed by a spate of surveys in the United States and abroad confirming the high prevalence of such unprofessional behaviors in undergraduate and graduate medical education (Sheehan et al. 1990; Silver and Glicken 1990; Uhari et al. 1994; Cook et al. 1996).

It is worth noting that, over time, many medical schools have moved away from viewing such negative behaviors, including sub-stance abuse and academic dishonesty, as uniquely characterological problems to be managed through the use of disciplinary action and honor codes. Instead, administrators have come to see that such forms of unprofessional behavior on the part of students and faculty need to be dealt with in the context of broad standards or codes of conduct, which in turn call for proactive educational programs promoting professionalism (Papadakis et al. 1999, 2001). This has reinforced the idea that behaving in a professional manner is best fostered by the recognition of a reciprocal covenant of expected and learned behaviors among students, faculty, and institutions. It is within this context that the need for and use of surveys in assessing professionalism in individuals, groups, and institutions must be examined.

Assessing Professional Behaviors and Attitudes

Interest in the direct assessment of "professionalism" as a distinct concept within the physician community is a fairly recent development. As indicated above, the earlier interest of social scientists was mostly in the process of professionalization (Vollmer and Mills 1966) and the achievement of "professional identity" (Bucher and Stelling 1977). Even the later empirical studies of physicians-in-training were largely driven by a "deficit" model, concentrating on identifying things that were wrong, or missing, such as the loss of ethical principles, or idealism (Eron 1955; Feudtner et al. 1994; Testerman et al. 1996). Viewed from this perspective, professionalism was somehow defined in the negative. Individuals were deemed as being professional to the degree that they were free from "unprofessional" attitudes and behaviors. Indeed, the first research report specifically using the term "professional" (as in "professional misconduct") for these events and behaviors surveyed medical students in one school concerning their observations of seven types of presented behaviors on the part of other students and faculty (Sheehan et al. 1990). It is of note that those persons believed to have exhibited such "professional misconduct" included faculty, residents, and nurses, as well as classmates. At the same time, this early empirical elaboration of unprofessional values, behaviors, and attitudes in some students and practitioners has served to provide a historical foundation for our current understanding of professionalism.

A more scientific and appropriate method of assessing professionalism requires the direct measurement of clearly defined dimensions that characterize professional thought and behavior. Thus, today we see professionalism not merely as the absence of negative attributes but as a set of identifiable positive qualities or behaviors. The truly professional physician will avoid doing bad (nonmalefi- cence) but also seek to do good (beneficence). Using this approach, scales can be developed and validated to target the essential dimen- sions of professionalism directly instead of by inference (Arnold et al. 1998; Rowley et al. 2000; Brownell and Côté 2001). Development of this type of standardized measure allows benchmarking and com- parison across individuals, groups, and institutions.

Using data from the General Social Survey, Bradburn (1969) has demonstrated that the assessment of positive and negative qual- ities takes place independently. Our internal conceptions of the world around us are multidimensional, allowing us to perceive both positive and negative qualities as existing in the same individual or the same situation. One possible conceptualization of professional- ism that includes both positive and negative dimensions is presented in Figure 6-1.

In this model, the truly professional physician achieves the best possible outcomes and uses the best means, or methods. The un- professional physician uses improper means, or methods, for im- proper purposes or to achieve negative outcomes. Note that it is also possible to use improper methods to achieve positive outcomes (think of the character Hawkeye Pierce in the movie *M*A*S*H*) or to insist on using proper methods only to achieve negative outcomes ("the operation was successful, but the patient died"). Viewed from this perspective, the assessment of professionalism requires an as- sessment of the outcomes achieved, *as well as* the means used to achieve them. Professionalism, as defined throughout this book, then, implies a foundation of clinical competence, ethical under-

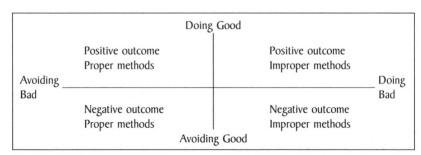

Figure 6-1 Measuring the Dimensions of Professionalism in Medicine.

standing, and communication skills upon which is built the aspiration to and wise application of humanistic principles that meet the health care needs of patients and communities.

The purpose of this discussion is to illustrate that, before we can measure anything, we must have a clear definition of what we are assessing. Historically, the goal has been to describe the values and behaviors of physicians, not to assess professionalism as we think about it today. Prior research has allowed us to infer some features of professionalism post hoc by aggregating reports of attitudes and behaviors collected for other reasons. However, as our sense of professionalism has changed, our methods of measuring it have changed, as well (Arnold 2002). Rather than targeting unprofessional behavior in a negative sense, with careful definition, we can now begin to assess professionalism in a positive sense.

The assessment of positive traits, such as professionalism, requires clear specification of the standard used to judge that trait. Traditionally, two types of standards for evaluative measurement are used: norm-referenced and criterion-referenced. Norm-referenced measurement gains meaning by comparing individuals to a reference group. This reference group can be a set of peers measured at the same time, or some standard population created to serve as a comparison group. A high score depends on being or doing better than the other people in the comparison group. Giving a passing score to the top 80% of the students in a class is an example of norm-referenced measurement.

Criterion-referenced measurement gains meaning by comparing individuals to some preset standard. Typically, this criterion is decided by an expert panel, which either sets a minimum passing level or defines some ideal to which all individuals should strive. A high score depends not on the responses of others but on achieving a preset criterion. Giving everyone in the class who scores 70% or better on a test a passing score is an example of criterion-referenced measurement.

Assessment of the positive qualities of professionalism means adopting one of these two measurement criteria. Benchmarking individuals relative to each other uses the norm-referenced standard. Certifying the absence of unprofessional behavior, or the degree to which the physician's behavior and attitudes are consistent with our ideal of professionalism, requires the use of the criterion-referenced standard.

To our knowledge, no completely satisfactory single scale or survey for assessing a comprehensive concept of professionalism in the

medical setting currently exists. This stems partly from the fairly recent transition to focusing on professional behaviors in the positive
sense, rather than measuring negative, or unprofessional, behavior.
It may also arise from the debate about whether we should be identifying only the very best and very worst of exemplars, or whether it
should be possible to scale the level of professionalism of every physician and physician-in-training. Finally, it probably is also due to the
ongoing, and as yet incomplete, efforts to arrive at a clear, specific,
consensual, and complete definition of professionalism.

Strengths and Weakness of Surveys as a Method

Surveys are most useful when the information sought is clearly defined and relatively straightforward. Each survey item poses a question and asks for a response. The information gained is based on
how individuals respond differently to the same presented items. This
process yields reliable and usable results only when all respondents
understand each item in a similar manner, *and* when the range of
possible answers can be presented succinctly. Such precision is
achieved only when there is a clear picture of what is being assessed.
Once this exists, surveys can increase our knowledge by providing a
number of essential types of information.

What Surveys Are Good For

Prevalence
Surveys are uniquely qualified for assessing the existence of and the
distribution of qualities within a population. A well-designed survey
will tell us not only that there is something out there but how much
of it there is. With survey results in hand, the discussion can be shifted
from descriptive to quantitative statements.

Focus on Subgroups
Surveys allow us to look at segments of the population, and how specific segments may differ from the whole. We can tell not only how
much of something there is, but also where it is concentrated. This
information lends topography to our understanding, allowing us to
map the peaks and valleys in a population rather than regarding all
members as the same.

Assessment of Variation

Surveys allow us to move beyond the consideration of the average and look at the distribution around that average. How similar or how different are the various individuals who make up the population in question? Understanding this variation protects us from simplistic generalizations based on averages and allows an appreciation of the range of possibilities that exist empirically.

Assessment of Subjective Experience

Surveys are better at allowing people to tell us what they think and feel about the world around them than they are at telling us what is incontrovertible fact. Because they are based on self-report, all such information provided is filtered through the respondents' subjective perspectives. This means that surveys are excellent tools for assessing subjects' beliefs and perspectives. Whether these reported impressions match objective reality is less important in guiding behavior than is the existence of the beliefs themselves. People act based on their impressions and beliefs. Subjective perceptions have a decisive impact on the ways we act and when we choose to act. To quote a famous aphorism, "That which we believe to be real is real in its consequences" (Thomas and Znaniecki 1995).

Broad Coverage

Surveys allow assessment of large segments of a population, or even a population in its entirety. (The AAMC's Annual Graduation Questionnaire attempts to survey the entire universe of graduating allopathic medical students in the United States.) This property protects us from the common cognitive mistake of assuming that some particular individuals are necessarily representative of the whole population.

Ease of Administration

When compared with other methodologies, surveys are relatively low cost and easy to administer. Although considerable expertise may be required in the creation of a survey, personnel with minimal training can actually conduct it. Survey administration can be made routine, fostering consistent delivery of questions and allowing planned periodic assessments. Costs can be controlled by varying sample size, the method of distribution, and the number of questions to match the available budget.

Multivariate Analysis
Surveys can measure a number of different things at the same time. This results in a rich data source amenable to multivariate statistical analyses. From these analyses, relationships among variables can be established and unanticipated patterns of covariation can be discovered.

Limitations of Surveys as a Method

Validation Issues
What people say about themselves or the world they live in may not reflect the objective reality of their circumstances. If surveys are used to report the behaviors of the respondent or others, efforts must be made to validate these self-reports against some more objective measure, such as direct observation. This can often be time-consuming, difficult, or even impossible.

Social Desirability Bias
Experience shows that respondents to surveys often try to give the answers that they think are expected rather than what reflects their actual experience or perspective. This is especially true when asking questions about behaviors that might elicit social disapproval or legal sanction.

Selection Bias
Although every effort should be made in administering a survey to gather responses from everyone in the target sample, 100% response rates are rarely if ever achieved. Bias may be generated by the fact that the people who do respond to the survey may be very different people, with different beliefs and attitudes, than those who do not respond. This problem can lead to false estimates of prevalence and cloud the interpretation of the amount of variation in the population.

Low Response Rates
The smaller the proportion of people in the sample who respond to a survey, the greater is the chance of selection bias. Surveys with response rates of less than 60% are generally suspect and need to be interpreted with caution.

Difficulty With Causal Interpretations
The analysis of survey data can tell what type of traits or behaviors occur together, but can shed little light about why that relationship

exists. Because the survey questions are all answered at the same time, the temporal sequence required for establishing the existence of a causal relationship is missing. Surveys tell us we have chickens and we have eggs, but cannot tell us which came first.

The Problem of the Question Not Asked

Each person who completes a survey is asked to respond to preset questions using the categories that are provided. Getting essential information from the survey depends on asking the right questions and providing options to allow respondents to say what they want to say. Surveys, therefore, are poor choices for early empirical investigations, because the right questions and the right response alternatives are very likely unclear or unknown. Survey development takes time and expertise and is usually preceded by observations, individual interviews, and focus groups with people from the target population. This initial, intensive groundwork helps to guide the investigator as to what to ask and how to ask it. Basic readings on survey design and administration can be found in such classic references as Bradburn and Sudman (1982), Converse (1986), Dillman (2000), Fink and Kosecoff (1985), Fowler (1993), Laurakas (1993), and Salant and Dillman (1994). However, an experienced consultant is highly desirable.

Assessing Professionalism by Means of Surveys

Using Surveys to Help Define Professionalism

The term "professionalism" is fundamentally an attributional construct. People may feel that they know it when they see it, but gaining a definition that is clear enough to allow measurement has proven elusive. Survey research can help to provide a working definition.

One method of achieving this is having people rate the degree to which presented characteristics are reflective of professional attitudes and values. Scheler (1913/1992) long ago stated that there is always a hierarchy or ranking of values. In the act of preferring, he claimed, one value is always rated above another. Values are generally viewed as higher, (1) the more they endure and are not transient; (2) the less they are divisible (as in a work of art that cannot be divided); (3) the more they serve as a foundation of another value, (4) result in a deeper experience of contentment or fulfillment, and (5) are related to absolute values—ones that exist in pure feeling or immediate intuition, such as love, holiness, and beauty. While this ranking of values might imply a simple comparative relativity, Scheler maintained that this method reveals the underlying "intuition" or "feeling" that determines the dimensions used to rate the values presented. The resulting rank order yields a set of gradients that can help define the concept of professionalism.

A survey by Rowley et al. (2000) asked practicing orthopedists rate a list of 20 descriptors or characteristics generally associated with professionalism and culled from lists prepared by several medical groups. When subjected to multidimensional scaling and/or factor analysis, such rankings provide a concrete representation of the dimensions used by the raters in their assessment of what it means to be a medical professional. In this particular study, qualities such as integrity and trustworthiness were found to be ranked at the top of the list, while altruism and virtue were at the bottom. Factor analysis, however, found that altruism and virtue formed an important secondary factor. At the very least, this work suggests that professionalism is multidimensional in the manner suggested at the beginning of this chapter. These ratings do not provide an empirical definition of professionalism, but do make clear the dimensions by which medical professionals make these judgments. Similarly, they can be used in determining differences and/or similarities between the preferences or behaviors of groups of subjects, for example, different specialties, or to track developmental changes in priorities as students and trainees progress in their development (Brownell and Côté 2001). One of us (D.C.B.) has used a revision of the list employed by Rowley et al. (2000) to determine if there are differences in the rank order of these descriptors by specialty (Baldwin 2003).

Using Surveys to Assess Professionalism

Once a clear definition of professionalism and the dimensions that define it have been established, surveys can help to assess those dimensions in a number of ways. The information generated from surveys depends on who is asked and what they are asked about. We can ask individuals about themselves, or their observations or perceptions of others, or the climate of their group or institution. Alternatively, we can ask institutional representatives to tell us what they know about their members or to describe the official policies that organize that institution. Table 6-1 lays out these options schematically.

Table 6-1   Use of Survey Data to Assess Dimensions of Professionalism

	Individual	Institution
Individual	Ask individual about individual E.g., Self-ratings (Baldwin et al. 2003)	Ask individual about institution E.g., Observations of others (Baldwin et al. 1998, 2003)
Institution	Ask institution about individuals E.g., Demographics and other aggregate data (Baldwin et al. 1995)	Ask institution about institution E.g., Policies and procedures (Kao et al. 2003; Rowley ˜n˒ Baldwin 1988; Hunt et al. 2001)

Ask Individuals About Themselves

These data can then be compared among individuals and their peers or aggregated to gain a picture of the group or institution. We have used this method extensively to ask students and physicians about substance use (Baldwin et al. 1991b; Hughes et al. 1991, 1992), cheating (Baldwin et al. 1996c), sleep deprivation (Baldwin and Daugherty 2004), gender discrimination and sexual harassment (Baldwin et al. 1996b; Nora et al. 2002), and working while ill or impaired (Baldwin et al. 2003). As noted above, the AAMC Annual Graduation Questionnaire uses this method to assess the educational experience of students at each of the medical schools in the United States. Based on these data, each medical school receives a report on their own students' responses that can be compared with the aggregated responses of students at other institutions (a norm-referenced measure).

Ask Individuals About Their Institutions or Environment

Rather than asking about their own attitudes and behaviors, individuals can be asked about what they perceive or have observed around them. Individuals are often much more willing to say that they have seen others doing something unacceptable than to admit that they have done it themselves. In this sense, such a question is projective, telling us something about an individual's own experience by asking him or her about the experiences of others. Data gathered in this way can be aggregated to sketch a picture of the institution as seen through the collective eyes of the participants. We have used this method extensively in our numerous assessments of students' reports of various types of mistreatment, or harassment and discrimination (Baldwin et al. 1991a, 1994, 1996b, 2003; Daugherty et al. 1998), as well as observations of unprofessional or unethical conduct by others (Sheehan et al. 1990; Arnold et al. 1998; Baldwin et al. 1998; Satterwhite et al. 1998).

Ask Institutional Authorities for Aggregated Data About Their Individual Members

This provides a summary of individual experiences and characteristics as known to the institutional authorities. We have used this method in our own national survey of withdrawal and extended leave from residency training (Baldwin et al. 1995), and violent events involving their students (Baldwin and Daugherty 1996a). Other interesting work has compared the responses collected from institutional authorities with those generated from direct questioning of individuals to highlight discrepancies (Chalasani et al. 2001).

Ask Institutional Authorities About Their Own Institution

These data can be used to monitor the existence of formal policies, practices, and procedures in different settings. This approach has been used in surveys of substance abuse policies (Rowley and Baldwin 1988) and by Swick et al. (1999) and Kao et al. (2003) in surveys concerning the teaching of professionalism in U.S. medical schools.

Types of Survey Tools

Surveys can be constructed for a wide variety of purposes and in a number of forms and formats. These include *questionnaires* that assess prevalence and subjective experience, such as those described above. They can be designed to assess values, attitudes, behaviors, knowledge, skills, and/or feelings and emotions, using direct or indirect questions, or prompts to elicit quantitative or qualitative responses from an identified group. Second, they can include the use of *semantic differentials,* which ask respondents to choose between paired descriptive adjectives, and can be used to generate descriptive ratings of persons, environments, and events. Third, *descriptive vignettes* can be used in assessing complex attitudes and values through posing of hypothetical dilemmas or actions aimed at eliciting deeper responses or judgments from respondents. Finally, subjective feelings and attitudes toward the environment can be assessed by means of *projective techniques.*

Questionnaires: Assessing Prevalence and Subjective Experience

In general, survey questionnaires are useful to establish the prevalence of, and/or to compile normative data about, a predetermined
array of experiences, behaviors, opinions, values, and attitudes presumed to be of relevance to an identified group of potential respondents. Since the reports are solicited from individuals and depend on the comprehension, understanding, and cooperation of
each respondent, they are, by definition, subjective in nature and
can never be checked immediately and directly. Consistency of reports over time, however, as in the use of sequential surveys, lends a
fairly high degree of confidence in such data (AAMC Annual Graduation Questionnaire; Daugherty et al. 1998; Baldwin et al. 2003;
Baldwin and Daugherty 2004). High response rates also provide assurance that the data obtained are representative of the population
under investigation (Defoe et al. 2001). Under the appropriate set
of conditions that assures anonymity, even questions involving in-
tensely subjective and/or potentially threatening issues, such as admitting to substance abuse, cheating, or medical errors, can provide
data which bear a relatively close correspondence to objectively obtained data collected by interviews and observation.

Behavior

If the correct categories can be clearly portrayed in question or statement form, and trust is high, most medical students and residents
will respond fairly accurately to questions requiring them to rate or
rank their knowledge, skills, and attitudes, and even their personal
characteristics and beliefs. Under the proper conditions, students
and residents will even admit to clearly unprofessional, unethical, or
immoral behavior (Baldwin et al. 2003).

There are many examples of how such survey "probes" can be
structured. We have used questions requiring personal reports of direct experience (e.g., "In general, how stressful was your current year
of residency?") using a Likert scale of 1, "not at all stressful," to 7,
"highly stressful." Questions on the same topic, such as "During this
year, how often, if ever, did you care for patients without what you
consider adequate supervision from an attending physician?" with
six options from "never" to "almost daily," and another asking residents, "Please rate your current year of graduate medical education
in terms of contact with attending physicians" on a 7-point scale, pro-

vide an opportunity to examine issues from more than one viewpoint. If prevalence of a certain behavior or event is desired, as well
as data concerning the source of such behavior, the question may
be structured as follows: "How often, if ever, did any of the following persons subject you to sexual harassment?" together with a list
of several possible sources, such as classmates or superiors, and several categories of frequency. Useful information also can be gleaned
from more general questions, such as "Please rate how much each
of the following contributed to your learning experience this year."
Any number of sources, including attending faculty, grand rounds,
other residents, and computer/internet, can be listed with ratings
ranging from 1, "not at all," to 5, "a great deal." Results can identify
learning patterns in different specialties and levels of training.

If the questions are aimed at eliciting reports of direct and personal observations of the behavior of others in the environment, they
can be phrased as "How often, if ever, did you observe any of the
following persons working in an 'impaired' condition during your
current year of residency?" Again, listing several categories of persons, as well as frequency, and presumed reasons for such behavior,
can expand upon the responses. Such questions can also set up follow-up queries of a more personal nature, such as, "How often have
you, yourself, worked in an 'impaired condition'?" with several categories of frequency and underlying reasons.

All of these questions can serve to establish prevalence for a particular individual or group at a particular level or stage of education
(Baldwin et al. 1995; Richardson et al. 1997), or responses can be
summed to look at how one school or institution is doing or ranks
with others. For example, with sufficient data, comparisons can be
made across schools, specialties, or even countries, as has been done
for cheating (Anderson and Obenshain 1994; Baldwin et al. 1996c),
substance use (Baldwin et al. 1991b; Hughes et al. 1991, 1992), and
mistreatment of students (Baldwin et al. 1991a; Cook et al. 1996; Elnicki et al. 1999; Uhari et al. 1994).

Knowledge

Examinations are basically surveys. By means of various types of questions, examiners attempt to sample and assess the expected knowledge of examinees, using either a criterion-based (if standards have
been established) or a norm-based referent for the group being
tested. More appropriate to this chapter, however, are the questions

concerning students' self-assessment of whether they received, or feel the need for, more, the same, or a lesser amount of a particular topic or subject, such as palliative care or family violence, which are asked of senior medical students in the AAMC's Annual Graduation Questionnaire. Such data can guide curriculum committees in their planning, as well as measure trends in student interest and subject content across time.

Attitudes

Attitudes can be assessed in several ways. The level or strength of agreement or disagreement with one or, preferably, a series of attitudinal statements can be assessed by asking respondents to rate each of a set of statements along a Likert scale of 5 or, better, 7 points (1, strongly disagree, to 7, strongly agree). Examples of such statements from our own work include "I would cheat if I were sure I would not get caught" and "Sleep deprivation has led me to make misjudgments in patient care." Means and norms for the group can then be established. These, in turn, can be followed over time by subsequent surveys to assess trends or following a planned intervention (Daugherty and Baldwin 1996). Attitudes toward academic dishonesty, for example, appear to shift away from more idealized positions as students progress in their training, suggesting an important effect of the institutional environment (Sierles et al. 1980; Simpson et al. 1989). At the same time, Baldwin et al. (1996c) found that cheating attitudes and behavior can shift in either direction depending on the environment experienced in a particular school.

An alterative method of assessing institutional environment is the use of semantic differential scales, as part or all of a survey (Osgood et al. 1957). These scales offer the respondent a set of opposing adjective pairs, such as "hard–soft," "strong–weak," and "rigid–flexible." Respondents are asked to indicate along a numerical or graphic scale which word best reflects their own perception of the environment or institution. Factor analyses of semantic differential adjective pairs show that they produce three underlying dimensions: (1) evaluation, good–bad; (2) potency, strong–weak; and (3) activity, active–passive. One of us (D.C.B.) has used this type of scale as a formative assessment instrument to track periodic changes in students' perceptions of their learning environment as they progressed through the first year of medical school. In this way, surveys can provide a way of assessing the professional climate of an institution. A systematic review of instruments to assess attitudinal changes in medical education can be found in Rezler and Flaherty (1985).

Vignettes: Assessing Complex Attitudes and Values

This method has been successfully used in a number of studies of values, behaviors, and attitudes deemed exemplary of professionalism. It consists of creating a series of (preferably) short, clinical or descriptive scenes or events in which a problem or dilemma is posed and an action either called for or described. These are usually arrayed around a particular theme or topic and designed to stimulate a decision-making response that reveals a complex attitude or value held by the respondent. The vignette has the advantage of placing the respondent within a situation with all of its nuances and contextual elements, so that the action or decision comes as close as possible to a real-life situation. Feudtner et al. (1994) have used vignettes successfully to elicit the ethical discomfort many medical students experience when placed in situations where their complicity is expected in a questionable "group" or team decision made by clinical superiors. Nora et al. (1993) also presented a set of 10 vignettes describing encounters between men and women in a variety of medical settings and asked students to rate the degree to which they perceived the scenario to represent sexual harassment and how uncomfortable they would feel in a similar situation. Green et al. (2000) also used vignettes to assess residents' use of deception with their colleagues, as did Rezler et al. (1990) to compare and contrast professional decisions and ethical values in medical and law students.

Future Developments

One method that shows promise for the assessment of professionalism of physicians, as well as students and residents, identifies and lists a series of specific, observable behaviors and/or actions considered to be professional on the part of personnel being evaluated. These are then distributed in survey form to patients, staff, and/or colleagues, and their responses are recorded as a scaled numerical score for each item (e.g., "makes eye contact when addressing me," "explains procedure thoroughly," "listens appropriately," "respects my opinion"). These scores are recorded for each of a list of such actions or behaviors for the individual being rated. After accumulating sufficient data on a series of individuals, say, in a particular class, specialty, or group, a mean score is determined for each item and is tentatively accepted as normative for that group. The latter can then be listed in a column next to the scores attained by the individual and compared. For a particular individual, this might look like table 6-2, with a low score indicating the need for improvement in a particular area.

It becomes clear, then, how each individual being assessed rates along side his or her colleagues, not only globally but also for each separate behavior. This allows for the institution of a highly specific remediation for the deficient behavior. If desired, standards or benchmarks for achievement may be set and progression toward these measured over time. Such data can be accumulated for all members of a generic class, such as students, in the same or a different class, or school, or in all schools. In similar fashion, the change or development of scores for all or a particular behavior may be followed across time, as with the expected changes for progression from student to resident. Variations on this method have been reported in several studies of physician communication skills and malpractice claims (Adamson et al. 1989, 2000). Several authors are currently working to construct and validate a series of student and resident professional behaviors that can be scored in this way.

Conclusions

No one survey instrument or method meets all needs. Readers are encouraged to become familiar with the alternatives and to select the resources and approaches that best meet their particular goals. That said, choosing a survey instrument that has been developed and used by others carries several advantages. First, an existing instru-

Table 6-2 Example Scores: Survey to Assess Professionalism of Physicians, Students, and Residents

Behavioral Item	Score (0–100)		
	Individual	Specialty	All Physicians
1. Makes eye contact when addressing me	73	85	81
2. Explains procedure thoroughly to me	83	80	78

ment cuts down on development time considerably and offers more assurance that the results will be valid. Second, any instrument that has already been used elsewhere provides a ready reference point to compare individuals and institutions. Third, use of a survey instrument in multiple settings allows the assessment of the impact of those settings. Finally, the repeated use of the same survey instrument across time allows a clean, simple way to track trends across time.

The early reports of cheating, substance abuse, sexual harassment, and student mistreatment referenced in this chapter were all secured by means of surveys. Each report has served to generate review and discussion, eventually resulting in administrative changes designed to prevent or eliminate such unprofessional behaviors. Over the years, their combined effect on the nature and quality of the teacher–learner relationship and the learning environment in medical education has been significant as indicated by position statements by the American Medical Association (1990) and AAMC (1992). While it may be impossible to completely eliminate such behaviors, there is growing evidence that the prevalence and severity of such "unprofessional" behaviors (usually on the part of superiors) are slowly but surely declining (Daugherty and Baldwin, unpublished data). In their turn, the identification and promotion of more positive and "professional" behaviors can help to establish a learning and working environment in which students and residents may expect to be treated with dignity and respect and to have the opportunity to observe and emulate more role models of exemplary "professional" behavior, as well as experience institutional interventions and cultures that promote professionalism.

Our hope is that with the passage of time, data can be accumulated from a set of convergent instruments which will allow the benchmarking of levels or stages of professionalism in both individuals and institutions (Baldwin 2003; Leach 2004). With this data pool as background, feedback can then be provided to each person that highlights both areas of strength and those that need improvement. As our experience increases, these data will become the standards by which we can track increases in individual professional behavior, as well as institutional cultures that promote professionalism.

References

AAMC. Reaffirming Institutional Standards of Behavior in the Learning Environment. Presidential Memorandum 92-38 [internal document]. Association of American Medical Schools, Washington, DC, July 28, 1992.

Adamson TE, Bunch WH, Baldwin DC Jr, Oppenberg A. The virtuous orthopaedist has fewer malpractice suits. Clin Orthoped 2000;378: 104–109.

Adamson TE, Tschann JM, Gullion DS, Oppenberg A. Physician communication skills and malpractice claims. A complex relationship. West J Med 1989;150:356–360.

American Medical Association. Teacher-learner relationship in medical education. AMA Policy H-295.955, Board of Trustees' Report ZZ, December 1990. In: AMA House of Delegates Policy Compendium [Internal document]. Chicago: American Medical Association 1997.

Anderson RE, Obenshain SS. Cheating by students: findings, reflections, and remedies. Acad Med 1994;69:323–331.

Arnold EL, Blank LL, Race KEH, Cipparrone N. Can professionalism be measured? The development of a scale for use in the medical education environment. Acad Med 1998;73:1119–1121.

Arnold L. Assessing professional behavior: yesterday, today, and tomorrow. Acad Med 2002;77:502–515.

Baldwin DC Jr. Toward a theory of professional development: framing humanism at the core of good doctoring and good pedagogy. In: Enhancing the Culture of Medical Education. Conference Proceedings, pp. 6–10. New York: Arnold P. Gold Foundation, January 17–19, 2003.

Baldwin DC Jr, Daugherty SR. Reports of violent events involving medical students. Advisor 1996a;16:3–6.

Baldwin DC Jr, Daugherty SR. Do residents also feel "abused?" Perceived mistreatment during internship. Acad Med 1997;72(suppl):S51–S53.

Baldwin DC Jr, Daugherty SR. Sleep deprivation and fatigue in residency training: results of a national survey of first and second year residents. Sleep 2004;27:217–223.

Baldwin DC Jr, Daugherty SR, Eckenfels E. Student perceptions of mistreatment and harassment during medical school: a survey of ten schools. West J Med 1991a;155:140–145.

Baldwin DC Jr, Daugherty SR, Eckenfels EJ, Leksas L. The experience of mistreatment and abuse among medical students. Proc Annu Conf Res Med Educ 1988;63:80–84.

Baldwin DC Jr, Daugherty SR, Rowley BD. Racial and ethnic discrimination during residency: results of a national study. Acad Med 1994;69(10): 19–21.

Baldwin DC Jr, Daugherty SR, Rowley BD. Sexual harassment and discrimination among medical students and residents. Acad Med 1996b; 71(suppl):S25–S27.

Baldwin DC Jr, Daugherty SR, Rowley BD. Observations of unethical and unprofessional conduct in residency training. Acad Med 1998;73: 1195–1200.

Baldwin DC Jr, Daugherty SR, Rowley BD, Schwarz MR. Cheating in medical school: a survey of 31 schools. Acad Med 1996c;71:267–273.

Baldwin DC Jr, Daugherty SR, Tsai R, Scotti M. A national survey of residents' self-reported work hours: thinking beyond specialty. Acad Med 2003;78:1154–1163.

Baldwin DC Jr, Hughes PH, Conard S, Storr CL, Sheehan DV. Substance use among senior medical students: a survey of 23 medical schools. JAMA 1991b;265:2074–2077.

Baldwin DC Jr, Rowley BD, Daugherty SR, Bay RC. Withdrawal and extended leave during residency training: results of a national survey. Acad Med 1995;70:1117–1124.

Bradburn N. The Structure of Psychological Well-being. Chicago: Aldine, 1969.

Brownell KW, Côté L. Senior residents' views on the meaning of professionalism and how they learn about it. Acad Med 2001;76:734–737.

Bucher R, Stelling JG. Becoming Professional. Beverly Hills, CA: Sage Publications, 1977.

Chalasani K, Nettleman MD, Moore SS, MacArthur S, Fairbanks RJ, Goyal M. Faculty misperceptions about how residents spend their call nights. JAMA 2001;286:1024.

Clark D, Eckenfels EJ, Daugherty SR, Fawcett J. Alcohol use patterns and alcohol abuse through medical school: a longitudinal study of one class. JAMA 1987;257:2921–2926.

Conard S, Hughes P, Baldwin DC Jr, Achenbach KE, Sheehan DV. Substance use by fourth year students at thirteen medical schools. J Med Educ 1988;63:747–758.

Cook D, Liutkus J, Risdon C, Griffith L, Guyatt G, Walter S. Residents' experiences of abuse, discrimination, and sexual harassment during residency training. Can Med Assoc J 1996;154(11):1657–1665.

Daugherty SR, Baldwin DC Jr. Sleep deprivation in senior medical students and first-year residents. Acad Med 1996;71(1):S93–S95.

Daugherty SR, Baldwin DC Jr, Rowley BD. Learning, satisfaction, and mistreatment during internship: a national survey of working conditions. JAMA 1998;279:1194–1199.

Defoe DM, Power ML, Holzman GB, Carpentieri A, Schulkin J. Long hours and little sleep: work schedules of residents in obstetrics and gynecology. Obstet Gynecol 2001;97:1015–1018.

Elnicki DM, Linger B, Asch E, Curry R, Fagan M, Jacobson E, et al. Patterns of medical students abuse during the internal medicine clerkship: perspectives of students at 11 medical schools. Acad Med 1999;74:S99–S101.

Eron LD. Effect of medical education on medical students' attitudes. J Med Educ 1955;30:559–566.

Feudtner C, Christakis DA, Christakis NA. Do clinical clerks suffer ethical erosion? Students' perception of their ethical environment and personal development. Acad Med 1994;69:680–689.

Green MJ, Farber NJ, Ubel PA, Mauger DT, Aboff BM, Sosman JM, et al. Lying to each other: when internal medicine residents use deception with their colleagues. Arch Intern Med 2000:160:2317–2323.

Hughes PH, Brandenburg N, Baldwin DC Jr, Storr CL, Williams KM, Anthony JC, Sheehan DV. Prevalence of substance use among U.S. physicians. JAMA 1992;267:2333–2339.

Hughes PH, Conard S, Baldwin DC Jr, Storr CL, Sheehan DV. Resident physician substance use in the United States. JAMA 1991;265:2069–2073.

Hunt DD, MacLaren C, Scott C, Marshall SG, Braddock CH, Sarfaty S. A follow-up study of the characteristics of dean's letters. Acad Med 2001;76:727–733.

Kao A, Lim M, Spevick J, Barzansky B. Teaching and evaluating students' professionalism in US medical schools. JAMA 2003;290:1151–1152.

Kassebaum DG, Cutler ER. On the culture of student abuse in medical school. Acad Med 1998;73:1149–1158.

Leach D. Professionalism: the formation of physicians. Am J Bioethics 2004;4:11–12.

McAuliffe WE, Rohman M, Santangelo S, Feldman B, Magnuson E, Weissman J. Psychoactive drug use among practicing physicians and medical students. N Engl J Med 1986;315:805–810.

Merton RK, Reader GG, Kendall P. The Student-Physician: Introductory Studies in the Sociology of Medical Education. Cambridge, MA: Harvard University Press, 1957.

Nora LM, Daugherty SR, Hersh K, Schmidt J, Goodman LJ. What do medical students mean when they say "sexual harassment"? Acad Med 1993;68:S49–S51.

Nora LM, McLaughlin MA Fosson SE, Stratton TD, Murphy-Spencer A, Fincher RME, German DC, Seiden D, Witzke DB. Gender discrimination and sexual harassment in medical education: perspectives gained by a 14-school study. Acad Med 2002;77:1226–1234.

Osgood, CE, Suci GJ, Tannenbaum PH. The Measurement of Meaning. Urbana, IL: University of Illinois Press, 1957.

Papadakis MA, Loeser H, Healy K. Early detection and evaluation of professional development problems in medical school. Acad Med 2001; 76:1100–1106.

Papadakis MA, Osborn EH, Cooke M, Healy K, and the University of California, San Francisco School of Medicine Clinical Clerkships Operation Committee. A strategy for the detection and evaluation of unprofessional behavior in medical students. Acad Med 1999;74:980–990.

Rezler A, Flaherty JA. The Interpersonal Dimension in Medical Education. New York: Springer, 1985.

Rezler AG, Lambert P, Obenshain SS, Schwartz RL, Gibson JM, Bennahum DA. Professional decisions and ethical values in medical and law students. Acad Med 1990;65:S31–S32.

Richardson DA, Becker M, Frank RR, Sokol RJ. Assessing medical students' perceptions of mistreatment in the second and third years. Acad Med 1997;72:728–730.

Rowley BD, Baldwin DC Jr. Datagram: substance abuse policies and programs at U.S. medical schools. J Med Educ 1988;63:759–761.

Rowley BD, Baldwin DC Jr, Bay RC, Karpman R. Professionalism and professional values in orthopedics. Clin Orthoped Rel Res 2000;378:90–96.

Satterwhite WM, Satterwhite RC, Enarson C. Medical students' perceptions of unethical conduct at one medical school. Acad Med 1998;73:529–531.

Scheler M. On Feeling, Knowing and Valuing: Selected Writings. Heritage of Sociology Series (Bershady H, ed.). Chicago: University of Chicago Press, 1992 (originally published 1913).

Sheehan KH, Sheehan DV, White K, Leibowitz A, Baldwin DC Jr. A pilot study of medical student "abuse": student perceptions of mistreatment and misconduct in medical school. JAMA 1990;263:533–537.

Sierles F, Hendrickx I, Circle S. Cheating in medical school. J Med Educ 1980;55:124–125.

Silver HK, Glicken AD. Medical student abuse: incidence, severity, and significance. JAMA 1990;263:527–532.

Simpson DE, Yindra KJ, Towne JB, Rosenfeld PS. Medical students' perceptions of cheating. Acad Med 1989;64:221–222.

Swick HM, Szenas P, Danoff D, Whitcomb ME. Teaching professionalism in undergraduate medical education. JAMA 1999;282:830–832.

Testerman JK, Morton KR, Loo LK, Worthley JS, Lamberton HH. The natural history of cynicism in physicians. Acad Med 1996;71:S43–S45.

Thomas WI, Znaniecki F. The Polish Peasant in Europe and America. Champaign, IL: University of Illinois Press, 1995.

Uhari M, Kokkonen J, Nuutinen M, et al. Medical student abuse; an international phenomenon, JAMA 1994;271:1049–1051.

Vollmer HM, Mills DL. (Eds.) Professionalization. Englewood Cliffs, NJ: Prentice-Hall, 1966.

General References on Survey Design and Administration

Bradburn N and Sudman, S. Asking questions: a practical guide to questionnaire design. San Francisco: Jossey Bass, 1982.

Converse J. Survey questions: Handcrafting the standardized questionnaire. Beverly Hills, CA: Sage Publications, 1986.

Dillman D. Mail and internet Surveys: the tailored design method. New York: Wiley, 2000.

Fink A and Kosecoff, J. How to conduct surveys: a step by step guide. Newbury Park, CA: Sage Publications, 1985.

Fowler FJ Jr. Survey Research Methods. 3rd. Edition. Thousand Oaks, CA: Sage Publications, Inc. 1993

Laurakas PJ. Telephone survey methods: Sampling, selection, and supervision (2nd ed.). Thousand Oaks, CA: Sage Publications,1993.

Osgood, CE, Suci GJ, Tannenbaum PH. The Measurement of Meaning. Urbana: University of Illinois Press, 1957

Salant P and Dillman, DA. How to Conduct Your Own Survey. San Francisco: John Wiley and Sons, 1994.

Telephone Survey Methodology. Eds. Groves RM, Biemer PP, Lyberg LE, Massey JT, Nicholis WL, Waksberg J. New York: John Wiley and Sons, 2001.

7

Measuring Specific Elements of Professionalism: Empathy, Teamwork, and Lifelong Learning

Jon Veloski and Mohammadreza Hojat

Professionalism concerns the aims, qualities, and behaviors that characterize a profession or the nature of one who practices such a profession, like medicine. Efforts to foster professionalism in medical education emphasize the qualities and attainments of physicians beyond the requisite medical knowledge and clinical skills. A growing consensus on what this set of personal attributes consists of has led to widespread agreement on the need to inspire professionalism throughout the continuum of medical education. In addition, there is recognition of the need to develop credible instruments to assure that this occurs.

In this chapter we recommend that a multiscore profile, depicting different elements of the multidimensional nature of professionalism, is the best way to move toward the goal of reinforcing and measuring professionalism. We assert that a global assessment cannot represent a complex and dynamic entity such as professionalism. In order to build the case for a multiscore profile we describe three representative elements of professionalism: empathy, teamwork with nurses, and lifelong learning. We provide details on the procedures used for development, including the empirical results of pilot studies for related scales that have been developed by our research team at Jefferson Medical College in Philadelphia, Pennsylvania. We provide tables of descriptive statistics and psychometric findings as evidence in support of their reliability and validity. Finally, we discuss the desirability of viewing the multidimensional and complex entity of professionalism from the vantage point of systems theory in which its elements (e.g., empathy, collaboration, lifelong learning) must operate in harmony to make the system fully functional.

Measuring Professionalism: Global Index or Multiscore Profile?

Leading organizations such as the American Board of Internal Medicine (ABIM), the Accreditation Council on Graduate Medical Education, and the Association of American Medical Colleges (AAMC) have approached professionalism either as a global construct or as a distinct facet of clinical competence. Although a global measure such as the scale reported by Arnold et al. (1998) is appealing and may be useful as a proxy for professionalism, we suggest that a multiscore profile has two important advantages. First, it can provide more complete information. An example of such an approach is the personality profile prepared for individuals who take the NEO PI-R (Personality Inventory—Revised, Costa and McCrea 1992), a 240-item personality inventory based on a five-factor model of personality. This profile, which describes scores on the five major dimensions of neuroticism, extraversion, openness, agreeableness, and conscientiousness, also includes scores on 30 distinct personality elements, or facets, within the five factors (Costa and McCrea 1992).

The second advantage of a multiscore profile is that it shows elements with high or low scores. Elements that may need attention can be identified in this profile. A global measure of professionalism derived from this model may not be meaningful because in this profile, a high score on one element (e.g., lifelong learning) cannot compensate for a low score in another element (e.g., empathy).

It is challenging to identify and define the elements of professionalism in medicine and to develop sound measures to quantify them. There are three recognized elements of professionalism: empathy, teamwork, and lifelong learning (Arnold 2002). Empathy is described as a fundamental attribute of the humanistic physician in chapter 1. Teamwork and interprofessional collaboration with nurses are behavioral examples of both respect and accountability to others on the health care team. Physician lifelong learning is a component of both excellence (maintenance of competence) and self-regulatory/accountable behavior to ensure quality of care.

Measuring Three Elements of Professionalism

In this chapter we discuss the development, psychometric properties, and findings reported in published studies for three instruments that our team at Jefferson Medical College has developed since 1985 (Hojat and Herman 1985). These include measures of physician empathy, physicians' attitudes toward interprofessional collaboration and teamwork with nurses, and physicians' lifelong learning.

Empathy: The Jefferson Scale of Physician Empathy

Empathy has been listed consistently as one of the key elements of professionalism (Arnold 2002). The importance of empathy as the foundation for positive relationships between patients and physicians has been discussed in medical education and health care research (DeMatteo 1979; Neuwirth 1997; Spiro et al. 1993; Zinn 1993). Despite its importance in enhancing these relationships (Bertakis et al. 1991; Levinson 1994) and in improving patient care (Jackson 1992; Hudson 1993; Nightingale et al. 1991), research on physician empathy has been limited for two reasons. First, the theoretical investigation of physician empathy has been hampered by ambiguity in its conceptualization and definition (Stephan and Finlay 1999; Thornton and Thornton 1995; Price and Archbold 1997). Second, empirical research on the topic has been limited by the absence of an instrument that would make it possible to gauge the empathy of medical students and physicians (Evans et al. 1993; Kunyk and Olson 2001).

The need to inculcate and assess empathy in both undergraduate and graduate medical education has been recommended universally. The ABIM (1983) has long recommended that residents' humanistic attributes, including empathy, be instilled and assessed. Both the Accreditation Council on Graduate Medical Education and the AAMC include empathy among their educational objectives by emphasizing that medical schools and residency programs strive to educate altruistic physicians who are compassionate and empathic in caring for patients and who can understand a patient's perspective through empathy.

Despite these recommendations, physician empathy remains largely an unexplored research area in medical education. Although the notion of empathy has been discussed in the medical education literature, there is no agreed-upon definition of the term. Because of the ambiguity in its definition, it has been suggested that the notion of empathy may not even exist and therefore should be eliminated from the language of psychology and replaced by a less ambiguous term (Levy 1997).

Definition of Empathy

Despite a lack of consensus on the definition of empathy, attempts have been made to describe it (Hojat et al. 2003b). The key element in these descriptions is the human capacity to understand the views, experiences, and feelings of another being without intensive emotional involvement. The desire to be understood by others is a basic human need (Kunyk and Olson 2001). Therefore, we propose that when an empathic relationship is established, a basic human need is fulfilled. Accordingly, physician empathy is built upon understanding the patient (Hudson 1993; Sutherland 1993). Such understanding is the backbone of relationships with patients (Levinson 1994). In summary, empathy involves an ability to "stand in a patient's shoes" without leaving one's own personal space. It is a capacity to view the world from a patient's perspective without losing sight of one's own personal role and responsibilities.

Therefore, the key component of a positive patient-physician relationship is understanding the patient through verbal and nonverbal communication involving empathic, interpersonal exchanges. This notion was elegantly described by Francis W. Peabody in his landmark article entitled "The Care of the Patient," originally published in 1927 and reprinted in 1984. Peabody proposed that "the practice of medicine in its broadest sense includes the whole relationship of the physician with his [her] patient." (Peabody 1984, p. 813) Similarly, Sir William Osler (1932) suggested, "It is as important to know what kind of a man [sic] has the disease, as it is to know what kind of disease has the man" (also cited in White 1991, p. 74). He advised physicians to "listen to the patient" because the patient is "telling you the diagnosis" (cited in Jackson 1992, p. 1630).

These descriptions and conceptualizations provided a framework for our definition of physician empathy: "A *cognitive* (as opposed to affective) attribute that involves an *understanding* of the inner experiences and perspectives of the patient, combined with a capability to *communicate* this understanding to the patient." (Hojat et al. 2002b, p. s58) In other studies we have indicated that the affective component of patient–physician relationship is more closely related to sympathy as opposed to empathy (Hojat et al. 2001b, 2002b, 2002c, 2003c). The key terms in italics are significant in the construct of empathy in patient care.

While a few research tools for measuring empathy in the general population do exist, none is specific to the health care environment. Three have been used in medical education research. The first is the Interpersonal Reactivity Index, developed by Davis (1983). Another research tool is the Empathy Scale, developed by Hogan (1969). The third research tool is the Emotional Empathy Scale, developed by Mehrabian and Epstein (1972).

We recognized a need for a tool to enable researchers to investigate empirically the development of physician empathy and its variation and correlates in the stages of medical education among groups of medical students and physicians. In response to this need, we developed the Jefferson Scale of Physician Empathy (JSPE; Hojat et al. 2001b, 2002c).

Validity

Construction of a test begins with developing a framework for understanding the concept that is to be measured. The usual first step is to conduct a literature review of the theories and observed tendencies, or behaviors, that describe the concept.

In the development of the physician empathy scale, as well as the other two scales that we describe further below, we first developed a long version of the instrument with items that appeared to have validity based on our review of the literature. In this step, a convincing theoretical argument must be presented to support the inclusion of every item. For example, in the development of the physician empathy scale we included items related to interest in literature and the arts based on the proposition that studying literature and the arts can improve one's understanding of human pain and suffering (Herman 2000; Hunter et al. 1995; McLellan and Jones 1996). Such interest would be relevant to physician empathy.

We drafted 90 items based on the literature review and used an abbreviated Delphi method to obtain independent judgments from our colleagues about the content and face validity of the items

(Hojat et al. 2001b). After several iterations and revisions to assure that the items reflected distinct and relevant aspects of empathy in patient-care situations, 45 of the original 90 items were retained in the instrument (Hojat et al. 2001b). Next, we probed for *content validity*, a term defined as that which provides evidence confirming that test items represent the domain of the concept that is being measured (Anastasi 1976, pp. 134–135). The content validity of the JSPE was examined by assuring that the test included a representative sample of the expected behaviors that fall within the domain of the concept of physician empathy as it had been defined.

Improving the clarity of the items was also requested from the expert judges in these preliminary steps of test development. Our goal was to assure that the items included a representative sample of attitudes and behaviors described in the definition of physician empathy. Occasionally new items would be suggested or some items were deleted when they were judged to be irrelevant. For example, the measurement of physician empathy included items measuring physicians' understanding of patients' experiences and perspective. This meant "perspective taking" was included as a factor.

Subsequently, 20 items were chosen for inclusion in the scale based on additional psychometric studies. These items are presented on a 7-point Likert-type scale, from 1 for strongly disagree through 7, strongly agree (Hojat et al. 2001b, 2002c).

The student version (S-Version) of the scale was originally developed to measure the orientation or attitudes of medical students toward physician empathy in patient-care situations (Hojat et al. 2001b). A second version, the health professional version (HP-Version), was developed to measure empathy among practicing physicians and other health professionals (Hojat et al. 2002c). In the HP-Version, minor modifications were made in the wording of some items to make them more relevant to the caregiver's empathic *behavior* rather than to empathic orientation or attitudes. For example, the following item appeared in the S-Version: "Because people are different, it is difficult for physicians to see things from their patients' perspectives" (Hojat et al. 2001b). This item was revised to read as follows in the HP-Version: "Because people are different, it is difficult for me to see things from my patients' perspectives." These modifications were also intended to make the scale applicable to other health care providers such as nurses and psychotherapists.

Construct validity is defined as the extent to which a test measures the theoretical constructs of the attribute that it purports to measure (Anastasi 1976, p. 151). Factor analysis examines if the dimensions of the underlying factors are consistent with those of the theoretical construct being measured. This enables the major dimensions characterizing the test score to be determined (Anastasi 1976, p. 154). The construct validity of the JSPE, determined by factor analysis, resulted in three reliable factors (Hojat et al. 2002c):

- Perspective taking, for example, "I try to understand what is going on in my patients mind by paying attention to their nonverbal cues and body language."
- Compassionate care, for example, "I try not to pay attention to my patients' emotions in history taking or in asking about their physical health."
- "Standing in the patient's shoes," for example, "Because people are different, it is difficult for me to see things from my patients' perspective."

All examples are taken from the HP-Version.

The factor structures of both the S- and HP-Version of the scale were stable when tested with medical students (Hojat et al. 2001b) and physicians (Hojat et al. 2002c). The stability of the factor structure across groups of medical students and practicing physicians provided support for the construct validity of both the S- and HP-Versions of the scale.

One approach to validation is to demonstrate high correlations between scores on the scale and conceptually relevant variables (convergent validity), accompanied by low correlations with irrelevant measures (discriminant validity; Campbell and Fiske 1959). When we correlated the JSPE scores with self-assessments of empathy on a 100-point scale, we found correlations of 0.37 and 0.45 for medical students and internal medicine residents, respectively (Hojat et al. 2001b). The convergent validity of the JSPE was also supported by statistically significant ($p \leq 0.05$) correlations between scores on the empathy scale and conceptually relevant measures, such as self-assessments of compassion (for residents, $r = 0.56$; for medical students, $r = 0.48$; Hojat et al. 2001b). Significant correlations were also observed between scores on the JSPE and the following subtest scores of the Davis Interpersonal Reactivity Index (Davis 1983): empathetic concern (for residents, $r = 0.40$; for medical students, $r = 0.41$), perspective taking (for residents, $r = 0.27$; for medical students,

$r = 0.29$), and fantasy (for residents, $r = 0.32$; for medical students, $r = 0.24$).

The moderate correlations with criterion measures in our studies suggest that empathy can be considered as a distinct personal attribute with limited overlap with compassion, concern, sympathy, perspective taking, imagination, warmth, dutifulness, tolerance, personal growth, trusting others, and communication (Hojat et al. 2001b). The discriminant validity of the JSPE was supported by a zero-order correlation between empathy and conceptually irrelevant measures such as self-protection ($r = 0.11$, nonsignificant; Hojat et al. 2001b).

Gender
We anticipated gender differences in empathy scores in the favor of women based on the presumption that women express more caring attitudes and are more receptive to emotions than are men. Recently, it has been proposed that female behavioral style is more "empathizing" than is that of men (Baron-Cohen 2003). We consistently observed in our studies that women scored higher than did men on the JSPE (Hojat et al. 2001b, 2002a). Female physicians scored higher than did male physicians not only on the total JSPE scores (Hojat et al. 2002c) but also on 17 items, of which six were statistically significant (Hojat et al. 2002b).

Academic Performance on Objective Written Examinations
There is no theoretical basis to link empathy with performance on knowledge tests. We examined the correlations between JSPE scores and measures of academic performance based on multiple-choice examinations, including scores on the Medical College Admission Test (biological sciences, physical sciences, and verbal reasoning scales), first- and second-year medical school grade-point averages, and scores on steps 1 and 2 of the U.S. Medical Licensing Examinations. None of the correlations was statistically significant (Hojat et al. 2002a).

Ratings of Clinical Competence in Medical School
We hypothesized that medical students who obtained higher scores on the JSPE would also obtain higher clinical competence ratings in medical school (Hojat et al. 2002a). This hypothesis was based on the notion that interpersonal skills are among the factors that are often considered in the assessment of clinical competence (Hojat et

al. 1986, 1988). It follows that empathy, built upon interpersonal relationships, would have significant overlap with the assessment of global clinical competence.

The hypothesis was confirmed in our study by observing that high scorers on the JSPE were more likely to obtain "high honors" ratings of global clinical competence, and low scorers on the JSPE were more likely to obtain marginal clinical competence ratings in six core clerkships (family medicine, internal medicine, obstetrics and gynecology, pediatrics, psychiatry, and surgery) in the third year of medical school (Hojat et al. 2002a).

Changes in Empathy During Medical School and Residency
Despite the good intentions of teaching faculty in undergraduate and graduate medical education, there has been a decline in humanistic qualities and an unfortunate increase in cynicism observed during medical education (Bellini et al. 2002; Sheehan et al. 1990; Silver and Glicken 1990; Kay 1990). We have observed a consistent decline in the empathy scores on the JSPE for internal medicine residents at progressive levels of training, but the decline did not reach the conventional level of statistical significance (Mangione et al. 2002). In another study (Hojat et al. 2004), a statistically significant decline in empathy scores was found among third-year medical students during their clinical clerkships.

Specialty
Because interpersonal relationships are the foundation of physician empathy, we predicted that physicians in the "people-oriented" specialties would score higher on the JSPE than those in the "procedure-oriented" or "technology-oriented" specialties. In three studies we found significant differences on scores of the JSPE between physicians in the two groups of specialties. For example, physicians in the "people-oriented" specialties (e.g., family medicine, internal medicine, pediatrics, obstetrics and gynecology, psychiatry, and medical subspecialties) had higher JSPE scores than did their counterparts in "technology-oriented" specialties (e.g., anesthesiology, radiology, pathology, surgery and surgical specialties; Hojat et al. 2001a, 2002b, 2002c).

When we examined each individual item of the JSPE, we noticed that those in the "people-oriented" specialties scored consistently higher than did those in the "technology-oriented" specialties on every item of the scale, and the differences in scores for 11 items were statistically significant (Hojat et al. 2002b). In another study, we found that psychiatrists obtained the highest mean score on the JSPE, and this average was significantly higher than mean scores for physicians in anesthesiology, general surgery, neurosurgery, orthopedic surgery, and obstetrics and gynecology. However, the psychiatrists' means were no different from those physicians in emergency medicine, family medicine, internal medicine, and pediatrics (Hojat et al. 2002c). It should be noted that the potential confounding effects of different fractions of women in these specialties were controlled when these comparisons were tested statistically.

It is important to emphasize that the differences in the empathy scores observed across specialties do not necessarily imply some deficiency in empathy in the low-scoring groups. This is primarily for two reasons. First, none of the indicators of clinical significance and practical importance (effect size estimates) was large enough to warrant a serious low score that was out of the normal range. Second, we presume that the duties involved in the "technology-oriented" specialties may not always demand the high degree of empathy that is required in the "people-oriented" specialties. It seems plausible that understanding the inner experiences and emotions of patients is more demanding in primary care than in, for example, the hospital-based specialties of anesthesiology, pathology, and radiology (Hojat et al. 2002b).

Reliability
Estimates of internal consistency reliability were calculated using Cronbach's coefficient alpha using data from single administrations of the scale to a sample of students, nurses, or physicians. Estimates of test-retest reliability were computed using test-retest reliability coefficients based on product-moment correlations when two sets of scores were available from administrations to the same sample at different points in time. The values of coefficient alpha for the S-Version were 0.89 for medical students and 0.87 for internal medicine residents (Hojat et al. 2001b). The coefficient alpha for the HP-Version was 0.81 for physicians, 0.85 for nurse practitioners, and 0.87 for registered nurses (Hojat et al. 2001c; Hojat et al. 2003a; Fields et al. 2004). The test-retest reliability coefficient for residents was 0.65, which suggests that the empathy scores were stable over time (Hojat et al. 2002c). The results of the psychometric studies and descriptive statistics are summarized in Table 7-1.

Table 7-1   Descriptive Statistics and Reliability Coefficients of the Jefferson Scales Measuring Three Elements of Professionalism in Medicine

Scales	No. items	Mean	SD	Median	Range	Reliability	
						Alpha	Test–Retest
JSPE[a]	20	120	12	121	20–140	0.81	0.65
JSAPNC[b]	15	48	4.9	48	15–60	0.78	NA
JSPLL[c]	19	61	8.6	62	19–76	0.89	0.91

NA, not available; SD, standard deviation.
[a]The Jefferson Scale of Physician Empathy (JSPE) includes 20 Likert-type items, answered on a 7-point scale (1 = strongly disagree, 7 = strongly agree). Sample included 704 physicians. [b]The Jefferson Scale of Attitudes Toward Physician–Nurse Collaboration (JSAPNC) includes 15 Likert-type items answered on a 4-point scale (1 = strongly disagree, 4 = strongly agree). Sample included 118 physicians. [c]The Jefferson Scale of Physician Lifelong Learning (JSPLL) includes 19 Likert-type items answered on a 4-point scale (1 = strongly disagree, 4 = strongly agree). Sample included 444 physicians. Note: Copies of the latest versions of the three scales are available from the authors.

Concluding Remarks on Physician Empathy

Failure to understand a patient's perspective can lead to suboptimal patient–physician relationships and can contribute to a patient's willingness to litigate (Beckman et al. 1994). Furthermore, research suggests that patient dissatisfaction due to miscommunication can lead to charges of malpractice *regardless* of the quality of medical care the physician renders (Hickson et al. 1994). Medical malpractice attorneys have indicated that more than 80% of malpractice suits are based on unsatisfactory patient-physician relationships (Avery 1985). These findings raise an important question regarding physician empathy and patient outcomes that requires empirical scrutiny in future research. The JSPE supported by psychometric evidence can be a useful tool to address issues related to physician empathy in future empirical research.

Interprofessional Collaboration: The Jefferson Scale of Attitudes Toward Physician–Nurse Collaboration

Teamwork and relationships built on interprofessional collaboration also represent an essential element of professionalism. Research suggests that interdisciplinary health care teamwork reduces patient death rates (Knaus et al. 1986), improves clinical care and patient satisfaction, and contains costs (Baggs et al. 1992; Blegen et al. 1995;

Fagin 1992; Gibson et al. 1994; Cook 1998; Kosper et al. 1994; Rubenstein et al. 1984; Warner and Hutchinson 1999). The most recent report from the Institute of Medicine on medical errors identified failures in communication as a key factor in medical errors. A recent study in Sweden showed that positive relationships between physicians and nurses had a beneficial effect on the improvement of behavioral disturbances among a large number of nursing home residents (Schmidt and Svarstad 2002). Another study found that malpractice claims were lower for those surgeons who had a nurse practitioner working in their offices (Adamson et al. 1997).

Professionalism promotes a mutually respectful collaboration between physicians and nurses and helps to counter some of the negative effects of a market-driven health care system. Better understanding of the principles of professionalism thus can enhance the capacity of both nurses and physicians to provide optimal care (Afflito 1997; Simon et al. 1990).

Social role theory asserts that individuals learn about their professional roles through processes of socialization. According to this theory, factors such as attitudes, personal orientation, and expectations play key roles in the development of collaborative relationships between physicians and nurses (Meleis and Hassan 1980; Ornstein 1990). For example, it has been reported that these relationships tend to be hierarchical in societies where nurses have little autonomy and physicians dominate patient-care decisions (Austin et al. 1985; Champion et al. 1987; Meleis and Hassan 1980). In contrast, interprofessional relationships tend to be "complementary" in societies where physicians and nurses share power and where their roles and responsibilities are viewed as complementary.

The hierarchical model places more emphasis on factors such as the gender divisions of labor in society (Sweet and Norman 1995), professional elitism, and gender role stereotypes (Blickensderfer 1996; Fagin 1992; McMahan et al. 1994; Prescott and Bowen 1985; Sprague-McRae 1996). This model naturally places medicine above nursing in patient-care responsibilities (Shein 1972). Correspondingly, the complementary model places more emphasis on the importance of education, common experiences, shared autonomy, and mutual authority. Attitudes toward interprofessional collaboration are expected to be more positive in societies in which a complementary model is promoted in the formal education of health professionals. Professionalism promotes complementary as opposed to hierarchical interprofessional relationships.

Definition of Physician–Nurse Collaboration

Physician–nurse collaboration is defined as "nurses and physicians working together cooperatively, sharing responsibilities for solving problems and making decisions to formulate and carry out plans for patient care" (Baggs and Schmitt 1988, p. 145). Based on this definition, we developed a measurement tool for physician–nurse collaboration. Despite the importance of the physician–nurse collaborative relationship in patient care, empirical research on the topic has not received sufficient attention. This is partly due to the fact that a psychometrically sound research instrument applicable to both physicians and nurses has not been available.

Although reports have been published on the physician–nurse collaboration, most have been based on anecdotal reporting or responses to short questionnaires lacking psychometric analysis. One comprehensive study of the attitudes of doctors and nurses toward interprofessional issues expressed in group discussions was reported by Weiss (1983). A health-role index was developed by Weiss and Davies (1983). Also, a brief instrument (six items) was developed by Baggs (1994) for measuring physician–nurse collaboration on patient-care decisions, but it is a unidimensional tool that cannot address the multifaceted nature of the concept. Any tool for assessing orientation toward such a relationship should take into consideration the complex and multidimensional nature of the relationships.

In response to a need for measuring attitudes toward physician–nurses collaborative relationships, we developed the Jefferson Scale of Attitudes Toward Physician–Nurse Collaboration (Hojat and Herman 1985; Hojat et al. 1997, 1999). The scale was originally developed to measure attitudes toward nurses and nursing services (Hojat and Herman 1985).

Validity

Based on a review of the literature, 59 statements about attitudes toward nursing services in health care were drafted and distributed to six experienced medical education and health care researchers, who were asked to judge the content validity of each for relevance to the measurement of attitudes about nursing and interprofessional collaboration. Based on their comments, 38 items were retained and modified to incorporate their suggestions (for a more detailed description of this preliminary version, see Hojat and Herman 1985).

Subsequently, these items were distributed to 20 reviewers: 15 registered nurses and 5 physicians. They were asked to review and judge the appropriateness of each item for its applicability to physician–nurse relationships in the context of hospital care. They were also encouraged to include additional items relevant to measuring attitudes toward physician–nurse collaborative relationships. Based on their recommendations, 25 items were included in the next version, of which 20 were retained after a preliminary psychometric analysis (Hojat and Herman 1985). These items were further modified to focus on attitudes toward physician–nurse alliance in patient-care situations (Hojat et al. 1997).

Further modifications were made in a another study to address physician–nurse collaboration specifically in areas of authority, autonomy, responsibility for patient monitoring, decision making, and role expectations (Hojat et al. 1999), in which 15 items of the previous version were retained after additional psychometric analyses.

The items in the final version of the Jefferson Scale of Attitudes Toward Physician–Nurse Collaboration (15 items) are answered on a 4-point Likert-type scale from strongly agree to strongly disagree. A higher total score reflects a more positive attitude toward collaborative relationships.

Results of an exploratory factor analysis (using data from 208 medical and 86 nursing students) provided support for the construct validity of this research tool. The prominent underlying factors of the Jefferson Scale of Attitudes Toward Physician–Nurse Collaboration (Hojat et al. 1999) included the following:

- Shared education and team work (seven items), for example, "During their education, medical and nursing students should be involved in teamwork in order to understand their respective roles."
- Caring as opposed to curing (three items), for example, "Nurses are qualified to assess and respond to psychological aspects of patients' needs."
- Nurse autonomy (three items), for example, "Nurses should be involved in making policy decisions concerning the hospital support services on which their work depends."
- Physician dominance (two items), for example, "The primary function of the nurse is to carry out the physician's orders."

The criterion-related validity of the scale was examined by using contrasted groups. In one study, we predicted that, in the absence of any targeted interdisciplinary educational programs, nursing students would obtain significantly higher scores on the scale than would medical students. This prediction was supported and provided evidence for the validity of the scale (Hojat et al. 1997, 1999).

In a cross-cultural study (Hojat et al. 2003d) we studied 2,522 physicians and nurses from four countries, the United States (118 physicians and 84 nurses), Israel (156 physicians and 446 nurses), Italy (428 physicians and 859 nurses), and Mexico (148 physicians and 287 nurses), to test the "principle of least interest" hypothesis (Waller and Hill 1951). This notion was introduced in the context of family relationship and predicts that those in a greater power position are less likely to express a desire for a collaborative relationship. Based on this prediction, we hypothesized that, if the scale is valid, then we would expect physicians to obtain lower scores than nurses regardless of the social-cultural professional roles. Our hypothesis was confirmed, although the attitudinal gap between physicians and nurses varied in different cultures (Hojat et al. 2003d). Similar results were found in another study in which American and Mexican physicians and nurses were compared (Hojat et al. 2001c).

In addition, based on socialization role theory (Austin et al. 1985; Champion et al. 1987; Conway 1978; Hardy and Conway 1978; Meleis and Hassan 1980; Ornstein 1990), we predicted that nurses from countries in which the complementary model of professional roles is prevalent (United States and Israel) would express more positive attitudes toward physician-nurse collaboration than would their Italian and Mexican counterparts, where a hierarchical model of professional roles is more common (Hojat et al. 2003d). The prediction was confirmed.

Reliability

We estimated the scale's internal consistency reliability by calculating the coefficient alpha for physicians and nurses in four diverse countries. The values of alpha were 0.76 for Italian physicians, 0.78 for American and Israeli physicians, and 0.86 for Mexican physicians (Hojat et al. 2003d). The values of alpha for this scale for medical and nursing students were 0.84 and 0.85, respectively (Hojat et al. 1999).

Concluding Remarks on Physician-Nurse Collaboration

A summary of results of psychometric studies and descriptive statistics is reported in table 7-1. The Jefferson Scale of Attitudes Toward

Physician–Nurse Collaboration can be used not only as an indicator of professionalism in medicine but also for the assessment of educational programs intended to promote a positive orientation toward physician–nurse collaboration (Hojat and Herman 1985), for the study of individual differences (Hojat et al. 1997, 1999), and for cross-cultural comparisons (Hojat et al. 2001c, 2003d).

Physician Lifelong Learning: The Jefferson Scale of Physician Lifelong Learning

Because of its relevance to patient care, lifelong learning is considered to be another important element of professionalism in medicine. Medical education is a learning process that begins in medical school, extends into graduate medical education, and continues throughout physicians' professional lives (AAMC 1999). The importance of preparing medical students to become lifelong learners has been evident in each of the three reports of the AAMC's Medical School Objectives Project (MSOP). In the practice of medicine, a commitment to rigorous learning throughout professional life has been described as an important element of "professionalism" (Nelson 1998).

Definition of Lifelong Learning

Despite the emphasis placed on physicians' lifelong learning, no universally accepted definition of the term has been recognized. Various terms such as self-directed learning, self-educative approach, self-initiative learning, active learning, independent learning, contextual learning, continuing education, and distance learning have been included in one terminological basket under the rubric of lifelong learning. Although these terms may share some common features, it would be difficult to measure lifelong learning without identifying its unique features (Miflin et al. 1999). According to some researchers, the key features of lifelong learning include personal motivation, recognition of needs that prompts an active search for knowledge, and information-seeking skills (Bligh 1993; Knowles 1975). Candy (1991) indicated that lifelong learning education equips people with competencies and skills to continue their self-education beyond the completion of their formal schooling.

Lifelong learning is a complex concept as reflected in the following definition:

Lifelong learning is the development of human potential through a continuously supportive process which stimulates and empowers individuals to acquire all the knowledge, values, skills and understanding they will require throughout their lifetimes with confidence, creativity and enjoyment in all roles, circumstances and environments. (Aspin et al. 2001, p. 592; also see Longworth and Davies 1996)

This definition could be considered broad. It is difficult to develop an operational measure embracing all the concepts described in this definition (e.g., human potential, continuously supportive process, stimulating, empowering, knowledge, values, skills, understanding, confidence, creativity, and enjoyment). For the purpose of our study, based on the reading of the literature and panel discussions in our pilot studies, we defined lifelong learning as a concept involving a set of *self-initiated activities* (behavioral aspect) and *information-seeking skills* (capabilities) that are activated in individuals with a sustained *motivation* (predisposition) to learn and the ability to recognize their own *learning needs* (cognitive aspect). The four key terms in this definition that are frequently described in the lifelong learning literature are printed in italics to underscore their significance in the construct of physician lifelong learning.

Despite the importance of lifelong learning in the profile of professionalism in medicine, no psychometrically sound tool has been developed to provide an operational measure of the concept and its empirically derived components among physicians. However, Guglielmino developed a Self-Directed Learning Readiness Scale (SDLRS; Guglielmino 1977) that contains 58 Likert-type items (e.g., "I love to learn."). A short version of the SDLRS (S-SDLRS) that includes only 28 items of the original scale was prepared by Bligh (1993). Another scale to identify predictors of self-directed learning was developed by Oddi (1986), but subsequent validity studies did not produce consistent supportive results (Six 1989; Oddi 1990). There was a need for a physician lifelong measuring tool with convincing psychometric support. The Jefferson Scale of Physician Lifelong Learning was developed in response to that need.

Validity
The first draft was developed based on a review of the literature and on two pilot studies by using the rational scale methodology (Reiter-Palmon and Connelly 2000) and a variation of the Delphi technique

(Cyphert and Gant 1970). In an early stage of development, 12 Jefferson Medical College faculty, members of the dean's medical education research team and involved in medical education research, met several times to draft a definition of lifelong learning and its associated features based on their review and discussion of relevant literature. Each was asked to draft statements to describe features of lifelong learning consistent with their reading of the literature. Forty statements were submitted by using the rational scale method of theory-based item selection (Reiter-Palmon and Connelly 2000).

Over three iterations, the faculty members were asked to judge the content validity of the items based on the definition of physician lifelong learning. They were also asked to make appropriate modifications, additions, or deletions to the items. After incorporating their suggestions, the first version of the instrument was developed. It consisted of 40 Likert-type items comprising a 4-point scale from 1, strongly disagree to 4, strongly agree.

In the next step, using an abbreviated Delphi technique (Cyphert and Gant 1970), faculty were asked to independently review the 40-item questionnaire. These faculty members were chosen from different departments and were known to the investigators for their involvement in medical education research. They were asked to judge if those items cover representative domains of behaviors or attitudes relevant to physician lifelong learning. In addition, they were asked to respond to each item and specify the relevance, clarity, and importance of each one in measuring lifelong learning among physicians.

Based on the respondents' feedback, we revised the questionnaire, including 37 items used in a pilot study with 160 physicians (Hojat et al. 2003e). After preliminary psychometric analyses in this pilot study, 19 items were retained in the final version of the Jefferson Scale of Physician Lifelong Learning (Hojat et al. 2003e). The higher the score on this scale, the greater the orientation toward lifelong learning. In a one-year study begun in 2003 with partial support from the National Board of Medical Examiners Edward J. Stemmler Medical Education Research Fund, the final 19-item scale was completed by 444 physicians (28% women). Exploratory factor analysis to examine the underlying components of the scale yielded four meaningful factors. The first was entitled "Professional Learning Beliefs and Motivation." The item with the highest coefficient on this factor was: "Rapid changes in medical science require constant updating on knowledge and development of new professional skills."

The second factor was a construct involving "Scholarly Activities." The item with the highest coefficient was: "I actively conduct research as a principle investigator or co-investigator." The third factor was entitled "Attention to Learning Opportunities." The item with the highest factor coefficient was: "I routinely attend grand rounds offered in my field regardless of whether a certificate for attendance is offered." Finally, the fourth factor was labeled "Technical Skills in Information Seeking." The item with the highest factor coefficient was: "My preferred approach in finding an answer to a question is to research the appropriate computer data bases."

These factors are conceptually relevant to the notion of lifelong learning and its unique features described by others (Bligh 1993; Candy 1991; Jennet and Swanson 1994; Knowles 1975; Nelson 1998). They are also consistent with the competencies and attributes of self-directed learning such as skills for information retrieval, motivation, and self-initiation (attention to learning opportunities, scholarly activities; described by Candy 1991) and identification of learning needs (e.g., professional learning beliefs and motivation; described by Jennet and Swanson 1994). These findings are consistent with the features of lifelong learning described in the literature and provide support for the construct validity of the scale.

We examined the criterion-related validity of the scale by correlating the physicians' scores with four criterion measures such as:

- Research activities (four items), for example, "I consider myself a researcher as well as a clinician."
- Need recognition and intrinsic motivation (four items), for example, "I can easily recognize what I need to learn with regard to the rapid advances in medicine."
- Computer skills (three items), for example, "I believe that the skill to surf websites to find out what's going on in medicine is important for all physicians in order to catch up with news and advances."
- Extrinsic motivation (two items), for example, "I am not interested in learning new things for the sake of learning, unless there is a need for it."

Correlational analyses showed that each factor of the physician lifelong learning scale yielded the highest correlation with a criterion measure that was conceptually more relevant to that factor. For example, factor scores of the "scholarly activities" of the scale yielded a higher correlation with the criterion measure of "research activities" ($r = 0.78$) than with any other criterion measure (e.g., the next highest correlation of this factor of the scale was with the criterion measure of "computer skills," $r = 0.42$). As expected, correlation between factor scores of "technical skills in information seeking" of the scale ($r = 0.57$) was higher than those for any other criterion measure (e.g., the next highest correlation of this factor was with the criterion measure of "research activities," $r = 0.37$).

The correlation of the total score on the physician lifelong learning scale with the four above-mentioned criterion measures ranged from a high of $r = 0.69$ (research activities) to a low of $r = 0.15$ (extrinsic motivation). The correlations between the total scale scores and the following global indicator of self-reported lifelong learning was $r = 0.53$: "On a scale from 1 (not committed to lifelong learning) to 10 (a tireless advocate of lifelong learning), you give yourself a rating of . . ."

Furthermore, examination of the mean scores of the lifelong learning scale in contrasted groups showed that physicians who published papers, presented research findings at professional meetings, or collaborated in the conduct of research obtained significantly higher mean scores on the Jefferson Scale of Physician Lifelong Learning than did those who were not involved in these types of activities. These findings were consistent with our expectations about lifelong learning activities and provided further evidence in support of the validity of the scale.

Reliability
The valued coefficient alphafor the pilot study for the entire scale (19 items) was 0.93 (Hojat et al. 2003e). In our 2003 study with 444 physicians, we found an alpha value of 0.89, and a test–retest reliability of 0.91 (~3 month interval between testing, $n = 71$ physicians with a second score on the scale). Reliability estimates of this magnitude are in the acceptable range for educational and psychological scales and therefore provide support for the internal consistency reliability and score stability of the Jefferson Scale of Physician Lifelong Learning.

Concluding Remarks on Lifelong Learning
Lifelong learning has become one of the most frequently discussed concept in professional education and is based on the notion that every professional person should be actively encouraged, motivated,

and able to learn throughout his or her professional life (McKenzie 2001). In our studies of physician lifelong learning, we attempted to conceptualize the multidimensional and complex notion of lifelong learning and develop an instrument to measure it specifically among physicians. To the best of our knowledge, this is the first instrument with supporting psychometric evidence designed to measure lifelong learning in physicians. The results of our studies, as summarized in table 7-1, suggest that it is feasible to assess lifelong learning among physicians as an element of the profile of professionalism in medicine.

Professionalism: A Systems-Theoretic Approach

Systems theory (Ackoff and Emery 1981) provides a framework that can be used to describe the multidimensional structure of complex entities such as medical professionalism. Professionalism in medicine can be viewed as a system with behavior outputs that can be measured by a set of psychometrically sound, relevant tools. The elements within the system must be identified to better understand the system and ultimately to assess the degree of professionalism for each individual physician. More than four decades ago, Allport (1960) suggested that human personality and its behavioral manifestations be viewed as a system, that is, as consisting of dynamic, interacting elements. The combined function of interacting elements generates a totality, or *gestalt* (Lilienfeld 1978), where the whole is greater than the sum of its parts. Such a system is fully functional only when there is harmony among all of its elements. Otherwise, the system becomes dysfunctional and the targeted outcome will not be produced.

The implication of systems theory is that a complete understanding of any total system requires an understanding of each of its elements. For example, in the context of family therapy, it has been proposed that if the family is viewed as a system, then an effective therapeutic intervention requires a complete understanding of all of the family's functions and the participation of all of its members in the therapeutic process (Bateson 1971).

One approach in applying systems theory to measuring professionalism is to identify the universe of elements of professionalism that should be included in the system based on the consensus of experts. Many attributes of physicians have been recommended for inclusion as elements of professionalism. These include altruism, attitudes, compassion, empathy, ethics, humanism, integrity, lifelong learning, noncognitive attributes, patient–physician relationships, personality, respect for others, and relationships with other members of the health care team (Arnold 2002). However, significant resources would be needed to develop an exhaustive set and achieve a consensus. Therefore, the approach that we have taken is to address each element one step at a time rather than to wait for a consensus on the complete set of elements that define professionalism.

Once a particular element of professionalism has been chosen for study, the initial step for development of a tool is to identify a representative sample of behaviors that can be measured by using an established methodology (e.g., self-reports, supervisor ratings, peer ratings, standardized patient check lists). For example, empathy, teamwork, and lifelong learning are the elements of professionalism that we address in this chapter. It is desirable to develop national norms for these scales in order to display an individual's multiscore profile of professionalism relative to a national group. It is also important to identify additional elements of professionalism in medicine and to develop tools for measuring them for inclusion in the profile of professionalism.

In closing, we mention some opportunities for medical schools and residency programs to use the three scales described in this chapter. These scales were designed to measure attitudes toward empathy, teamwork, and lifelong learning rather than individual behavior. Although some may view this as a limitation in that the scales fall short of measuring observable behavior, it is well documented that attitudes and preferences, sometimes referred to as the covert dimension of personality, play a key role in the generation of behavior, which is the overt component of personality (Fishbein and Ajzen 1975). Therefore, because attitudes exert significant influences on an individual's behavior, attitudes and behavior are by necessity related (Rosenberg and Hovland 1960). Evidence in support of the criterion-related validity of the scales, such as the relationship between lifelong learning scores and research productivity, suggests that a link exists between scores on the scales and behavioral manifestations of the attribute measured by the scale. Some readers may question the practical value of self-reports because it seems uncertain that individuals with deficiencies will provide truthful responses if they know that the data will be used for their own evaluation. However, self-reports produce valid measures of attitudes and are much more efficient than observational rating scales and other instruments that require the effort of trained independent observers. In addition, evidence in support of criterion-related, discriminant and convergent validity suggests that these self-repeat scales are valid measures of what they purport to measure and that social desirability does not distort the expected pattern of findings.

How can a clerkship coordinator or residency program director use these scales in the assessment of professionalism? The scales are well adapted for the measurement of groups of students or residents. For example, they could be used as baseline assessments at the beginning of a clerkship or in the first year of a residency program to gauge the relative standing of a peer group. The distribution of scores and array of responses to each item could be used as a basis for discussions with trainees in outlining the goals of clerkship or residency program. The instruments can also be used as an assessment tool at different levels of medical education to examine changes or to evaluate the effectiveness of targeted educational programs or remedies in pretest–posttest evaluation design.

In conclusion, professionalism in medicine is a complex system consisting of humanistic, accountability, and excellence subsystems, each containing elements that need to be operationally defined and empirically measured. This is a challenging agenda for future research on professionalism in medicine.

Acknowledgments

We wish to express our sincere appreciation to Caryl Johnston and Bethany Brooks who assisted with the preparation of the manuscript and who provided expert editorial assistance. Nevertheless, the authors assume full responsibility for its accuracy.

References

ABIM Evaluation of humanistic qualities in the internist: by subcommittee of evaluation of humanistic qualities in the internist of the American Board of Internal Medicine. Annals of Internal Medicine, 1983; 99: 720–724.

Ackoff RL, Emery PE. On Purposeful Systems. Seaside, CA: Intersystems, 1981.

Adamson TE, Baldwin DC Jr, Sheehan TJ, et al. Characteristics of surgeons with high and low malpractice claim rates. Western Journal of Medicine, 1997; 166: 37–44.

Afflito L. Managed care and its influence on physician-patient relationships: Implications for collaborative practice. Plastic Surgical Nursing, 1997; 17: 217–218.

Allport GW. The open system in personality theory. Journal of Abnormal and Social Psychology, 1960; 61: 301–310.

Anastasi A. Psychological Testing. New York: Macmillan, 1976.

Arnold EL, Blank LL, Race KEH, et al. Can professionalism be measured? The development of a scale for use in the medical environment. Academic Medicine, 1998; 73: 1119–1121.

Arnold L. Assessing professional behavior: yesterday, today and tomorrow. Academic Medicine, 2002; 77: 502–515.

Aspin D, Chapman J, Hatton, M, Sawano Y, eds. International Handbook of Lifelong Learning, 2001 (Parts 1 and 2). London: Kluwer Publishing.

AAMC. Contemporary issues in medicine—medical informatics and population health: report 2 of the Medical School Objectives Project. Academic Medicine, 1999; 74: 130–141.

Austin J, Champion V, Tzeng OCS. Cross-cultural comparison on nursing image. International Journal of Nursing Studies, 1985; 22: 231–239.

Avery JK. Lawyers tell what turns some patients litigious. Medical Malpractice Review, 1985; 2: 35–37.

Baggs JG, Ryan S, Phelps CE, Richardson JF, Johnson JE. The association between interdisciplinary collaboration and patient outcomes in a medical intensive care unit. Heart and Lung, 1992; 21: 18–24.

Baggs JG, Schmitt MH. Collaboration between nurses and physicians. Image: Journal of Nursing Scholarship, 1988; 20: 145–149.

Baggs JG. Development of an instrument to measure collaboration and satisfaction about care decisions. Journal of Advanced Nursing, 1994; 20: 176–182.

Baron-Cohen, S. The Essential Difference. New York: Basic Books, 2003.

Bateson G. A systems approach. International Journal of Psychiatry, 1971; 9: 242–244.

Beckman GB, Markakis KM, Suchman AL, et al. The doctor-patient relationship and malpractice: Lessons from plaintiff depositions. Archives of Internal Medicine, 1994; 154: 1365–1370.

Bellini LM, Baime M, Shea JA. Variations of mood and empathy during internship. Journal of the American Medical Association, 2002; 287: 3143–3146.

Bertakis KD, Roter D, Putman SM. The relationship of physician medical interview style to patient satisfaction. Journal of Family Practice, 1991; 32: 175–181.

Blegen MA, Reiter RC, Goode CJ, et al. Outcomes of hospital-based managed care: A multivariate analysis of cost and quality. Obstetrics and Gynecology, 1995; 86: 809–814.

Blickensderfer L. Nurses and physicians: creating a collaborative environment. Journal of Intravenous Nursing, 1996; 19: 127–131.

Bligh J. The S-SDLRS: A short questionnaire about self-directed learning. Postgraduate Education for General Practice, 1993; 4: 121–125.

Campbell DT, Fiske DW. Convergent and discriminant validation by the multitrait-multimethod matrix. Psychological Bulletin, 1959; 56: 81–105.

Candy PC. Self-Direction for Life-Long Learning: A Comprehensive Guide to Theory and Practice. San Francisco, CA: Jossey-Bass, 1991.

Champion V, Austin J, Tzeng OCS. Cross-cultural comparison of images of nurses and physicians. International Nursing Review, 1987; 34: 43–48.

Conway ME. Theoretical approaches to the study of roles. In Hardy and Conway, eds. Role Theory: Perspectives for Health Professionals (pp. 17–27). New York: Appleton-Century-Crofts, 1978.

Cook TH. The effectiveness of inpatient case management: fact or fiction? Journal of Nursing Administration, 1998; 28, 36–46.

Costa PT Jr, McCrea RR. Revised NEO Personality Inventory (NEO PI-R) and NEO Five-Factor Inventory (NEO-FFI): Professional Manual. Odessa, FL: Psychological Assessment Resources, 1992.

Cyphert FR, Gant WL. The Delphi technique: a tool for collecting opinions in teacher education. Journal of Teacher Education, 1970; 31: 417–425.

Davis MH. Measuring individual differences in empathy: Evidence for a multidimensional approach. Journal of Personality and Social Psychology, 1983; 44: 113–126.

DeMatteo MA. A social-psychological analysis of physician-patient rapport toward a science of the art of medicine. Journal of Social Issues, 1979; 35: 12–33.

Evans BJ, Stanley RO, Burrows GD. Measuring medical students' empathy skills. British Journal of Medical Psychology, 1993; 66: 121–133.

Fagin CM. Collaboration between nurses and physicians: no longer a choice. Academic Medicine, 1992; 67: 295–303.

Fields SK, Hojat M, Gonnella JS, Mangione S, Kane G. Comparisons of nurses and physicians on an operational measure of empathy. Evaluation & the Health Professions 2004; 27: 81–94.

Fishbein M and Ajzen I. Beliefs, Attitudes, Intention and Behavior: An Introduction to Theory and Research. Reading, MA: Addison-Wesley, 1975.

Gibson SJ, Martin SM, Johnson MB, et al. CNS directed case management: Cost and quality in harmony. Journal of Nursing Administration, 1994; 24: 45–51.

Guglielmino LM. Development of the Self-Directed Learning Readiness Scale. Doctoral dissertation, University of Minnesota, 1977. Dissertation Abstracts International, 38, 6467A.

Hardy ME, Conway ME, eds. Role Theory: Perspectives for Health Professionals. New York: Appleton-Century-Crofts, 1978.

Herman J. Reading for empathy. Medical Hypothesis, 2000; 54: 167–168.

Hickson GB, Clayton EW, Entman SS, et al. Obstetricians' prior malpractice experience and patients' satisfaction with care. Journal of the American Medical Association, 1994; 272: 1583–1587.

Hogan R. Development of an empathy scale. Journal of Consulting and Clinical Psychology, 1969; 33: 307–316.

Hojat M, Borenstein BD, Veloski JJ. Cognitive and non-cognitive factors in predicting the clinical performance of medical school graduates. Journal of Medical Education, 1988; 63: 323–325.

Hojat M, Fields SK, Veloski JJ, et al. Psychometric properties of an attitude scale measuring physician-nurse collaboration. Evaluation and the Health Professions, 1999; 22: 208–220.

Hojat M, Fields SK, Gonnella JS. Empathy: comparisons of nurse practitioners and physicians. Nurse Practitioner, 2003a; 28: 45–47.

Hojat M, Fields SK, Rattner SL, et al. Attitudes toward physician-nurse alliance: comparisons of medical and nursing students. Academic Medicine, 1997; 72(suppl): S1–S3.

Hojat M, Gonnella JS, Nasca TJ, et al. Physician empathy: definition, components, measurement, and relationship to gender and specialty. American Journal of Psychiatry, 2002c; 159: 1563–1569.

Hojat M, Gonnella JS, Erdmann B, Vogel V. Medical students' cognitive appraisal of stressful life events as related to personality, physical well-being, and academic performance: a longitudinal study. Personality and Individual Differences, 2003b; 35: 219–235.

Hojat M, Gonnella JS, Mangione S, et al. Empathy in medical students as related to academic performance, clinical competence, and gender. Medical Education, 2002a; 36: 522–527.

Hojat M, Gonnella JS, Mangione S, et al. Physician empathy in medical education and practice: experience with the Jefferson Scale of Physician Empathy. Seminars in Integrative Medicine, 2003c; 1: 25–41, at 178.

Hojat M, Gonnella JS, Nasca TJ, et al. Comparisons of American, Israeli, Italian and Mexican physicians and nurses on the total and factor scores of the Jefferson scale of attitudes toward physician-nurses collaborative relationships. International Journal of Nursing Studies, 2003d; 40: 427–435.

Hojat M, Gonnella JS, Nasca TJ, et al. The Jefferson Scale of Physician Empathy: further psychometric data and differences by gender and specialty at item level. Academic Medicine, 2002b; 77: S58–S60 (Suppl).

Hojat M, Gonnella JS, Xu G. Gender comparisons of young physicians' perceptions of their medical education, professional life, and practice: a follow-up study of Jefferson Medical College graduates. Academic Medicine, 1995; 70: 305–312.

Hojat M, Herman MW. Developing and instrument to measure attitudes toward nurses: preliminary psychometric findings. Psychological Reports, 1985; 56: 571–579.

Hojat M, Mangione S, Gonnella JS, et al. Empathy in medical education and patient care. Academic Medicine, 2001a; 76: 669–670, at 185.

Hojat M, Mangione S, Nasca TJ, et al. The Jefferson Scale of Physician Empathy: development and preliminary psychometric data. Educational and Psychological Measurement, 2001b; 61: 349–365.

Hojat M, Mangione S, Nasca TJ, et al. An empirical study of decline of empathy among third-year medical students. Medical Education 2004; 38: 934–941.

Hojat M, Nasca TJ, Gonnella JS, et al. An operational measure of physician lifelong learning: its development, components, and preliminary psychometric data. Medical Teacher, 2003e; 25: 433–437, at 198, 201.

Hojat M, Nasca TJ, Cohen MJM, et al. Attitudes toward physician-nurse collaboration: a cross-cultural study of male and females physicians and nurses in the United States and Mexico. Nursing Research, 2001c; 50: 123–128, at 194.

Hojat M, Veloski JJ, Borenstein BD. Components of clinical competence of physicians: an empirical approach. Educational and Psychological Measurement, 1986; 46: 761–769.

Hudson GR. Empathy and technology in the coronary care unit. Intensive and Critical Care Nursing, 1993; 9: 55–61.

Hunter KM, Charon R, Coulehan JL. The study of literature in medical education. Academic Medicine, 1995; 70: 787–794.

Jackson SW. The listening healer in the history of psychological healing. American Journal of Psychiatry, 1992; 149: 1623–1632.

Jennet PA, Swanson RW. Lifelong, self-directed learning: why physicians and educators should be interested. Journal of Continuing Education in Health Professions, 1994; 14: 69–74.

Kay J. Traumatic deidealization and future of medicine. Journal of the American Medical Association, 1990; 263: 572–573.

Knaus WA, Draper EA, Wagner DP et al. An evaluation of outcome from intensive care in major medical centers. Annals of Internal Medicine, 1986; 104: 410–418.

Knowles, M. Self-Directed Learning: A Guide for Learners and Teachers. New York: Association Press, 1975.

Kosper KG, Horn PB, Carpenter AD. Successful collaboration within an integrative practice model. Clinical Nurse Specialist, 1994; 8: 330–333.

Kunyk D, Olson JK. Clarification of conceptualizations of empathy. Journal of Advanced Nursing, 2001; 35: 317–325.

Levinson W. Physician-patient communication: a key to malpractice prevention. Journal of the American Medical Association, 1994; 273: 1619–1620.

Levy J. A note on empathy. New Ideas in Psychology, 1997; 15: 179–184.

Lilienfeld, R. The Rise of Systems Theory: An Ideological Analysis. New York: Wiley, 1978.

Longworth N, Davies WK. Lifelong Learning: New Visions, New Implications, New Roles for Industry, Government, Education and the Community in the 21st Century. London: Kogan Page, 1996.

Mangione S, Kane GC, Caruso JW, Gonnella JS, Nasca TJ, Hojat M. Assessment of empathy in different years of internal medicine training. Medical Teacher, 2002; 24: 371–374.

McKenzie P. How to make lifelong learning a reality: implications for the planning of educational provision in Australia. In Aspin D, Chapman J,

Hatton M, Sawano Y, eds. International Handbook of Lifelong Learning (pp. 367–378). London: Kluwer, 2001.

McLellan MF, Jones AH. Why literature and medicine? Lancet, 1996; 348: 109–111.

McMahan E, Hoffman K, McGee G. Physician-nurse relationships in clinical settings: a review and critique of the literature, 1966–1992. Medical Care Review, 1994; 51: 83–112.

Mehrabian A, Epstein, NA. A measure of emotional empathy. Journal of Personality, 1972; 40: 525–543.

Meleis AI, Hassan HS. Oil rich, nurse poor: the nursing crisis in the Persian Gulf. Nursing Outlook, 1980; 28: 238–243.

Miflin BM, Campbell CB, Price DA. A lesson from the introduction of a problem-based, graduate entry course: the effects of different views of self-direction. Medical Education, 1999; 33: 801–807.

Nelson AR. Medicine: business or professionalism, art or science? American Journal of Obstetrics and Gynecology, 1998; 174: 755–758.

Neuwirth ZE: Physician empathy: Should we care? Lancet, 1997; 350: 606.

Nightingale SD, Yarnold PR, Greenberg MS. Sympathy, empathy, and physician resource utilization. Journal of General Internal Medicine, 1991; 6: 420–423.

Oddi F. Construct validity of the Oddi continuing learning inventory. Adult Education Quarterly, 1990; 40: 139–145.

Oddi F. Development and validation of an instrument to identify self-directed continuing learners. Adult Education Quarterly, 1986; 36: 97–107.

Ornstein HJ. Collaborative practice between Ontario nurses and physicians: is it possible? Canadian Journal of Nursing Administration, 1990; 3: 10–14.

Osler W. Aequanimitas, With Other Addresses to Medical Students, Nurses, and Practitioners of Medicine. 3rd ed. Philadelphia: Blakiston, 1932.

Peabody FW. The care of the patient. Journal of the American Medical Association, 1984; 252: 813–818 (originally published JAMA, 1927; 88: 887–882).

Prescott PA, Bowen SA. Physician-nurse relationships. Annals of Internal Medicine, 1985; 103: 127–133.

Price V, Archbold J. What's it all about, empathy? Nursing Education Today, 1997; 17: 106–110.

Reiter-Palmon R, Connelly MS. Item selection counts: a comparison of empirical key and rational scale validities in theory-based and non-theory-based item pools. Journal of Applied Psychology, 2000; 85: 143–151.

Rosenberg MJ, Hovland CI. Cognitive, affective, and behavioral components of attitudes. In Hovland CI, Rosenberg MJ, eds. Attitude Organization and Change (pp. 1–14). New Haven, CT: Yale University Press, 1960.

Rubenstein LZ, Josephson KR, Weiland GD, English PA, Sayer JA, Kane R. Effectiveness of geriatric evaluation unit. New England Journal of Medicine, 1984; 311: 1664–1670.

Schmidt IK, Svarstad BL. Nurse-physician communication and quality of drug use in Swedish nursing homes. Social Science and Medicine, 2002; 54: 1767–1777.

Sheehan KH, Sheehan DV, White K, Leibowitz A, Baldwin DC Jr. A pilot study of medical student 'abuse': student perceptions of mistreatment and misconduct in medical school. Journal of the American Medical Association, 1990; 263: 533–537.

Shein, E. Professional Education. New York: McGraw-Hill, 1972.

Silver HK, Glicken AD. Medical student abuse: incidence, severity, and significance. Journal of the American Medical Association, 1990; 263: 527–532.

Simon SR, Pan RJD, Sullivan AM et al. Views of managed care: a survey of students, residents, faculty, deans at medical schools in the United States. New England Journal of Medicine, 1990; 340: 928–936.

Six, J. The generality of the underlying dimensions of the Oddi continuing learning inventory. Adult Education Quarterly, 1989; 40: 43–51.

Spiro HM, Curnen MGM, Peschel E, St. James D. Empathy and the Practice of Medicine: Beyond Pills and the Scalpel. New Haven, CT: Yale University Press, 1993.

Sprague-McRae JM. The advanced practice nurse and physician relationship: Considerations for practice. Advanced Practice Nursing Quarterly, 1996; 2: 33–40.

Stephan WG, Finlay KA. The role of empathy in improving inter-group relations. Journal of Social Issues, 1999; 55: 729–743.

Sutherland JA. The nature and evolution of phenomenological empathy in nursing: an historical treatment. Archives of Psychiatric Nursing, 1993; 7: 369–376.

Sweet SJ, Norman I. The nurse-physician relationship: a selective literature review. Journal of Advanced Nursing, 1995; 22: 165–170.

Thornton S, Thornton D. Facets of empathy. Personality and Individual Differences, 1995; 19: 765–767.

Waller W, Hill R. The Family: A Dynamic Interpretation. New York: Dryden, 1951.

Warner, PM, Hutchinson C. Heart failure management. Journal of Nursing Administration, 1999; 29: 28–37.

Weiss SJ. Role differentiation between nurses and physicians: implications for nursing. Nursing Research, 1983; 32: 133–139.

Weiss SJ, Davies HP. The health role expectation under measurement of alignment, disparity and change. Journal of Behavioral Medicine, 1983; 6: 63–76.

White KL. Healing the Schism: Epidemiology, Medicine, and the Public's Health. New York: Springer-Verlag, 1991.

Zinn W. The empathetic physicians. Archives of Internal Medicine, 1993; 153: 306–312.

8

Faculty Observations of Student Professional Behavior

John Norcini

Faculty observation of students' professional behavior can be designed to have many of the characteristics of an effective assessment as described in chapter 1. First, it can incorporate the judgments of multiple experts as they observe an individual's natural behavior across multiple situations in time. Second, the evaluation will be made in a realistic setting, and this is important given the context-dependent nature of medical practice. Third, this form of evaluation will include the conflicts that arise naturally in an educational setting. Finally, transparency can be assured by including and informing students of the assessment system's design, implementation, and feedback. In this chapter I address these characteristics by (1) describing approaches to collecting faculty judgments, (2) presenting the issues affecting faculty observation, (3) providing practical examples, and (4) outlining steps in administering a program of faculty evaluation.

Approaches to Collecting Faculty Judgments

Faculty members have been asked to make judgments about the professionalism of students in a variety of different ways, just as peers have (Norcini 2003). For purposes of this chapter, the approaches to collecting faculty judgments will be classified along two dimensions. The first dimension relates to the grounds on which they are being asked to make their assessment: performance in a single encounter or impressions of routine performance. The second dimension relates to the type of judgments the faculty members must make: occurrence, quality, or suitability.

Grounds for the Judgment

Single Encounter

In these forms of evaluation, the faculty members are asked to make a judgment about a single specific performance. The mini–Clinical Evaluation Exercise (mini-CEX) is an example of this form of assessment (Norcini et al. 2003). A faculty member observes a resident or student as he or she interacts with a patient in a brief clinical encounter. The faculty member then provides ratings, along a number of dimensions, of the student's performance with that patient. Typically, several different encounters are aggregated to generate an overall evaluation of a student, but the assessment is ultimately grounded in judgments about specific performances.

Judgments grounded in an evaluation of a single task have the advantage of focusing faculty on a particular performance and ensuring that the student has been observed. However, it has been repeatedly demonstrated that physician performance is task or case specific, meaning that performance on one case or task does not predict performance on another (Elstein et al. 1978). Consequently, to obtain reliable results, students' overall assessments must be based on several different tasks or encounters with patients.

Routine Performance

It is more common to ask faculty members to base their judgments on the impressions they have formed rather than on single encounters. Specifically, they are asked to consider a student's actions over a period of time and to ground their judgments in the student's routine performance. For example, Davis et al. (1986) developed a 14-item rating scale that was administered at the end of each clinical rotation in a general pediatrics training program. It assessed medical knowledge, interpersonal and professional relationships, and attitudes toward education. Similarly, Reisdorff et al. (2003) developed an 86-item global assessment form for emergency medicine residents. The form covered all aspects of competence, including professionalism, and it is appropriate for residents in all three years of training.

Judgments grounded in an assessment of routine performance have the advantage of being based on observations of a student across a number of different activities and this should accrue to their reliability. However, these judgments have often been rendered even if the evaluator has not directly observed the student engaged in the behavior being evaluated (Day et al. 1990). Moreover, they tend to be influenced by the faculty members' general impression of the student rather than his or her skill in the specific competence being assessed.

Types of Judgment

Faculty members have been asked to make judgments about whether particular behaviors have occurred, the quality of performances, or whether the performances are suitable for a particular purpose.

Occurrence

Faculty members have often been asked to report when they observe an occurrence of particular unprofessional behavior or critical incidents. For example, Papadakis et al. (1999) describe an evaluation system based on reporting instances of unprofessional behavior. Faculty use the Physicianship Evaluation Form to evaluate students who have engaged in inappropriate behavior and to specify the nature of their transgression (e.g., "The student misrepresents or falsifies actions and/or information").

Quality

Faculty members are more frequently asked to judge the quality of the students' performance. These judgments are often captured on a several-point rating form. For example, the attending rating form of the American Board of Internal Medicine (ABIM) captures ratings of professionalism on a 9-point scale ranging from "below expectations" to "exceeds expectations" (copies of the form can be found in ABIM 1994).

Key to the worth of these judgments is the number of faculty members engaged in the rating process. There is good evidence in the literature that faculty evaluators differ in stringency even when observing exactly the same performance (Noel et al. 1992). Therefore, evaluations from several faculty members are needed to produce reliable results. For example, Carline et al. (1992) report that reliable ratings of students' overall clinical skills require a minimum of seven faculty observations. More observations are needed for the interpersonal aspects of clinical performance, and these results were unaffected by rater experience and clerkship setting. Similar results were achieved by Kreiter et al. (1998).

Suitability

Faculty members are most often asked to make two judgments simultaneously: the quality of the performance and whether it was good enough for a particular purpose. For example, the professionalism ratings gathered on the mini-CEX evaluation form of the ABIM have the anchors "unsatisfactory," "satisfactory," and "superior" (Norcini et al. 2003). This requires faculty to both judge the quality of the performance and then decide whether it is better or worse than their standards for first year residents.

These simultaneous judgments are well suited to the academic environment, where decisions about advancement are needed. However, both judgments contain various errors and combining them makes an evaluator's judgments unclear. For example, a performance can be judged unsatisfactory when it was of reasonable quality but the evaluator had very high standards. Where it is practical to do so, separating the judgments will enhance both reliability and validity.

Issues Affecting Faculty Observations

Although faculty observation is an essential component of an assessment of professionalism, three issues influence the quality of the results, especially if the assessment is used for summative evaluation: role conflict, stakes, and equivalence.

Role Conflict

The nature of the relationship of faculty and students is complex. Faculty members are directly responsible for student learning on the one hand and assessment on the other. In the case of summative high stakes assessment for example, these two roles can be directly in conflict. To the extent that they are, the quality of both education and faculty observation will be adversely influenced.

There is no way to avoid this conflict, although there are at least two ways to lessen its effects. First, it is helpful where possible to use faculty observers who are not directly involved in the teaching of the students being assessed. This removes faculty from the position of assessing the outcomes of their own educational efforts, although they are now assessing the outcomes of their colleagues' work. Second, it may be helpful to maintain the anonymity of the faculty evaluators since it shields them to some degree from the interpersonal consequences of making adverse judgments.

Stakes

Although there is no definitive research on the influence of the stakes of an assessment on its quality, it is reasonable to assume that faculty observations could be affected by the use to which they will be put. Specifically, faculty may be less likely to provide adverse assessments when the consequences to the student are significant.

There is no way to completely avoid this issue, but again, it may help to ensure the anonymity of the evaluators. It may also be useful to limit faculty judgments to occurrences or the quality of a performance rather its suitability for a particular purpose. Judgments of suitability are necessarily of higher stakes, so setting standards may be better done at a distance from the judgments about quality or occurrence.

Equivalence

One of the assumptions inherent in the use of faculty observation is that the assessments of all students are equivalent. However, there are at least two threats to this assumption. First, the activities students undertake while they are being judged may not be the same and therefore not of the same complexity. This is almost certainly the case in the clinical setting where the patient problems vary naturally. Second, as previously mentioned faculty members differ in stringency so the assessment of the exact same performances by different faculty members may be different. Both of these issues lead to scores that may not comparable.

Again, there is no way to completely avoid these issues. Increasing the number of faculty members making judgments about the students across a broader range of activities, however, should lessen their effects. In addition, training and calibrating the faculty will have the effect of reducing some of the stringency differences among them.

Practical Examples

Evaluation Program

An evaluation program that keeps track of students or residents who have specific behavioral problems in the area of professionalism focuses on what students actually do in the context of training. A good example can be found in the assessment system developed and used at New Mexico School of Medicine (Phelan et al. 1993). The purpose of the system was to provide ongoing evaluation of professional traits that complemented the assessment of cognitive and clinical skills.

The school developed an evaluation form that allowed faculty to quantify their impressions of students who had difficulties. Seven traits were included in the evaluation: (1) reliability and responsibility, (2) maturity, (3) critique, (4) communication skills, (5) honesty and integrity, (6) respect for patients, and (7) shows signs of chemical dependency or mood disorder. Within each trait were three or more observable behaviors. For example, under maturity there was (1) behaves respectfully, (2) accepts blame for failure, (3) takes steps to correct shortcomings, and (4) is abusive and critical during times of stress. For each, faculty rated students on a 5-point scale from "acceptable" to "severe problem."

When a faculty member identified a student with deficiencies, he or she submitted a completed form to the assistant dean. To protect the student and institution, no action was taken unless a different faculty member submitted a second form expressing concerns about the student's behavior. After discussion among the assistant dean, chair of the student progress committee, and the student a remediation program was designed. If the remediation program was not completed satisfactorily, the institution's academic disciplinary procedure was applied and the student's problems were documented for the academic record.

During a 3-year period, 32 students (6%) received at least one report of unprofessional behavior. Of these, 22 students had only one report and no action was taken. The remaining 10 students had 2 to 14 reports with an average of more than 4. Of the 10, one student was ultimately dismissed, and the remainder graduated, although three did not make regular progress through the curriculum.

Mini-CEX

The mini-CEX is an example of a method that demonstrates whether students can behave in a professional manner. It is designed to assess the clinical skills of students and residents as they interact with real patients (Norcini 2003; Kogan et al. 2003). For each mini-CEX encounter, a faculty member observes the student or resident conduct a brief clinical encounter in an inpatient, outpatient, emergency department, or other setting. After asking the student for next steps, the faculty member completes a rating form that includes an assessment of professionalism.

The evaluation of humanistic qualities/professionalism is captured on a 9-point scale where 1–3 is unsatisfactory, 4 is marginal, 5–6 is satisfactory, and 7–9 is superior. Humanistic qualities/ professionalism are described as "shows respect, compassion, empathy, establishes trust; attends to patient's needs of comfort, modesty, confidentiality, information.

The mini-CEX has been applied experimentally to first-year residents in 21 internal medicine training programs (Norcini et al. 2003). The results indicated that the highest ratings among the clinical skills were given to professionalism and that these ratings increased over the year of training. Roughly four encounters were sufficient to generate reasonable confidence in the final results for all but residents who were marginal. The mini-CEX assessed residents in a broad range of clinical situations and offered the residents more opportunity for observation and feedback than they might have otherwise gotten. Similar results were achieved with medical students by Kogan et al. (2003).

Steps in Administration

There are at least five steps in administering a process for the assessment of professionalism: specifying the purpose, developing assessment criteria, training the faculty and informing the students, monitoring the program, and providing routine feedback.

Specify the Purpose

The first step in the administration process is to specify the purpose of the assessment in writing. For example, the purpose may be formative assessment (e.g., to give students feedback), summative assessment (e.g., to make a decision about students' professionalism), or program evaluation (e.g., whether a course in professionalism is effective). All decisions about content, construction, standards, and analysis flow from the purpose and its specification guides these decisions. In addition, it makes it more difficult for the assessment to take on an implicit purpose for which it is not designed.

The same assessment program often has more than one aim (e.g., to give students feedback and to assure that they are competent). When this occurs and it is feasible, it is best to develop a separate assessment procedure for each purpose. Faculty and students will approach an evaluation intended for feedback differently than, for example, one intended for grading purposes and the amount and nature of the data collected will differ. Using the same assessment device to fulfill both purposes will entail compromises that render neither ideal.

The purpose(s) should be communicated to all participants, along with the expectations of their performance as evaluators and as the objects of evaluation. This is particularly important for high stakes assessment since it will significantly impact the performance of students and faculty.

Develop Assessment Criteria

The second step in the process is the development of assessment criteria. Starting with a definition of professionalism, this includes specification of exactly what aspects of the domain will be assessed as part of the evaluation process, which students will be assessed, when they will be assessed, which faculty and how many need to be included in the process, what contributes to the quality of a performance, and what constitutes an acceptable standard if the purpose is to determine suitability.

From these criteria will flow the details of the assessment process. For instance, the method and nature of data collection will become apparent, as will the exact content to be addressed, the method for aggregating the results, the level of reporting, and the other pieces of the process.

Train the Faculty and Inform the Students

As discussed elsewhere in this book, there are a number of different definitions of professionalism, and intuitive understandings of the concept vary. Consequently, it is important to train faculty so that they have a shared understanding of what is being assessed and what standards of performance are being applied. This can be accomplished in any number of ways ranging from the provision of written material, to training workshops, to sessions in which the faculty are calibrated on the instruments being used.

Although training is important, it is not a substitute for ensuring that students are evaluated by more than one faculty member. Increasing the number of faculty brings different perspectives into the evaluation process and thus adds to its validity. It also has a larger impact on reducing errors of measurement than increasing the amount of faculty training. Where it is feasible, having assessments from three or four faculty members is often sufficient, with additional numbers not likely to make a sizable difference.

Just as faculty requires training, students need an understanding of what is expected of them. The validity of the assessments will hinge on whether they have been educated as to the definition of professionalism, the purpose of the assessment, and the criteria being employed. The assessment process should be made transparent to them and mechanisms for appeal should be provided.

Monitor the Program

Once underway, the results of the assessments should be monitored regularly. This should include feedback about the entire assessment process from faculty and students. Where appropriate, their input should lead to changes in data collection strategies and assessment devices, further training of faculty, and/or additional information and instruction for students.

Similarly, it will be important routinely analyze the psychometric aspects of the assessment process. Data may support or contradict the assertions of students and faculty or they could identify areas of concern independent of the input of the system's users. Included should be reliability, item analyses, and checks on the validity of the assessments.

Provide Routine Feedback

Feedback should be provided routinely to all participants. It would be most helpful if faculty received summary data on their evaluations, ideally comparing them (anonymously) with other evaluators to identify those who are too stringent or lenient. Provision of this information is usually sufficient to draw outliers to the middle. For those few faculty members who persist, more intense efforts may be needed.

Similarly, students should receive feedback over time concerning their performance. Specifically, it would be useful if they were apprised of the ratings and reports gathered throughout the process. Ideally, feedback to students would be given in a fashion that enables comparisons (anonymously) with peers and interactions with faculty. This is especially important for students who are having difficulties, since it offers them the opportunity to improve and guidance on how to do so.

Summary

Faculty observations about the professionalism of students can be classified along two dimensions. The first dimension relates to the grounds on which they are being asked to make their assessment: performance in a single encounter or impressions of routine performance. The second dimension relates to the type of judgments the faculty members must make: occurrence, quality, or suitability.

Three issues influence the quality of the results: role conflict, stakes, and equivalence. A critical incidents approach to assessing professionalism focuses on what students actually do. The mini-CEX is an example of a method designed to assess whether students know and can show how to demonstrate professional behavior.

The steps in administering a process for the assessment of professionalism are (1) specifying the purpose, (2) developing assessment criteria, (3) training the faculty and informing the students, (4) monitoring the program, and (5) providing routine feedback.

References

ABIM. Project Professionalism. Philadelphia: American Board of Internal Medicine, 1994.

Carline JD, Paauw DS, Thiede KW, Ramsey PG. Factors affecting the reliability of ratings of students' clinical skills in a medicine clerkship. J Gen Intern Med. 1992;7(5):506–510.

Davis JK, Inamdar S, Stone RK, Inter-rater agreement and predictive validity of faculty ratings of pediatric residents. J Med Educ. 1986;61:901–95.

Day SC, Grosso LG, Norcini JJ, Blank LL, Swanson DB, Horne MH. Residents' perceptions of evaluation procedures used by their training program. J Gen Intern Med. 1990;5:421–426.

Elstein AS, Shulman LS, Sprafka SA. Medical problem-solving: an analysis of clinical reasoning. Cambridge, MA: Harvard University Press, 1978.

Kogan JR, Bellini LM, Shea JA. Feasibility, reliability, and validity of the mini-clinical evaluation exercise (mCEX) in a medicine core clerkship. Acad Med. 2003;78(10 suppl):S33–S35.

Kreiter CD, Ferguson K, Lee WC, Brennan RL, Densen P. A generalizability study of a new standardized rating form used to evaluate students' clinical clerkship performances. Acad Med. 1998;73(12):1294–1298.

Noel GL, Herbers JE, Caplow MP, Cooper GS, Pangaro LN, Harvey J. How well do internal medicine faculty members evaluate the clinical skills of residents? Ann Intern Med. 1992;117:757–765.

Norcini JJ. Peer assessment of competence. Med Educ. 2003;37:539–543.

Norcini JJ, Blank LL, Duffy FD, Fortna G. The mini-CEX: a method for assessing clinical skills. Ann Intern Med. 2003;138:476–481.

Papadakis MA, Osborn EH, Cooke M, Healy K. A strategy for the detection and evaluation of unprofessional behavior in medical students. Acad Med. 1999;74:980–990.

Phelan S, Obenshain SS, Galey WR. Evaluation of the noncognitive professional traits of medical students. Acad Med. 1993;68:799–803.

Reisdorff EJ, Hayes OW, Reynolds B, Wilkinson KC, Overton DT, Wagner MJ, et al. General competencies are intrinsic to emergency medicine training: a multicenter study. Acad Emerg Med. 2003;10(10):1049–1053.

9

Using Critical Incident Reports and Longitudinal Observations to Assess Professionalism

Maxine Papadakis and Helen Loeser

This chapter completes the transition from measures of professionalism that are completed by the individual being evaluated through
observers outside of the clinical context, to observations of individuals in the daily environments of medical practice. Evaluations in
context naturally have greater face validity, because there is no need
to extrapolate performance in an artificial setting to the real context
of care. Using the analogy from George Miller's pyramid of assessment presented in chapter 2 (see figure 2-2), this chapter begins to
describe observations of what a student "does" rather than "knows,
knows how, or shows how."

Evaluations in context either can be one-time snapshots (critical incidents) of performance or can require faculty to reflect on student behaviors over a longer period (1 month or more) of performance. Individual faculty members often have such close and
lengthy attachments to students that such longitudinal assessments
can be made (see chapter 8). More often in today's hectic clinical
environment, faculty have only brief attachments to students, and
therefore are more likely to provide snapshots of student perform-

ance. One-time critical incidents can provide very detailed descriptions of specific sentinel events—particularly useful for students at the extremes of performance. While some systems of assessment described in this book allow for comparison among all students, the critical incident system is particularly directed to the extreme outliers of behavior—students with whom educational leaders spend an inordinate amount of time.

The technique of assessing critical incidents as a retrospective evaluation of actual events, focusing on purpose and consequence of behaviors, was introduced by Flanagan (1954). This technique was subsequently applied in developing the National Board of Medical Examiners' definition of step III clinical competencies and level of performance (Hubbard et al. 1965). More recently, it has been used as a curricular tool with which students can process important and challenging experiential learning at the interface of empathy and acculturation (Branch et al. 1993). It has been used to promote professionalism, triggering transformative learning through reflection on behaviors, particularly underlying reasons and assumptions (Lichstein and Young 1996); and to study factors underlying changes in clinical behavior and practice (Allery et al. 1997; Baernstein and Fryer-Edwards 2003). Thus, a critical incident system appears useful to evaluate professionalism. It affords assessment of individual, observed events in context, and allows detailed description, effectively "lowering the radar" for professional behaviors. This is particularly important since students can have multiple observers for variable periods of times, evaluators can feel uncertain about the veracity of their observations or fear retribution, students experience different stressors and cultures as they rotate through various specialties, and individual clerkships may not take ownership of the professionalism competency realm.

A critical incident system also allows for the possibility that single events do not necessarily define professionalism, which is consistent with our definition and understanding of professionalism as a set of behaviors rather than a dichotomous dimension—and one in which every professional has a range of behaviors, including lapses. Furthermore, because the critical incident technique allows individual behaviors to be observed, it does not necessarily engender the often mistaken generalization from professional behaviors to "professional character."

Ultimately, the ability of medical faculty to promote professionalism relies on the ability to collect specific information on student performance over time. The fact that many medical schools are incorporating more small-group experiences, collaborative learning projects, and community-based experiences provides new opportunities to observe professional development. Faculty observations in these setting are particularly compelling because the behavior of problematic students is more obvious in group settings. The identification of these issues early in a student's medical career allows more time to incorporate feedback into their professional development. Longitudinal tracking of critical incidents is also an excellent means through which to monitor the effectiveness of remediation strategies.

The University of New Mexico pioneered a critical incident system that assesses students' professional traits of responsibility, reliability, maturity, self-assessment, communication, honesty, integrity, and respect for patients and peers in order to identify students who have problems in these areas (Phelan et al. 1993). This system allows for reporting of problematic behavior longitudinally while protecting both the student and the evaluator. Candid documentation of even a single incident is possible with a measured response so that a single occurrence is not "blown out of proportion." Individual faculty members complete a form that describes the student's negative behavior, and the form is submitted to the dean's office. If a student receives at least two forms from different individuals, a meeting occurs between the chair of the student progress committee and the assistant dean. The meeting and the remediation strategy that is developed are documented. If the student fails the remediation program, the school's standard academic disciplinary procedure is implemented and documentation is placed in the student's academic record. Most of these reports have been generated by basic science faculty in the first 2 years of medical school (Phelan et al. 1993).

The University of California at San Francisco Physicianship Evaluation System

Our critical incident method of assessing professionalism began in 1995, when the School of Medicine at the University of California at San Francisco (UCSF) adopted a physicianship evaluation system that monitors students' critical incident reports longitudinally and has academic consequences for patterns of unprofessional behavior (Papadakis et al. 1999, 2001). The standard physicianship evaluation criteria are ability to meet professional responsibilities, ability to improve and adapt, and ability to establish adequate relationships with faculty and administrative personnel.

Remediation is central to this process and the flow of information is key. Our system takes advantage of the separation between the offices of curricular and student affairs. Notably, students' academic performance records are maintained in the office of curricular affairs, which also generates their medical student performance evaluation (MSPE—formerly known as the "dean's letter"). This separation of offices provides two levels of reporting for faculty and therefore creates a system with a graded level of response to professionalism issues. Critical incidents are initially managed by the office of student affairs, allowing faculty to report even minor professionalism incidents without concern that these events will necessarily lead to dismissal. Multiple incidents over time trigger a more formal response that may include notification of the office of curricular affairs. This separation thus allows for faculty to have a lower threshold for the reporting of professionalism issues. The process is described below.

Faculty Reporting System

A faculty member who has concerns about a student's professional behavior during a course or clinical rotation reports that behavior to the course or clerkship director. This individual makes inquiries about the student's behavior. Such inquiries usually include direct communication with a preceptor, small-group leader, or lecturer. If the course or clerkship director is convinced that the student has deficiencies in professional development, this individual meets with the student to provide feedback and review the contents of the UCSF Physicianship Evaluation Form (figure 9-1). The Physicianship Evaluation Form provides cues for faculty members to identify the specific area of professional behavior of concern, invites open-ended descriptions, and ensures that the faculty and student have discussed the issue and initiated a plan or remediation. The student is asked to sign the form, acknowledging the opportunity to discuss its contents with the course or clerkship director. The form also includes a section for the student to include optional comments. The student may provide information that refutes the Physicianship Evaluation Form, and the course director may choose to retract the form. More often, the form is submitted to the associate dean for student affairs. The deadline for such a submission is 8 weeks into the student's next course or rotation.

Student Name _____   Course _____

Course Director _____   Course Director Signature _____

Date this form was discussed with the student _____

The student has exhibited one or more of the following behaviors that need improvement to meet expected standards of physicianship:

This student needs further education or assistance with the following: (circle)

1. **Reliability and responsibility**
   a. Learning how to complete assigned tasks (1st–2nd year)
   b. The student misrepresents or falsifies actions and/or information (3rd–4th year)
   c. The student does not complete essential responsibilities by the prescribed deadline (institutional)

2. **Self-improvement and adaptability**
   a. Accepting constructive feedback (1st–2nd year)
   b. The student demonstrates arrogance (3rd–4th year)
   c. The student is abusive or critical in times of stress (institutional)

3. **Relationships with students, faculty, staff, and patients**
   a. Relating well to fellow students in a learning environment (1st–2nd year)
   b. The student inadequately establishes rapport with patients or families (3rd–4th year)
   c. The student does not respect professional boundaries in interactions with administrative faculty or staff (institutional)

4. **Upholding the Medical Student Statement of Principles (1st–2nd year only)**

5. **Diminished relationships with members of the health care team (3rd–4th year)**

6. **Please comment on the appropriate plan of action to pursue when counseling this student:**

_____

_____

This section is to be completed by the student:
I have read this evaluation and discussed it with my course/clerkship director.

Student signature _____   Date _____

My comments are:

_____

Figure 9-1   USCF Physicianship Evaluation Form (Sampled from Preclinical, Clinical, and Institutional forms). Complete forms available from UCSF website: http://medschool.ucsf.edu/professional_development/professionalism/index.aspx

The UCSF Associate Dean for Student Affairs is informed that a physicianship form has been filed by the clerkship or course director. The student may discuss the evaluation with the associate dean, ask for additional review of the physicianship form by his/her advisor, or request a review by the Student Welfare Committee, an ad hoc committee of students and faculty appointed by the faculty council. In all cases, if the evaluation is found invalid, the issue will be dropped and the evaluation amended. In the clinical years, students may also be given a nonpassing grade in the clerkship for failing to demonstrate appropriate personal and professional attributes required for a physician.

In most cases, the associate dean meets with the student to identify the problematic issues, to counsel, and to attempt remediation. She facilitates referrals to appropriate substance abuse and psychiatric counseling, where appropriate. At the quarterly academic screening (promotions) committee meetings, course and clerkship directors are asked about the student's progress in professional growth. Course or clerkship directors are notified of the student's educational needs so that the most appropriate preceptor or clerkship site can be chosen to help that student. The faculty member in charge of a course or clerkship can submit only one Physicianship Evaluation Form about a student. If a course is given throughout the academic year—for example, Foundations of Patient Care—a Physicianship Evaluation Form can be submitted once for each quarter that the course is offered.

In order to enhance early recognition and remediation of problematic behaviors, the academic consequences of receiving a Physicianship Evaluation Form in the first or second year of medical school differ from those in the third or fourth year. In the first 2 years, the Physicianship Evaluation Form is not made part of the student's official file.

In the clinical years, if a student receives one physicianship evaluation, it is not referred to in the MSPE. Reports of subsequent physicianship evaluations are mentioned in the MSPE, along with any teaching plans that were developed to assist the student. Students who receive two or more Physicianship Evaluation forms are placed on academic probation and can be referred to the Academic Standards Committee for review of the deficiencies. The Academic Standards Committee can recommend dismissal. Recommendations from the Academic Standards Committee are forwarded to the dean for final action. Dismissal appeals may be made to the faculty council, in accordance with School of Medicine policy.

In addition, if a student receives two or more Physicianship Evaluation Forms (from two or more courses) during the first 2 years, and receives a subsequent form in the third or fourth year from a clerkship or rotation, this indicates a persistent pattern of inappropriate behavior. The academic consequences are the same as if two clerkships had submitted Physicianship Evaluation Forms in the third and fourth years.

Institutional Reporting System

Students are expected to demonstrate adequate professional and personal attributes both within and outside the boundaries of a course or clerkship. If inadequate professional behaviors are noted outside of course work or clinical experiences, students may receive a Physicianship Evaluation Form from the central administration.

Examples of the behavior that would warrant an institutional physicianship evaluation include the following: a student falsifies financial information in order to procure student loans; a student does not respond in a reasonable manner to multiple communications from the Offices of Curricular or Student Affairs; a student does not meet the requirements that are in place to progress to clinical responsibility, including but not limited to receiving required immunizations, and scheduling and completing the U.S. Medical License Examination, steps 1 and 2, by the required dates.

Concerns are summarized and the form will be completed by the Associate Dean for Curricular or Student Affairs, rather than by course or clerkship directors. Therefore, this category of physicianship evaluation is called "institutional physicianship." The evaluation describes areas in which improvement in professional performance is needed and is parallel to and includes the standard physicianship evaluation criteria. The grievance process for the institutional physicianship evaluation is similar to the process used to grieve physicianship forms that are submitted by course and clerkship directors. The academic consequence of receiving an institutional physicianship evaluation is the same as receiving a physicianship evaluation from a course or clerkship director.

Description of UCSF's Experience

In addition to the routine longitudinal course and clerkship evaluation forms, in 1995 UCSF began its physicianship evaluation critical incident system. Through 2003, 75 Physicianship Evaluation Forms have been submitted on 59 third and fourth-year medical students (table 9-1). Twelve first and second-year students have received Physicianship Evaluation Forms since 1999, when the system was expanded to include them. These students represent less than one percent of the student body. Only one student received a Physicianship Evaluation Form during the first 2 years of medical school and then another during the last 2 years of medical school. However, this may be something of a distortion given the differing time frame in which physicianship evaluation forms have been used. In the first 2 years of medical school, all but one form was submitted from courses that taught clinical skills in small groups. The most common reason for submitting a form in the third and fourth years of medical school is unmet professional responsibility (75% of forms), followed by lack of effort toward self-improvement and adaptability (40%), and diminished relationship with members of the health care team (40%). Only 12% of students were critiqued as having diminished relationships with members of the health care team. (Students can be cited in multiple categories on the Physicianship Evaluation Form.) A typical scenario under the category of unmet professional responsibility is a student who is repeatedly late to morning rounds or has unexcused absences in preceptorship sessions. Most commonly, students who are critiqued for "lack of effort toward self-improvement and adaptability" were defensive in accepting criticism, unaware of inadequacies, resistant in making changes, and/or arrogant. Students who received the category of "diminished relation-

Table 9-1   Physicianship Evaluation Form Distribution in 59 Third- and Fourth-Year Students

Clerkship/Course	Number of Students	Male	Female
OB-GYN	21	13	8
Psychiatry	9	6	3
Pediatrics	5	2	3
Medicine	9	8	1
Senior medicine	4	2	2
Neurology	6	3	3
Surgery	1	1	0
Family medicine	7	3	4
Other	13	8	5
Total	75	46	29

ships with members of the heath care team" had difficulty fitting into a health care team setting, displayed rudeness, or challenged the hierarchical structure.

Of interest, Physicianship Evaluation Forms were not randomly distributed throughout clerkships. The core clerkship of obstetrics-gynecology submitted the most forms, while the core clerkship of surgery submitted the least number of forms. Yet these clerkships share many similarities. They are principally inpatient clerkships in a surgical field that take place in multiple sites; students are observed for prolonged intervals at their assigned site. The disparity in the number of forms submitted may center around "the culture" of each specialty, given that different environments and stressors bring out different behaviors in students and different priorities in their evaluators. The greater proportion of male students identified as displaying problematic behavior in obstetrics-gynecology is consistent with these theories.

In their meetings with the associate dean for student affairs, students consistently respond that this is the first time they are hearing about deficient behaviors and complain that they have not heard previously from the faculty about these concerns. They also concur that the issues identified are mainly appropriate but feel that the criticisms are out of proportion. Typically, they do not believe that their behaviors warrant a Physicianship Evaluation Form or the academic consequences that ensue but do accept the physicianship evaluation strategy and criteria as they apply to other medical students.

In contrast to the University of New Mexico's experience, we have had numerous forms submitted during third- and fourth-year rotations. In the past, we have been impressed that students who had not been identified in the first 2 years as having unprofessional behaviors were identified in the third and fourth years. However, with the opportunities for closer and more longitudinal observations by faculty that are afforded in our new curriculum, we believe this pattern may shift. These faculty also come from clinical departments and are more experienced in documenting less than satisfactory behaviors. There remain two options for documenting unsatisfactory behavior at our institution.

We strongly believe that students who have received more than one physicianship form have significant deficits in professional development (table 9-2). These students, when discussed in promotions committees, are well known to course directors, and these educators generally agree on their deficiencies. Without a physicianship eval-

Table 9-2   Outcome of 11 Students With Two or Three Physicianship Evaluation Forms in Third & Fourth Year

Mentioned in dean's letter	2
Notification of residency programs after the match	1
Withdrawal	1
Dismissal	2
Negotiated leave of absence	2
Other*	3

*Initially, no administrative action during policy development

uation system, our institution would have continued to promote and graduate these students. In addition, we believe that a disproportionate number of these students do not accept responsibility or "ownership" for the problems identified but, rather, believe that the evaluators are unfair or inaccurate. Students also relate that they have never received feedback about the behaviors identified; thus, the paper trail of previous physicianship reports helps to reinforce the persistent nature of their deficiencies. In two instances, the physicianship evaluation system has been particularly helpful in encouraging students to take a leave of absence for health reasons when they had initially not been inclined to do so. The ability to tell these students that they could be dismissed from medical school based on the multiple physicianship reports was a catalyst for them to take a medical leave of absence to address their mental health care needs or to take the time to assess the decision to become a physician in a mature fashion. If unprofessional behavior persists upon their return to medical school, they are likely to be dismissed.

Reliability and Validity of Critical Incident Reports

The most reliable observations are based on different evaluators simultaneously observing and evaluating the same behavior similarly. That seldom occurs in the real world of medical education. Also, studies have shown that physician performance varies from one patient to the next, so a reliable assessment requires information from multiple encounters (Norcini 2003). Ramsey et al. (1993) estimated that reliable peer assessment required 11 peers to assess performance in order to achieve a reliability coefficient of 0.70. Whether these data are applicable to the evaluation of professionalism in students is not clear. A more realistic model for valid observations of professionalism allows evaluators to observe similar behavior over time, which is built into the UCSF system. In addition, individual evaluators cannot submit a Physicianship Evaluation Form; rather, these forms can only be submitted by course or clerkship directors after they have investigated the veracity of the observations of unprofessional behavior. This process increases the validity of the observation. Nonetheless, the validity of the observations is not certain. Thus, a graded response has been built into the system; at least two Physicianship Evaluation Forms are needed if there will be punitive academic consequences.

To validate the UCSF physicianship evaluation system, we examined variables in medical school performance of UCSF medical students dating back to the 1940s that were associated with subsequent disciplinary action by a state medical board. The threshold was whether unprofessional comments in the students' files were of a level that the student would have generated a Physicianship Evaluation Form, had that system been in place. We also examined whether the more traditional variables of medical school performance, such as undergraduate grade-point average (GPA), Medical College Admission Test (MCAT) scores, ability to pass medical school courses on the first attempt and the U.S. Medical License Examination step 1 scores were associated with subsequent disciplinary action by a state medical board. We found no relationship between these students' professionalism skills and the more traditional academic realms of fund of knowledge or test taking. That is, students identified through physicianship forms are no more likely to have deficiencies in fund of knowledge or clinical skills than were other students. We found that students whose unprofessional behavior reached the threshold of a Physicianship Evaluation Form were more than twice as likely to be subsequently disciplined by a state medical board than were the other students (table 9-3; Papadakis et al. 2004). This finding adds

Table 9-3   Predictors of Disciplinary Action

Predictor	Odds Ratio	CI (95%)	P Value
Male sex	2.24	0.87–5.77	0.09
Undergraduate GPA	0.76	0.32–1.78	0.53
MCAT lowest quartile	0.75	0.34–1.65	0.47
Did not pass ≥1 medical school course	1.53	0.66–3.55	0.33
Professionalism severity ranking of Physicianship Evaluation Form	2.32	1.22–4.44	0.01

validity to UCSF's system of professionalism evaluation and, more important, adds validity to the conviction that the competency of professionalism must be mastered for a student to graduate from medical school. Unprofessional behavior in medical school is an early warning sign for subsequent unprofessional behavior by physicians. This finding highlights the need for far greater study of remediation strategies during medical school and their outcomes.

The Legal Context of Professionalism Assessment

According to our physicianship evaluation system, there is a graded response to the problems identified; two students have been dismissed principally because of the physicianship evaluation system, and another student most likely would have been dismissed but was allowed to withdraw from medical school. In David Irby and colleagues' important reviews of legal issues pertaining to dismissal, they clarify that dismissal proceedings from medical school can be either academic or disciplinary (Irby et al. 1981; Irby and Milam 1989).

Academic dismissals involve the professional evaluation of a student's academic or clinical performance. In *Horowitz* (1978), decided by the U.S. Supreme Court, factors other than grades were found to be sufficient grounds for an academic dismissal. "Personal hygiene and timeliness may be as important factors in a school's determination of whether a student will make a good medical doctor as the student's ability to take a case history or diagnosis an illness" (Irby and Milam 1989, 641; *Horowitz* 1978). Disciplinary dismissals include fact-finding about violations of the school's regulations or policies, and share similarities with criminal court proceedings. Academic dismissals are treated differently by the courts than disciplinary dismissals; the courts focus on the institution's professional academic judgment in academic dismissals and focus much less on due process issues. Disciplinary dismissals must adhere to stricter due process requirements and hearing procedures. The physicianship evaluation system and any dismissals that may result from that are treated as academic dismissals, since attainment of physicianship skills is one of the core competencies of the academic curriculum. The physicianship evaluation system provides for the legal issue of fair and equitable treatment, and our experience (and that of our legal counsel) is that the physicianship evaluation system amply meets the due process requirements for academic dismissals. Our physicianship evaluation system has been in place for 8 years, and grievances and hearings have taken place. This set of experiences provides institutional precedent that we can refer to when new students with problematic behavior are identified. Thus, students receive fair and equitable treatment based not only on policy but also on precedent.

Lastly, faculty may question whether documentation of unprofessional behavior can lead to a finding of defamation of character by the court. The court has found that negative evaluations are not defamatory (Irby and Milam 1989; *Kraft v. William Alanson* 1985). "The faculty members were protected by an absolute privilege because there was implied consent on the part of the student to have the evaluations used within the school, because the statements were relevant to the evaluation, and because publication of the results was limited to persons with a need to know" (Irby and Milam 1989, 642). The court stated that

> a person who seeks an academic credential and who is on notice that satisfactory performance is a prerequisite to his or her receipt of that credential consents to frank evaluation by those charged with the responsibility to supervise him. . . . Candid evaluations of student performance will be protected if they are good-faith exercises of professional judgment, not communicated to third persons outside the school, and not made with malicious intent. (Irby and Milam 1989, 642; *Kraft v. William Alanson* 1985)

There is also the recurrent vexing issue of clerkship or course directors receiving verbal information about unsatisfactory performance by a student from a faculty member who is unwilling to put that observation into writing. Irby and Milam (1989)

> encourage directors to write a file memorandum describing the faculty member's comments, and send a copy to the faculty member. This information is as valid for making academic decisions as are rating forms signed by the observing faculty member—because the decision is rooted in the professional judgement of the faculty and based upon the entire record. All relevant information counts and is helpful. (Irby and Milam 1989, 642)

Lessons Learned From the UCSF Experience

We continue to learn from this process and to refine our collective approach. One of the biggest challenges remains the timely collection of pertinent information at the course director level. This problem has improved since we have extended the deadline for submission of a Physicianship Evaluation Form to 8 weeks into the next course and have implemented an online evaluation system. We have also clarified with course directors that the submission of a Physicianship Evaluation Form can precede the completion of the course evaluation. Because we have many students in extended curricular plans, we recognize the importance of clarifying their status as medical students and our expectations of their behavior, whether they are actually enrolled or on leave and undertaking, for example, additional international experience, laboratory-based research, or participation in community program development.

Having firmly established physicianship evaluation at the student level, our next challenge is to advance this set of standards and consequences to residents and faculty. It is also the responsible next step to our students. For starters, we have inserted the following two items into every evaluation completed by students on individual residents and faculty teachers: (1) "I was treated with respect by this attending physician (or resident)", and (2) "I observed others (students, residents, staff, patients) being treated with respect by this attending physician (or resident)."

A Roadmap to Establishing a Critical Incident Reporting System

Institutions that wish to establish a similar evaluation system must take several critical steps. First, articulation that this is a core value of the school by the leadership is fundamental. Second, the process is likely to be more rapidly implemented if a sentinel event or an exemplar student propels consensus. Third, clarity from leadership about responsibility and ownership is key. Fourth, there must be broad course leadership and student involvement throughout this process. Finally, in addition to disseminating the criteria and guidelines for this evaluation system, key aspects of faculty development must address the following potential barriers: multiple sites with different educational cultures, multiple evaluators, late submission of evaluations, evaluators' reluctance to document negative performance, and evaluators' uncertainty regarding the validity of their subjective observations.

References

Allery LA, Owen PA, Robling MR. Why general practitioners and consultants change their clinical practice: a critical incident study. BMJ 1997; 314: 870.

Baernstein A, Fryer-Edwards K. Promoting reflection on professionalism: a comparison trial of educational interventions for medical students. Acad Med 2003; 78: 742–747.

Branch W, Pels RJ, Lawrence RS, Arky R. Becoming a doctor-critical incident reports from third-year medical students. N Engl J Med 1993; 329: 1130–1132.

Flanagan JC. The critical incident technique. Psychol Bull 1954; 51: 327–358.

Horowitz, 435 U.S. 78, 91 n.6 98. T. 948, 955–6 n.6, 1978.

Hubbard JP, Lefit EJ, Schumacher CF et al. An objective evaluation of clinical competence: new techniques used by the National Board of Medical Examiners. N Engl J Med 1965; 272: 1321–1328.

Irby DM, Fantel JI, Milam SD, Schwarz MR. Legal guidelines for evaluating and dismissing medical students. New Engl J Med 1981; 304: 180–184.

Irby DM, Milam S. The legal context for evaluating and dismissing medical students and residents. Acad Med 1989; 64: 639–643.

Kraft v. William Alanson White Psychiatric Foundation. 498 A.2d 1145–1149 (D.C. App.), 1985.

Lichstein PR, Young G. "My most meaningful patient." Reflective learning on a general medicine service. J Gen Intern Med 1996; 11: 406–409.

Norcini JJ. Peer assessment of competence. Med Educ 2003; 37: 539–543.

Papadakis MA, Hodgson CA, Tehranni A, Kohatsu ND. Unprofessional behavior in medical school is associated with subsequent disciplinary action by a state medical board. Acad Med 2004; 79: 244–249.

Papadakis MA, Loeser H, Healy, K. Early detection and evaluation of professional development problems in medical school. Acad Med 2001; 76: 1100–1106.

Papadakis MA, Osborn EH, Cooke M, Healy K, and the University of California, San Francisco School of Medicine Clinical Clerkships Operation Committee. A strategy for the detection and evaluation of unprofessional behavior in medical students. University of California, San Francisco School of Medicine Clinical Clerkships Operation Committee. Acad Med 1999; 74: 980–990.

Phelan S, Obenshain SS, Galey WR. Evaluation of the noncognitive professional traits of medical students. Acad Med 1993; 68: 799–803.

Ramsey PG, Wenrich MD, Carline JD, Inui TS, Larson EB, LoGerfo JP. Use of peer ratings to evaluate physician performance. JAMA 1993; 269: 1655–1660.

IO

Content and Context of Peer Assessment

Louise Arnold and David Stern

In the current climate of clinical medical education, medical teachers have less time to spend in direct contact with students and residents. Thus, opportunities for learners to demonstrate a wide variety of professional and unprofessional behaviors are more likely to occur among peers who spend more time with one another and work closely together as a team. Moreover, the professional behaviors of responsibility, effective communication, interprofessional respect, thoroughness, and altruism either have a direct impact on peers or reflect values that peers might be able to infer and observe more easily from the actions of their counterparts than would faculty or other supervisors.

For the purpose of this chapter, peers are individuals who have attained the same level of training or expertise, exercise no formal authority over each other, and share the same hierarchical status in an institution. It is these nonhierarchical relationships among peers that can promote both authentic behavior and genuine feedback among peers while reducing the biasing influence of social desirability. As opposed to sociometry, which directs peers to evaluate their own feelings toward each other, peer assessment is a technique that asks peers to judge each others' characteristics or behaviors relevant to an evaluation task (Kane and Lawler 1978).

Emerging in the 1920s, peer assessment aroused considerable interest during World War II as a method to identify leaders among groups of servicemen. In subsequent decades, civilian work organizations, under pressure to improve performance appraisals, recognized the utility of peer assessment, as well. Peer assessment of behavior has been shown to be particularly useful in situations in which (1) peers are afforded a unique view of one another's behavior, (2) peers are capable of accurately perceiving and interpreting one another's behavior, and (3) there is a need to improve the effectiveness of assessment of group members' behavior (Montgomery 1986). Peer assessments have been used at all levels of education for the evaluation of group participation skills, writing skills, presentation skills, and professional skills (Topping 1998). Peer assessment found its way into medical education in the mid-1950s when medical students rendered their judgments about peers' clinical performance at two institutions (Kubany 1957; Small et al. 1993). Although peer assessment could be used for performance appraisal in many domains, the purpose of this chapter is to explore how peer assessment can make a positive contribution to the evaluation of professionalism among medical students, residents, and physicians in practice.

We first identify the principles of professionalism addressed in peer assessment and then turn to the research on peer assessment, including its unique perspective, the methods used to elicit peer assessments, their psychometric properties, and implications of those properties for the use of peer assessment. We describe examples of peer assessment that are a standard part of the assessment process of medical students, residents, and physicians in practice and close with an exploration of the crucial context of peer assessment.

Principles of Professionalism in Peer Assessment

Peer assessment of professionalism in medicine has most often been part of a more comprehensive assessment of the performance of learners and practitioners, rather than a characterization of a specific set of professional behaviors or even of professionalism as a single domain. These assessments have used, or more typically result in, a bifurcated description of competence: technical knowledge and skills versus nontechnical, interpersonal, humanistic qualities and skills. Examples of these nontechnical traits, skills, or behaviors examined by peers include integrity, responsibility and conscientiousness, interest in self-improvement, concern for the profession, patient rapport, compassion, empathy, respect, interpersonal skills, humanistic communication, and management of psychosocial aspects of illness. These qualities that comprise the nontechnical dimension of competence relate to the principles of professionalism described as central to the definition of professionalism in chapter 2. Occasionally, peer assessment revolves around generalized descriptors of classmates' competence (e.g., suitability for a desirable residency) that might offer insight not only into technical competence but also into the principles of professionalism (Small et al. 1993; McCormack 2004). Alternatively, a global item at the end of an instrument simply directs evaluators to assess the professionalism of a peer, as a way to summarize their judgments of specified technical and nontechnical aspects of competence (Dannefor 2003).

A 1998 review of peer assessment in medicine concluded that peer assessment appears to complement other information about learners' performance, specifically in the areas of professionalism and humanism (Holmboe and Hawkins 1998). The accuracy of this generalization and potential reasons underlying it are issues to which we now turn.

Research Supporting the Use of Peer Assessment

Peers' Unique Perspective

One promise of peer assessment lies in the unique perspective that peers can bring to the evaluation process. Peers not only observe different behaviors but also provide a different perspective on the same behaviors observed by others (Borman 1978). Research on applicants to medical school, medical students, residents, and practicing physicians has documented that peer ratings of performance can provide information about personal characteristics and interpersonal relationships that are independent from, or complement, other measures of medical knowledge or skills (Leape et al. 1976; Schumacher 1964; Linn et al. 1975; Kegel-Flom 1975; Thomas et al. 1999; DiMatteo and DiNicola 1981; Ramsey et al. 1993). More specifically, in one study of peer involvement in the admissions process, the quantitative and qualitative information provided through peer assessment supplemented information about applicants that came from premedical advisory committees, college faculty, and premedical grades (Leape et al. 1976). A study of medical student achievement found that a majority of the measures, such as grades across the curriculum, board scores, and senior students' peer ratings, tapped a single medical knowledge dimension (Schumacher 1964). However, it noted, too, that peer ratings and to some extent fourth-year grades also loaded on a second dimension, skill in patient relationships. The study thereby concluded that peers are a likely source of information about interpersonal skills of medical students. At the graduate medical education level, peer assessment of residents' interpersonal skills shared an average of only 3% of their variance with ratings from faculty, patient, and self-evaluations (DiMatteo and DiNicola 1981). A study of peer assessment of physicians in practice found that ratings of peers' humanistic qualities were only weakly related to board certification scores, while ratings of peers' knowledge were moderately related to these same scores (Ramsey et al. 1993).

On the other hand, several works question whether peers do offer a unique perspective about their counterparts' behavior. One study noted that peer ratings of resident physicians bore a positive linear relationship with faculty ratings, regardless of the performance areas judged, including interpersonal skills (Davis 2002). Other research, in exploring the uniqueness of peer assessment, found that medical students' peer assessments did not explain the variance in students' subsequent performance in residency, while grades and faculty ratings based on the same form did (Arnold et al. 1981).

For the most part, however, data do provide evidence that peers—across career stages—have unique information about the performance of each other, particularly about behaviors relevant to professionalism. Whether this unique information derives from more opportunities to observe behavior or from a truly unique perspective remains an issue of some contention. In one study, assessments by faculty who worked closely with the same group of students over the course of 4 years had greater predictive validity than did other assessments from faculty who presumably had more episodic contact with students (Arnold et al. 1981). Several studies of peer assessment in fields other than medicine also questioned the power of peers to provide unique information about their peers' performances (Hollander 1978; Lewin et al. 1971). Indeed, one showed that it is access to observing the performances of other people, rather than any unique perception, that can make peers useful in the assessment of each other.

In addition to the evidence from researchers, medical students themselves have advanced the notion that they have an edge in evaluating their counterparts' behavior precisely because they have better access to observing students' performances than do faculty (Arnold et al. 2004). Students comment that they are on their best behavior in the presence of faculty but let their guard down when they are alone with peers. They view themselves as more likely to experience firsthand the consequences of peers' irresponsibility because they have to cover for them or "pick up the slack." They note that the structure of clinical work itself serves as a barrier to faculty and resident observation of medical students since the former are more deeply engrossed in patient care. They agree with the previously described research evidence that students have the opportunity to see each other in variety of contexts not available to faculty such as informal extracurricular events (Hundert et al. 1996).

However, students caution that peers' advantage in observing each other has limits (Arnold et al. 2004). They admit they might not notice unprofessional behavior such as inappropriate language because it commonly occurs. Thus, according to students, peers must be motivated to make observations about their fellows' actions. Although they sense that their observational expertise in assessing technical skills does not surpass that of faculty or residents, students contend that they can better observe behaviors relevant to such principles of professionalism as honesty and integrity (e.g., cheating on tests), responsibility (e.g., being a team player), respect (e.g., mocking patients), and caring and helping (e.g., teaching other students; Arnold et al. 2003a).

In short, with appropriate access and motivation, peer assessment appears to be a useful avenue for exploring the assessment of professionalism in medicine, because it offers information about performance that complements other evaluators' judgments.

Methods of Peer Assessments

Ratings, nominations, rankings, voting, and qualitative comments have all been used for peer assessment. Ratings involve each group member rendering a judgment about other members on a specified set of behaviors, performances, or characteristics by using a scale. Nominations consist of each group member naming a certain number of group members as the best along a particular performance dimension or quality. Ranking entails each group member ordering all other group members from best to worst on specific behavioral dimensions or characteristics. A peer voting technique assigns learn-ers a number of votes equal to the number of small-group members and directs learners to apportion their votes across the group mem-bers according to the degree to which each member exhibits a be-havior or quality relevant to the evaluation.

Ratings are by far the most frequently used method to elicit peer feedback across all stages of a medical career. Nominations, nomi-nations or ratings converted to ranking, and voting have been used with medical students (Kubany 1957; Small et al. 1993; McCormack 2004; Frank and Katcher 1977)—albeit infrequently. Medical peer assessment relying exclusively on ranking (DiMatteo and DiNicola 1981; Reiter et al. 2002) or qualitative comments (Wendling and Hoekstra 2002) has been rarely used in medicine.

Evaluation forms most often require respondents to provide global assessments of performance of peers in small groups and/or in clinical settings (Norcini 2003), frequently based on Likert-type scales. Occasionally, judgments of peers' performances of specific tasks, such as communication skills demonstrated in a taped patient interview, are sought (Rudy et al. 2001). Forms such as these can di-rect peers to judge whether their counterparts have exhibited cer-tain characteristics or behaviors, what the quality of their counter-parts' performances have been, and/or whether their characteristics or behaviors have been suitable for the purpose at hand (Norcini 2003).

Psychometric Characteristics of Peer Assessments

Ratings

Of all methods for peer assessment, ratings are the most common and most supported with evidence of reliability and validity. More than half of the 18 studies on peer ratings in medicine reported re-liability statistics. Interrater reliability, derived from intraclass corre-lation analysis, ranges from moderate levels of 0.5 and 0.52 in work on medical students (Arnold et al. 1981) to high levels of 0.9 with respect to specific ratings of interpersonal skills of residents (Davis 2002). Generalizability analyses indicate between six (Violato et al. 1997) and 11 physician peers (Ramsey et al. 1993) are necessary to achieve reliability coefficients of 0.7. Peer rating instruments used by medical students, residents, and practicing physicians appear to demonstrate high internal consistency of items with coefficient alphas of 0.93–0.96 (Arnold et al. 1981; Thomas et al. 1999; Violato et al. 1997). However, the strength of these coefficients may also indicate the presence of a halo effect (i.e., students who perform well on some dimensions, e.g., clinical knowledge, being given higher ratings in other domains, e.g., professionalism, when no association necessarily exists). Test–retest reliability over the course of 2 weeks was high at 0.9 for ratings of both peers' knowledge and relationship skills (Linn et al. 1975). On balance, peer ratings in medicine appear to be acceptably reliable.

The results of studies of bias in peer ratings in medicine yield a rather optimistic picture. Research on peer assessment among medical students found no relationship between peer ratings and the race, gender, geographical origin, or social class of the ratees (Arnold et al. 1981). On the other hand, among practicing physicians, peer ratings were related to the length of time peers had shared patients and to the size of their medical practice, although the magnitude of statistically significant relationships was low (Lipner et al. 2002). Not surprisingly, the number of patient referrals a peer rater had made to the ratee was the most powerful predictor variable of peer ratings (Ramsey et al. 1993). The role of friendship and likeability in medical peer ratings has not been studied.

On the whole, peer ratings appear to have acceptable face, content, construct, concurrent, and predictive validity. More than half of the reviewed work on peer ratings either described or reproduced the items that comprised the peer-rating instrument. At least one-third based their work on instruments that were previously studied for reliability and validity or were carefully developed by experts and/or participating faculty (e.g., Arnold et al. 1981; Linn et al. 1975; Davis 2002; Davis and Inamdar 1988; Ramsey et al. 1993; Violato et al. 1997). Most often, construct validity was established through factor analysis of the peer ratings of students, residents, and practicing physicians. The analysis typically resulted in a two-factor solution of a knowledge/technical skill dimension explaining the larger portion of variance in the ratings (40–75%) and an interpersonal, humanistic, relationship, integrity dimension (Linn et al. 1975; Thomas et al. 1999; Ramsey et al. 1993; Schumacher 1964).

Concurrent validity of peer ratings has been examined through relating those ratings with other performance indicators, including grades, standardized tests, certifying examinations, faculty ratings, and nurse ratings measured around the same time as the peer assessments were gathered. As expected, the relationship between peer ratings of students' relationship skills and their grades or standardized test scores is weak (Linn et al. 1975), and the relationship between residents' peer ratings and their standardized test scores was nonexistent (Van Rosendall and Jennett 1994). Of particular note are the moderate to high relationships found between peer ratings of residents and faculty ratings of specific principles of professionalism such as responsibility, interpersonal relationships, and humanism (Davis and Inamdar 1988; Risucci et al. 1989; Thomas et al. 1999). Peer ratings and nurse ratings of practicing physicians are moderate to high, including a moderate relationship for ratings of responsibility and a strong relationship for ratings of compassion (Ramsey et al. 1993).

Predictive validity of peer ratings has been infrequently researched, with a focus only on peer ratings of medical students. These studies (Arnold et al. 1981; Korman and Stubblefield 1971) found weak to moderate relationships between peer ratings of medical students and faculty ratings of clinical performance, including principles of professionalism, when these students became interns or residents.

Interpretations of these data patterns offered as evidence of validity are various and contradictory. Low relationships between peer ratings and other measures have been cited in support of the validity of peer ratings as a unique or complementary measure of performance. Moderate relationships have been interpreted as a sign that each measure brings something special to the assessment process. Strong relationships between peer ratings and other measures have been seen as grounds for strong validity but have raised the issue of the need for peer ratings. Several of the researchers responsible for these data patterns, along with the authors of this chapter, query the practice of relating peer ratings to other measures as an appropriate test of concurrent validity. The practice of attributing validity to peer ratings because they bear weak or no relationship to other measures appears especially suspect, since the absence of a relationship proves nothing. Further, the rise in the strength of relationships between peer ratings and other measures as peer ratings are elicited from physicians with increasing experience (students compared to residents compared to physicians) raises the issue of the impact of the socialization process in the use of peer assessments (Arnold et al. 1981; Morton and MacBeth 1977; Rudy et al. 2001; Sullivan et al. 1999; Davis and Inamdar 1988; Risucci et al. 1989;

Thomas et al. 1999; Davis 2002). This issue may be particularly relevant when faculty use peer assessment to gain unique information about professionalism among learners whom they have already chosen to engage in the profession. Ultimately, we believe that there is no gold standard against which to compare the validity of peer assessment; the contribution of peer assessment provides a unique view into the professional behaviors of physicians.

Nominations

The nomination of peers for outstanding professional behavior has been a longstanding and common practice for graduation awards, but research on its psychometric properties is less mature than for peer ratings. Of five peer nomination studies in medical education, three examine principles of professionalism as part of a more comprehensive evaluation of clinical competence (Kubany 1957; Small et al. 1993; McCormack 2004), one focuses on leadership qualities (Frank and Katcher 1977), and the third on professionalism as a set of specific behaviors (Panszi et al. 2000). In three studies reporting interrater reliability, peer nominations resulted in coefficients averaging 0.89 (Kubany 1957) or identified 10–15% of the graduating class as competent physicians-to-be, with a high degree of agreement—although differentiation among the rest of the class did not occur (Small et al. 1993; McCormack 2004). In one preliminary study where positive and negative nominations were converted into a single numeric score for each student, generalizability theory indicated that six peer assessments could provide estimates with a reliability of 0.75 (Panszi et al. 2000). Internal consistency of items on the peer nomination instruments and test–retest reliability were not described.

Two of the studies examined the presence of bias among peer nominations by medical students in their senior year (Kubany 1957) and in a first-year anatomy course (Frank and Katcher 1977). One found that peer assessments were relatively independent of friendship and acquaintanceship (Kubany 1957), while the other established gender stereotyping among men students judging their peers' leadership qualities (Frank and Katcher 1977).

With respect to validity, two studies offered factor analysis results supportive of construct validity of peer nominations among senior medical students (Small et al. 1993; McCormack 2004). This work also obtained a significant relationship between an earlier peer assessment and the senior year peer assessment as well as weak relationships and/or nonsignificant relationships between the peer assessments and basic science grade-point average, National Board of Medical Examiners (NBME) part I scores, and admissions data (Small et al. 1993). Concurrent validity statistics, available in two of the studies, show moderate correlations at a statistically significant level between the peer assessments and other measures of performance such as clinical grade-point average ($r = 0.40$; Small et al. 1993) and instructors' ratings of clinical performance ($r = 0.44$; Kubany 1957). At the same time, the correlation between peer assessments and NBME part II scores was relatively weak ($r = 0.28$; Small et al. 1993). Whether the most appropriate index of the validity of peer nominations is the size of its correlation with test scores, grades, and instructors' ratings is a recurring issue, especially if other research and comments from peers themselves are correct with respect to their unique perspective on behaviors.

The task of nominating one's peers is relatively easy for assessors to complete, but the technique is more challenging to administer and score than ratings. Recent developments in computerized nomination forms and associated programs for data analysis hold promise for making this process more generally accessible (McCormack 2004).

Ranking

Peer assessments using a ranking method are a rarity in medicine. One study of residents in multiple specialties has relied upon ranking to gather peer assessments (DiMatteo and DiNicola 1981). Results from this work show that peer rankings are reliable, and that they have construct validity derived from factor analysis, which generated the typical two-factor solution of a technical skill dimension and an interpersonal skill dimension, where the latter explained the larger part of the variance in the peer assessments. This result contrasts with factor analysis of peer ratings where the technical dimension explains most of the variance. Low correlations (ranging from 0 through 0.33) between residents' peer rankings and assessments by faculty and patients again bring into question the practice of gauging concurrent validity of peer assessments against evaluations from faculty and other sources. But for this study, few data are available to support the proposition that ranking is a reliable and valid means for assessing peer performance in medicine. Further, the evaluator's task of comparing performance in a ranking of more than a few peers is technically challenging, except at the extremes. With large numbers of students, it is possible that ranking converges to high and low nominations, with little differentiation possible at the center of the distribution.

Voting and Qualitative Comments

Information about the psychometric properties of voting and qualitative comments as methods for peer assessment is scarce. One study of medical students voting for their counterparts who had most helped them learn microbiology found that these peer judgments, made in the basic science years, were the measures most closely related, albeit moderately, to peer assessments of competence in the senior year (Small et al. 1993).

Implications of Psychometric Characteristics for Use of Peer Assessment in Medicine

Research on peer assessments suggests they can be reliable. While the dissatisfaction with criterion variables to establish the validity of peer assessment calls for creative ways to characterize and understand their independent validity, peer assessments may be moderately valid and can bring a complementary perspective to the assessment task of professionalism. The methods themselves differ primarily in the degree of discrimination they can make among groups of peers.

Peer ratings are the method of choice when specific information about each group member is desired. Because information about all individuals in a group can be obtained, ratings are the most useful peer assessment method for formative assessment providing feedback (Kane and Lawler 1978). Compared to other methods, ratings may be most sensitive to peer information that is accessible to other group members only. They may have less validity than other methods because peers are judging their counterparts across the entire range of performances or qualities. They are subject to problems of bias that attend rating scales of a global nature. Behaviorally anchored scales and training of assessors may help to address these issues.

Peer nominations are best for identifying group members at the extreme positive and negative ends of a continuum (Kane and Lawler

1978). As a result, they do not provide information about the performance or characteristics of all individuals in a group, and the technique has little use as a feedback mechanism to all participants. They may be subject to acquaintance or friendship bias that becomes problematic when these considerations are irrelevant to the performance or quality being evaluated.

Peer rankings, by definition, allow for judgments that discriminate across the entire range of performance levels of group members. However, they have been infrequently studied and present a challenge to evaluators of more than a few individuals to discriminate beyond the margins. Similarly whether the technique of relative ranking would be useful for peer assessment in the future awaits additional study.

Regardless of method used, caution is advised in making cross-group comparisons of peer assessments since the size of a peer group and the culture of a group can affect ratings in various ways (Kane and Lawler 1978). In medicine, for example, one study noted that negative peer assessments occurred more frequently in some student groups than others, depending on the leadership style of the attending physician (Arnold et al. 1981).

Moreover, the use of peer assessments may well affect their validity. Peer assessment as part of a high-stakes evaluation, it has been suggested, could result in inflated judgments of performance (Hay 2003). Empirical evidence lends credence to this view. Most practicing physicians received high ratings from their peers, and few received low ratings (Ramsey et al. 1993; Hall et al. 1999). Peers typically awarded their resident colleagues ratings in the middle of the scale, even though the evaluation did not involve high stakes (Kegel-Flom 1975; VanRosendall et al. 1994). On the other hand, peer ratings are lower than faculty ratings, including areas relevant to principles of professionalism (Van Rosendall and Jennett 1994).

Practical Examples

Peer assessments as a standard operating procedure of evaluation occur in small groups in the early years of the curriculum at some medical schools. For example, in a pharmacology course, students rate the participation of their peers in small groups formed to complete required projects (Cuddy et al. 2001). At the close of the course, each student receives a computerized profile summarizing his or her peer ratings that contribute to the student's final grade. In a microbiology course, students rate the cooperative learning skills of peers with whom they have worked in small groups (Small et al. 1993). The purpose of their confidential assessment is formative, and negative comments are not shared with administrators or other faculty but may be used to help students address their problems.

For more than 30 years at the University of Missouri–Kansas School of Medicine, students in the obstetrics-gynecology clerkship and in a required annual internal medicine rotation have evaluated their peers (Arnold et al. 1981). Since students take the internal medicine rotation annually for 3 years, they receive from the peer assessments a longitudinal picture of their technical and professional development. Initially, the assessments were anonymous, but more recently students have been asked to sign the evaluations to prevent capricious and malicious reports. Two years ago, the clinical performance evaluation form that peers (and faculty) complete was modified to include rating scales specifically based on the American Board of Internal Medicine (ABIM) definition of professionalism. Since that time, most of the negative reports of professional behavior that the student promotion committee has received have come from peers.

Another peer assessment system of long standing, at the University of Florida College of Medicine, is designed to evaluate the professional competence of rising seniors and seniors (Small et al. 1993). The system, based on nominations, identifies 10–15% of the class as outstanding. The information appears in the dean's letter of these top students. According to the authors, some residency programs have taken special note of these peer assessments, which in turn has enabled some students to get more desirable residencies than they would have otherwise. Within the past few years, the system has been expanded to include items describing humanistic qualities of students. These evaluations are being used to select students for the Arnold P. Gold Humanism Honor Society at a growing number of U.S. medical schools.

A family medicine residency program uses a discussion format, led by a faculty facilitator, to gather peer assessments of residents from peers who are not at the same year level (Wendling and Hoekstra 2002). From the peer comments, the faculty facilitator prepares a report on each resident who discusses it individually with the faculty facilitator on a timely basis. The report is placed in the resident's file. The monthly formal written rotation evaluation contains peer perceptions and comments regarding changes in a resident's performance in response to peer feedback.

As part of the ABIM recertification process, practicing physicians may elect to participate in a peer assessment module that provides a comparison of at least 10 peer ratings with patient and self-ratings on a set of professional characteristics (Lipner et al. 2002). There is no passing standard for this module; its intent is to assist candidates in reflection upon and improvement of patient-care quality.

The Context of Peer Assessment

The process of peer assessment provides one of the clearest examples of why considerations of context are critical in assessment. The reactions of learners and practitioners to peer assessment and the procedures used for initiating, maintaining, and reporting peer assessments can affect the integrity of evaluations reported by peers. For example, raters may be reluctant to provide genuine evaluations if the consequences of peer assessment lead to possible dismissal from medical school or from practice.

Reactions of participants in the process of peer assessment vary, from positive to indifferent to negative. Medical students have expressed interest in the process (Linn et al. 1975). They have indicated their willingness to participate as long as a number of their concerns about peer assessment are addressed (Arnold et al. 2003b). Indeed, medical students have provided feedback to their peers (Rudy et al. 2001; Cuddy et al. 2001; Arnold et al. 1981; Small et al. 1993; McCormack 2004). Residents who participated in peer assessment saw its value (Thomas et al. 1999; Wendling and Hoekstra 2002). Three-fourths of practicing physicians in a peer assessment study thought that the technique should be used in the assessment of humanism, communication, and psychosocial management of patients. ABIM diplomates have elected to undergo peer assessment during the recertification process although their numbers (356 between 1999 and 2002) are not impressive. On the other hand, medical students have declined to participate in research on peer assessment (Linn et al. 1975). Marked refusal to participate and a low response were difficulties also encountered in a study of peer assessment of residents (Thomas et al. 1999). Another study of residents encountered strong resistance to peer assessment even though it was not part of their grade and was anonymous (Van Rosendall and Jennett 1992). Residents' failure to be critical of each other in yet another study might have been a sign of their reluctance to conduct peer assessment (Davis 2002).

Understanding the grounds for reluctance is important if peer assessment is to become an important tool for assessing professionalism. Students have expressed a more general cultural antipathy toward "whistle blowing" (Rennie and Crosby 2002) and "ratting out on each other" (Arnold et al. 2003a). Along with residents, they fear that peer assessment can upset the delicate but crucially supportive relationships among peers on health care teams (Van Rosendall and Jennett 1992; Arnold et al. 2003a). Practicing physicians have been shown to be reluctant to criticize peers or aggressively self-regulate out of concerns that might threaten another physicians' livelihood (Friedson 1970).

Close attention to the environment and administrative processes surrounding the assessment may diminish participants' reluctance to participate in peer assessment. Medical students are more likely to participate in good faith if assessment occurs in the context of a supportive environment, including school responsiveness to peer reports, behavioral standards on professionalism that faculty consistently enforce, and student groups whose members are amenable to teaching each other and to exploring professionalism issues (Arnold et al. 2003b). Close relationships between students and faculty, approachable administrators who trust students, and a value placed on assessment aimed at learners' improvement, are also part of an environment conducive to peer assessment, according to students. In addition, students remark, education that explores the meaning of professionalism, specifies expectations for professional behavior, provides training for feedback on professionalism and conflict resolution, highlights the importance of peer assessment, and provides for faculty modeling of peer assessment would promote students' willingness to assess their peers (Arnold et al. 2003a).

Further, students' interest in participation depends upon who is involved in the evaluation; its use, content, anonymity, timing; and whether the evaluation is required (Arnold et al. 2003a). Anonymity and the impact of peer assessment on ongoing relationships between students and teamwork are crucial for their honest participation. Moreover, if peer assessment covers areas in which peers see themselves as particularly perceptive, students would be more inclined to evaluate each other. Addressing the environment and the education for peer assessment along with characteristics of the peer assessment process is more important to students than are the details of the peer assessment form. In short peer assessment must reflect the ideas and the lives of those who will participate in the system.

Students' comments echo advice from researchers in the field. In designing a system, for example, the features of groups and situations to which such methods are applied are paramount, not the methods themselves. Thus, peer assessment must focus on the needs and capabilities of the peer group that will be evaluated (Kane and Lawler 1978). Further, if it is to provide unique information, then the dimensions set for assessment must be specifically defined (Kane and Lawler 1978) and focused on characteristics or behaviors that peers can best observe and interpret.

In implementing a peer assessment process, it has been suggested, the purpose of the assessment should be stated in writing (Norcini 2003). Assessment criteria must be identified and publicized to all participants. Training should be offered. Results of the assessments should be monitored, and feedback given to all participants. The process should be studied continuously to ensure that its purpose is being met.

Summary

In any comprehensive program of professionalism assessment, peer assessment should play a significant role. Reliability and validity of the available instruments are sufficient to warrant their inclusion. In particular, the use of a nomination instrument to identify those individuals with outstanding performance in domains of professionalism appears to be appropriate and useful for rewarding those who demonstrate excellence. This type of evaluation could also be used to identify poor performers, as well, although this use has been less well studied. A nomination system would not work for all individuals in a group; rating scales would be more appropriate in this setting. While somewhat less psychometrically sound, a rating system for peer assessment also seems possible. In either case, the system of evaluation must be acceptable to peers and so must adapt to their concerns that peer assessment should be used best either for rewarding excellence or for formative feedback. The use of peer information for summative decisions is not likely to be successful, since peers are generally unwilling to participate in such high-stakes evaluations.

A process for incorporating peer assessment into an educational system should begin by identifying stakeholders and involving the individuals to be assessed. Early decisions on the uses and anonymity of peer assessments will help assuage participant concerns. If peer assessments are to be used for more than one purpose—for example, both formatively and summatively—entirely separate systems are suggested, since the use of peer data so strongly affects participant response. Stakeholders, especially peers who will be evaluated, can also provide information on the kinds of professional behaviors they can observe in specific settings, to assure the assessment instruments have a high degree of relevance. Process concerns, about the frequency of evaluation, feedback to participants, and administrative oversight, should be fully addressed prior to implementation. Finally, linking assessment back to curriculum is essential, so that those being assessed are aware of expectations and understand the system being used to monitor and encourage their professional behavior.

References

Arnold L, Kritt B, Shue C, Ginsburg S, Stern DT. Towards Assessing Professional Behaviors of Medical Students through Peer Observations. Research in Medical Education Conference, Washington, DC, 2003a.

Arnold L, Kritt B, Shue C, Ginsburg S, Stern DT. Toward Assessing Professional Behaviors of Medical Students through Peer Observations. Final Report to the Stemmler Fund for Medical Education, National Board of Medical Examiners, Philadelphia, PA, July 30, 2003b.

Arnold L, Kritt B, Shue C, Ginsburg S, Stern DT. Peer assessment provides unique insight into professional behavior: the students' perspective. Research In Medical Education Conference, Association of American Medical Colleges, Boston, MA, November 2004.

Arnold L, Willoughby L, Calkins V, Gammon L, Eberhart G. Use of Peer Evaluation in the Assessment of Medical Students. J Med Educ 56; 1981: 35–42.

Borman WC. The Rating of Individuals in Organizations: An Alternate Approach. Org Behav Hum Perform 12; 1974: 105–124. Quoted in: Kane JS, Lawler EE III. Methods of Peer Assessment. Psychol Bull 85; 1978: 555–586.

Cuddy P, Oki J, Wooten J. Online Peer Evaluation in Basic Pharmacology. Acad Med 76; 2001: 532–533.

Dannefor E. Ways to Identify and Assess Humanism in Applicants, Medical Students, Residents, and Practicing Physicians: Assessing Humanistic Growth and Mission. Presented at the Arnold P. Gold Foundation Barriers to Humanism in Medicine Symposium VI New York, NY, January 17–20, 2003.

Davis JD. Comparison of Faculty, Peer, Self, and Nurse Assessment of Obstetrics and Gynecology Residents. Obstet Gynecol 99; 2002: 647–651.

Davis JK, Inamdar S. Use of Peer Ratings in a Pediatric Residency. J Med Educ 63; 1988: 647–649.

DiMatteo MR, DiNicola DD. Sources of Assessment of Physician Performance: A Study of Comparative Reliability and Patterns of Intercorrelation. Med Care 19; 1981: 829–842.

Frank HH. Katcher AH. The Qualities of Leadership: How Male Medical Students Evaluate Their Female Peers. Hum Rel 30; 1977: 403–416.

Friedson E. Profession of Medicine: A Study of the Sociology of Applied Knowledge. New York, Dodd, Mead, and Co, 1970.

Hall W, Violato C, Lewkonia R, Lockyer J, Fidler H, Toews J, Jennett P, Donoff M, Moores D. Assessment of Physician Performance in Alberta: The Physician Achievement Review. CMAJ 161; 1999: 52–57.

Hay JA. Tutorial Reports and Ratings. In: Shannon S, Nocterm G, eds. Evaluation Methods: A Resource Handbook. Hamilton, Ontario: McMaster University (1995). Reprinted in: Norcini JJ. Peer Assessment of Competence. Med Educ 37; 2003: 539–43.

Hollander EP. Peer Nominations on Leadership as a Predictor of the Pass-Fail Criterion in Naval Air Training. J Appl Psychol 38; 1954: 150–153. Quoted in: Kane JS, Lawler EE III. Methods of Peer Assessment. Psychol Bull 85; 1978: 555–586.

Holmboe ES, Hawkins RE. Methods for Evaluating the Clinical Competence of Residents in Internal Medicine: A Review. Ann Int Med 129; 1998: 42–48.

Hundert EM, Douglas-Steele D, Bickel J. Context in Medical Education: The Informal Ethics Curriculum. Med Educ 30; 1996: 353–364.

Kane JS, Lawler EE III. Methods of Peer Assessment. Psychol Bull 85; 1978: 555–586.

Kegel-Flom P. Predicting Supervisor, Peer, and Self Ratings of Intern Performance. J Med Educ 50; 1975: 812–815.

Korman M, Stubblefield RL. Medical School Evaluation and Internship Performance. J Med Educ 46; 1971: 670–673.

Kubany AJ. Use of Sociometric Peer Nominations in Medical Education Research. J Appl Psychol 41; 1957: 389–394.

Leape LL, Palubinskas AL Steindler J, Wild B, Dalrymple W. Peer Evaluation of Applicants to Medical School. J Med Educ 51; 1976: 586–588.

Lewin A, Dubno P, Akula W. Face-to-face Interaction in the Peer Nomination Process. J Appl Psychol 55; 1971: 495–497. Quoted in: Kane JS, Lawler EE III. Methods of Peer Assessment. Psychol Bull 85; 1978: 555–586.

Linn BS, Arostegui M, Zeppa R. Performance Rating Scale for Peer and Self Assessment. Br J Med Educ 9; 1975: 98–101.

Lipner RS, Blank LL, Leas BF, Fortna GS. The Value of Patient and Peer Ratings in Recertification. Acad Med 77; 2002: S64–S66.

McCormack WT. Can Peer Assessments Serve as a Tool to Provide Consistent Measures of Humanistic Qualities? Available at: http://www.pathology.ufl.edu/~mccormac/MedEduc.html. Accessed August 20, 2004.

Montgomery BM. An Interactionist Analysis of Small Group Peer Assessment. Small Group Behav 17; 1986: 19–37.

Morton JB, MacBeth WAAG. Correlations Between Staff, Peer, and Self Assessments of Fourth-Year Students in Surgery. Med Educ 11; 1977: 167–170.

Norcini JJ. Peer Assessment of Competence. Med Educ 37; 2003: 539–543.

Panszi S, Gruppen L, Grum C, Stern DT. What Do Peers Know About Professionalism? Presented at the Research in Medical Education Conference, Group on Educational Affairs, Association of American Medical Colleges Annual Meeting, Chicago, IL, November 1, 2000.

Ramsey PG, Wenrich MD, Carline JD, Inui TS, Larson EB, LoGerfo JP. Use of Peer Ratings to Evaluate Physician Performance. JAMA 269; 1993: 1655–1660.

Reiter HI, Eva KW, Hatala RM, Norman GR. Self and Peer Assessment in Tutorials: Application of a Relative-Ranking Model. Acad Med 77; 2002: 1134–1139.

Rennie SC, Crosby JR. Students' Perceptions of Whistle Blowing: Implications for Self-Regulation. A Questionnaire and Focus Group Survey. Med Educ 36; 2002: 173–179.

Risucci DA, Tortolani AJ, Ward RJ. Ratings of Surgical Residents by Self, Supervisors, and Peers. Surg Gynecol Obstet 169; 1989: 519–526.

Rudy DW, Fejfar MC, Griffith CH III, Wilson JF. Self- and Peer Assessment in a First-Year Communication and Interviewing Course. Eval Health Prof 24; 2001: 436–445.

Schumacher CF. A Factor-Analytic Study of Various Criteria of Medical Student Accomplishment. J Med Educ 39; 1964: 192–196.

Small PA, Stevens B, Duerson MC. Issues in Med Educ: Basic Problems and Potential Solutions. Acad Med 68; 1993: S89–S98.

Sullivan ME, Hitchcock MA, Dunnington GL. Peer and Self Assessment During Problem-Based Tutorials. Am J Surg 177; 1999: 266–269.

Thomas PA, Gebo KA, Hellmann DB. A Pilot Study of Peer Review in Residency Training. J Gen Int Med 14; 1999: 551–554.

Topping K. Peer Assessment Between Students in Colleges and Universities. Rev Educ Res 68; 1998: 249–275.

UCSF. Professionalism. Available at: http://medschool.ucsf.edu/professional_development/professionalism/index.aspx. Accessed June 20, 2005.

Van Rosendall GMA, Jennett PA. Resistance to Peer Evaluation in an Internal Medicine Residency. Acad Med 67; 1992: 63.

Van Rosendall GMA, Jennett PA. Comparing Peer and Faculty Evaluations in an Internal Medicine Residency. Acad Med 69; 1994: 299–303.

Violato C, Marini A, Toews J, Lockyer J, Fidler H. Feasibility and Psycho-
    metric Properties of Using Peers, Consulting Physicians, Co-workers, and
    Patients to Assess Physicians. Acad Med 72; 1997: S82–S84.
Wendling A, Hoekstra L. Interactive Peer Review: An Innovative Resident
    Evaluation Tool. Family Medicine 34; 2002: 738–743.

I I

Using Reflection and Rhetoric
to Understand Professional Behaviors

Shiphra Ginsburg and Lorelei Lingard

Preceding chapters in this book have addressed important issues in the assessment of ethical understanding, communication skills, and the aspiration to humanism and accountability. Chapters 8–10 on critical incident reports and faculty and peer observations all propose methods by which individuals might observe and assess professional behaviors. But professionalism entails not only the ability to uphold the principles and values of the profession but also the ability to negotiate between competing values in a specific context. As Coles (2002) stated, professional practice involves practitioners in finding not so much the "right" answer (which may not exist in an absolute sense) but rather in deciding what is "best" in the situation in which they find themselves (3). Understanding the nature of such negotiations requires asking more than "What did the student *do?*" or "What choice did the student *make?*" Instead, we must ask, "Why did the student choose that action?" or "How did they justify their actions?" (Rest and Narvaez 1994; Burke 1969).

What are the advantages of exploring reflection as a way to understand students' professional behaviors? First, reflection can provide insight into students' attitudes about the medical profession and their sense of developing identity in relation to their new community and its expectations. It can also expose their patterns of reasoning as they approach challenging professional dilemmas. Exploring the reasoning behind behaviors is important because the choices made by an individual are not necessarily evident in the outcome we observe. For example, a student who fails to disclose a diagnosis to a patient because her attending physician told her not to may be acting dishonestly, but is she withholding the truth from the patient because she's concerned about her evaluation from the attending physician, or because she realizes she can't answer all the patient's inevitable questions, and thus may cause unnecessary distress before she can find someone more senior to talk to the patient (Ginsburg et al. 2004)? The behavior—lying to the patient—does not tell us *why* the student acted. What methods are available to understand the reasoning strategies of this student? How could we measure those strategies and decide if one is better than another?

The literature addressing reflection as a window onto professionalism can be broadly divided into two schools: those studies that elucidate students' professional attitudes and identity formation, and those that probe reasoning and phronesis, that is, the application of knowledge and attitude to form judgments in situations requiring action. Following a description of these two domains, we briefly describe the means through which these kinds of reflections could be used for assessment.

Student Attitudes, Identity, and Perception

How do medical students and residents view their own development, and what can this tell us about their developing professionalism? Many studies have involved self-reports of attitude changes during medical training (Rezler 1974; Wolf et al. 1989; Flaherty 1985; see also chapter 3). Students have reported increased cynicism and have felt that their ethical principles have become eroded or lost as medical school progressed (Feudtner et al. 1994; Testerman et al. 1996; Satterwhite et al. 2000). However, at least one study has also shown an increase in some positive attitudes, such as feeling more helpful or having more concern for patients, and one that used standardized moral reasoning tests showed that there may be no change at all (Feudtner et al. 1994; Patenaude et al. 2003; see also chapter 5).

One group also assessed gender differences and found that women graduates were more likely than their male counterparts to feel that they had achieved some of the "ideal attributes" of a physician (Clack and Head 1999). An interesting study involving primary care residents showed a shift in narrative attitude when essays were collected over different points in time: These residents began their training searching for core values and a professional identity; this shifted in second year toward disillusionment and despair, but by the third year some glimmers of hope and reconciliation were evident (Brady et al. 2002).

These studies have been very helpful in documenting attitude changes during training and suggest that the education process itself might actually have some unintended negative effects on students' professional development. However, since most of these studies are retrospective reviews, end-of-training surveys, or involved essays as course requirements, they may be biased in what students report. In addition, much of this work has looked at groups, rather than individuals, so it is difficult to draw conclusions about particular students for the purposes of evaluation.

However, interesting work by Niemi and colleagues provides some insight into how individual medical students think of themselves as professionals. In one study, the author used learning logs written by first-year students and "professional identity status" interviews based on a preexisting protocol (Niemi 1997). The clearest views of the profession were held by the "committed reflectors" who were more certain about their professional choice than were the other groups. On the other hand, students who reported only scant and diffuse information in their logs were more likely to consider quitting medical school, and their interviews reflected an avoidance of professional and educational commitment. In a subsequent study, the same authors reported on first-day medical students' representations of themselves as professionals, based on essays written on the first day of medical school (Niemi et al. 2003). These essays were categorized along several axes, for example, reflective versus foreclosed, idealistic versus realistic. The students who viewed the profession as having high status, unquestioned expertise, and authority were also likely to have more idealistic expectations for future success. The authors postulated that these students might have more difficulties adjusting when faced with the reality of medicine on the teaching wards, but follow-up data have not yet been published. These approaches have not been explored by others, and there is some question as to the validity of dichotomizing otherwise complex constructs, but their data do suggest an important potential link between what students write about and their views of themselves as professionals. The connection between these self-perceptions and actual behaviors remains a fruitful area for further inquiry.

In contrast with Niemi and colleagues' focus on the ideal professional, our research group has focused on students' perceptions of "lapses" in professionalism, and these studies give us some insight into what students think constitutes professional or unprofessional behavior. In one study, medical students in focus groups were asked to discuss lapses in professionalism that either they had witnessed or in which they had participated (Ginsburg et al. 2002). Grounded theory analysis of the focus group transcripts revealed that students' descriptions of lapses could be easily sorted into six categories, which focused on the *action* in the lapse, for example, communicative violation, objectification of patients, or accountability. Their reports did not map easily onto the standard definitions or elements of professionalism often espoused, which use abstract terms such as respect, honesty, and altruism.

As an illustration of this approach, consider the following passage from one focus group:

> I saw a nurse start talking about law suits, and suggesting that "You know, this is very important because this woman could end up dying here and then the doctor could get sued . . ." and starts talking about this in front of the patient. And discussing possible death in front of the patient, and it turned out that that woman's husband was an attorney who defends malpractice . . . and [the nurse] actually got terminated and then reinstated because he threatened to launch another lawsuit against the university.

This description of a lapse could be classified as a lack of respect for others, reflecting the nurse's failure to respect both the student and patient. But if we focus on the student's own language, we get a different picture—he uses words such as "talking," "suggesting," and "discussing," which direct our attention to the action—communication—in the lapse. This approach—focusing on behaviors rather than definitions, and grounding the framework in students' own words—operationalizes the abstract and is perhaps more reflective of students' own reality. By framing professionalism in terms of behaviors rather than abstractions, we may approach a more context-bound, realistic framework for understanding professional behavior (Ginsburg and Stern 2004).

This behavior-based framework was developed using clerkship students' reflections and has subsequently been validated in a study of preclerkship (second-year) students (Ginsburg et al. 2005). Interestingly, we found several key differences between these two groups. For example, the junior students seemed more willing to report on lapses committed by their peers, which was not seen at all in the clerkship data, but at the same time they often failed to consider the broader context involved that may have contributed to a lapse.

Consider the following example in which a female medical student, who was accidentally separated from her partner during a visit to an addiction and treatment centre, was left alone with a group of male patients who began to ask her personal questions:

> And she's sooo nice, that she thought, ok, I'm just going to talk to them. . . . And the conversation progressed and progressed, . . . and it got to the point where . . . they started asking her out on dates. And I could not believe that she had let it go that far. Because she had divulged so much information about her personal life. . . . So she came out of there extremely, extremely disappointed, and she was scared. She was scared. (Ginsburg et al. 2005)

In reporting this incident, the narrator sees the student as having committed a major lapse, by divulging personal information about herself to patients. But rather than considering the context and situation that led to the lapse, or even placing some responsibility with the supervisor that left the students alone, he blames the student. In fact, he states that a lot of people in the class "couldn't believe what she did." In this relatively myopic view, students may not see the wider context and framework in which lapses can occur. This tendency to blame individuals often comes at the expense of a more reflective analysis. In addition, preclerkship students tended to have a more "generic" view of professionalism, in which school teachers and other health care workers were also considered, rather than a "medicine-specific" viewpoint. They seemed to see themselves as one group of professionals among many, which is a concept that appears to diminish as training progresses.

This difference in perception at different stages is important for educators to acknowledge, because without taking the stage of training into account, we will not be able to appropriately teach and assess students' professional development. These differences have also been shown in several other studies. For example, preclerkship students in one study emphasized different elements of professionalism than did other groups when asked to consider how a first-year student might display professionalism (Rudy et al. 2001). For this group, dedication to learning was the most important element, followed by respect (including toward classmates), confidentiality, listening, dress, courtesy, and teamwork, which accurately reflects their status as very junior students. In contrast, medical residents listed competence first, followed by respect, empathy, honesty, and responsibility (Brownell and Cote 2001). A group of practicing orthopedic surgeons listed integrity, trustworthiness, and responsibility (Rowley et al. 2000). Surprisingly, the residents listed altruism at 26th on a list of 28 elements (Brownell and Cote 2001), the orthopedic surgeons listed it 19th out of 20 (Rowley et al. 2000), and the students didn't mention it at all (Rudy et al. 2001). Other differences have also been noted. Preclerkship students have been shown to display more sensitivity to professional and ethical issues than do their senior colleagues, who have been reported to lose their sense of professionalism along the way (Satterwhite et al. 2000; Testerman et al. 1996). Preclerkship students have also demonstrated more willingness and responsibility toward self-regulation and "whistle blowing" (Rennie and Crosby 2002; Ginsburg et al. 2003a). In terms of education and assessment, then, it seems that not only must we understand what our learners think of as "professional," we must also pay attention to what they omit and ensure that we have adequate education to fill the gaps.

This body of work taken as a whole gives us very useful insights into students' attitudes about the medical profession and their sense of developing identity in relation to their new community. For example, students' and residents' attitudes are seen to shift throughout the education process, students' writings may be linked to their identity status, and students' perceptions of lapses in professionalism provide a useful framework for understanding the student reality. However, these studies were not designed to demonstrate a direct link between self-perceptions and actual behaviors, and this remains an important area for further research.

Reasoning and Phronesis

The other major domain of research in student reflection explores how students reason through professional dilemmas and how these reasoning processes illustrate dimensions in a developing sense of applied professional judgment or phronesis. Phronesis refers to the practical wisdom that individuals use to determine appropriate ends and the means of attaining them.

For the past 5 years, our research program has taken this approach to studying professionalism, analyzing students' oral and written stories of reasoning and decision making in the face of professional dilemmas. This approach offers a method of connecting thought and action, of getting underneath the visible, concrete behaviors that students may exhibit during clinical training to the complex web of attitudes, arguments, and motivations that students draw on as they talk themselves into or out of particular actions. To provide a theoretical foundation for this approach, we discuss briefly the tenets of rhetorical theory that underlie our focus on reasoning and reflection.

The science of rhetoric provides tools for excavating and analyzing students' reasoning strategies (Lingard and Haber 1999). Rhetoric has been used for millennia as a method of explicating the means of persuasion through argument (Aristotle 1984; Toulmin 1964; Burke 1945).[1] The common notion of rhetoric as "persuasion" arises from a vast scholarly project that seeks to understand the structures of logic by which social beings talk themselves—and others—into things. The relevance of rhetoric to the project of assessment is strong; after all, Aristotle's students were learning to assess their own and their philosophical opponents' argumentative skill. While its application to the assessment of professionalism is in a nascent phase, there is good potential that rhetoric can illuminate critical and complex aspects of professional reasoning. As linguistic beings, our perceptions and behaviors are dependent on language—without it, we can neither interpret nor participate in our world (Burke 1966). We act in response to how we "story" our social surroundings: Language both reflects and shapes our reality. Students' stories of professional dilemmas, therefore, provide a window onto their perception—and construction—of their roles in the medical world. These stories reflect their growing database of practical wisdom—their phronesis—as they talk themselves into, and out of, professional actions (Pellegrino and Thomasma 1993).

Rhetorical theory considers the patterns that underlie processes of persuasion: both the persuasion of self and the persuasion of others. Language, particularly narrative and symbolic language, is a key ingredient of persuasion among social and literate beings. To study students' reflections is to explore the means of persuasion they employ as they story themselves as medical professionals (Burke 1969). The patterns of narrative—the way they portray their stories, the way they build their arguments in defense of or against particular actions—suggest the logics that produce student action. Two rhetorical concepts are especially important here: the function of "motives" and the role of "terministic screens."

Kenneth Burke makes the critical connection between logics of "motive" and human action, arguing for a theory of action that recognizes the influence of attitudes, emotions, and ideologies on the possible actions that individuals perceive as available to them. In doing so, he reinforces Richards' notion of "attitude as incipient action" (Burke 1969), which expresses the power of attitudes not only to shape action but also to *substitute* for action. As an example of this, consider a description written by a student for a research study, in which a procedure was almost performed without proper patient consent. This student observed in horror, "disturbed to realize that, rather than being dismissed, this notion was being actively entertained by the group!" The student himself didn't intervene in the lapse, substituting for action the attitude of "horror" that the professional lapse was occurring (Lingard et al. 2001).

Another key dimension of the rhetorical theory of motives is the complex ways in which arguments or logics can emphasize one motive over another, or select one motive from a cluster of related motives, as a way of simplifying the argument and increasing persuasive force (Burke 1969). Where decision making is complex, we often simplify the story, focusing attention on one dimension or another and thus shaping our actions and interpretations accordingly. For example, one study found that supervisors, when judging their students' behaviors, often considered the presumed motives behind the actions (Lavine et al. 2004). From their point of view, if students were thought to be acting for the sake of patient care, for the sake of their own learning, or for the sake of their team, the behavior was judged positively, but if students were thought to be avoiding work or acting for the sake of appearances, the same behavior was judged negatively. These quick and frequent judgments supervisors make of students in part reflect the fundamental attribution error, that is, the tendency to underestimate the impact of the situation and over-estimate the extent to which a behavior reflects an individual's traits and attitudes; but they also remind us that motives—expressed or attributed—are readily simplified and invariably persuasive as we judge choices among possible arguments and actions.

The second concept, that of "terministic screens," focuses our attention on the role of language in human reasoning. Burke argues that how language-using beings name things influences how they perceive them and how they act in relation to them (Burke 1966). This argument for the constructive nature of language directs our attention to how important student stories about professionalism can be. For, in the telling of such stories and reflecting on them, students are not only describing, they are constructing—constructing their professional personae, their dominant motives, their arguments, their phronesis or practical wisdom for application in future instances of professional dilemmas. Consider the following example from one of our studies, in which a student reported being very upset that no one had told a patient that his prognosis had worsened; however, when asked why she didn't tell the patient herself, she said "I'm the student! That's totally not my place!" (Ginsburg et al. 2002). The screen of "student" is a key part of the construction of this event for the student-narrator—after all, she could have used the screen of team member, or patient advocate instead, which would have radically changed her self-constructed position in the story. By using the metaphor of "terministic screens," our attention is directed to the rhetoric underlying *any* choice of terminology, for no single term can capture all the nuances of a situation. All terms, all choices students make when they tell their stories, act to "select, reflect, and deflect" reality.

In this regard, the concepts of terministic screens and motives are related ideas. Consider the following example taken from another student's essay: "These final events occurred on the last day of the rotation, and I didn't feel that I had the emotional restraint to argue the point with my intern." The posited reasoning—the student stated that s/he would "explode" if s/he confronts his/her resident—may conceal another reason suggested by the reference to "the last day of the rotation": the student's fear that his/her evaluation will be affected if s/he confronts the resident (Lingard et al. 2001). Indeed, this passage was coded as an example of "deflection." As students select the terms of their stories, they select some aspects over others, they reflect certain attitudes and beliefs, and they try to deflect attention from dimensions of the situation that they desire to downplay. These actions of selection, reflection, and deflection can provide enormous insight into students' impressions of what is sanctioned and valued—or unsanctioned and forbidden—in medicine.

As alluded to in the examples above, based on the theories described we conducted several studies designed to explore and understand how students think, by examining the reasoning strategies they engage in when faced with professionally challenging situations. Our initial work involved a rhetorical analysis of essays that clerkship students submitted, each of which described a single lapse in professionalism that a student had witnessed or participated in (Lingard et al. 2001). The framework developed was validated using a slightly different sample of essays, ones that were written anonymously specifically for our study, rather than as a course requirement for purposes of grading (Ginsburg et al. 2003b). In both of these studies, we found that when students report their experiences, they invoke reasoning strategies that enable them to "re-story" the dilemmas that they have encountered. In almost all cases, students "dissociated" from the lapse they had written about, by condescending (e.g., becoming outraged, or washing their hands of the situation) or by invoking "identity mobility" (oscillating between two or more potential roles, for example, student and caregiver). Condescension is another strong example of the substitution of an attitude for an action, while students' language choices around identity mobility illustrate their selection of some orientations toward a professional dilemma and deflection of other orientations. This dissociation is understandable, because it allows students the maneuvering room and psychological distance required to re-story the lapse and/or their idealistic framework to be less discordant. Interestingly, the students in this study also often "engaged" in the lapse in some way, sometimes to interrupt a lapse in progress, or more often to deal with the consequences of a lapse (e.g., comforting a patient, reporting the situation to the administration). These data further illustrate that although students may feel discomfort or disempowerment in these situations (Clever et al. 2001), they often act despite their feelings, emerging as professional actors rather than passive bystanders. Students' preference for dealing with the consequence of the lapse after the fact rather than interrupting the lapse suggests their balancing of sometimes conflicting motivations: to do the right thing and to protect themselves as vulnerable members of the team.

These sorts of studies, then, can provide us with insight into what Schön (1983) might have called students' "reflection *on* action" rather than "reflection *in* action," in other words, students' post hoc rationalizations or justifications of actions that had already taken place. However, because of the retrospective nature of this type of analysis, what we are assessing is students' reasoning strategies at a "rehearsed" level, since they have had ample time to reflect and rationalize by the time they chose to write their essays. They may also have selectively reported only those "lapses" in which they feel they had ultimately behaved appropriately, which can skew our understanding. Nevertheless, the language patterns used in their arguments invariably provide insight into their reasoning process, because terministic screens such as "I'm just the student" illustrate students' selections and deflections of reality. And, since the stories were self-selected, there is no way to standardize across students. Our next set of studies are attempting to minimize these problems of hindsight bias by investigating what factors students weigh when considering action in the moment. An understanding of students' "real-time" motivations is essential for the development of effective feedback and evaluation.

In one recent study, students were shown five videotaped segments each depicting a student who is placed in a difficult professional situation in which he or she must act (Ginsburg et al. 2003a). One example is of a student who is just told by her attending surgeon not to tell a patient her diagnosis; in the next scene, the patient asks the student what her tests show. The students in the study were asked to discuss what they would do next and why. An analysis of the actions they suggested revealed that students do see many options available to them, many of which they considered plausible in real life. However, what was more interesting was the reasons they gave for their suggestions. Further, grounded theory analysis from the perspective of students' *motives* revealed that students were motivated to consider actions by making reference to a principle (an abstract or idealized concept, e.g., honesty), an affect (a feeling or emotion), or an implication (a potential consequence of action, for the patient, the student, or others). While some of these principles and implications are avowed as ideals of the profession (e.g., honesty, self-regulation), others, such as obedience or deference to one's attending physician, could be considered "unavowed." These principles, although not openly expressed, are clearly recognized by students, can be considered legitimate, and they may even be crucial to success in the clerkship and in the profession. However, they are certainly not discussed openly as part of our explicit professional or educational agenda. Yet they should be, because rhetorical theory asserts that motives directly shape attitudes, which shape—and sometimes substitute for—actions themselves.

When we looked further at what specific "implications" motivated students, we found a third category—students often considered implications for *themselves* when deciding how to act, which is not simply unavowed but is actively *disavowed*, or denounced by our profession as being inconsistent with the ideal of altruism. Attention to core motives, and the tensions among them, is an important variable for consideration in assessing student reasoning in professionally challenging situations. We suggested that instead of denying the existence of these unavowed and disavowed influences, we should aim to devise assessment strategies that elicit the impact of these influences on student reasoning, which would bring us closer to an authentic assessment of students' developing professional judgment.

This study has been replicated using faculty attending physicians in internal medicine and surgery, to determine what they think students should do (and why) in these same dilemmas (Ginsburg et al. 2004). Analysis is still under way, but preliminary results suggest that faculty also see many options available for students, and they also make reference to similar principles, affects, and implications. What appears to be different is faculty's reliance on students to "know" what is right and wrong and to have the strength of character to go with their gut feelings. This perspective suggests that faculty implicitly understand the role of motivation and attitude in producing action.

Heuristics for Assessing Reasoning

How can these concepts be used in a practical way to assess learners' professionalism? Again, although there is very little research that has looked at this explicitly, some of the theoretical literature may be relevant, along with research conducted in other (i.e., non-healthcare) settings.

For example, some authors have theorized that there may be a hierarchy of the types of judgments professionals make in practice. Coles (2002) suggests four broad ways in which professionals make judgments: intuitive, which relates to "What do I do now?"; strategic, or "What might I do now?"; reflective, or "What could I do now?"; and deliberative, or "What ought I do now?" Although there is a hierarchy involved, these types of judgments do not necessarily progress in stages, from novice to professional. A practitioner may still find situations in which intuitive judgment is best (e.g., a medical emergency), and novices may be able to demonstrate deliberation when appropriately challenged. To our knowledge, this framework has not been used as a means of assessment as yet, but it may be a useful way to capture how students are making decisions in professionally challenging situations.

Another area that may be quite relevant is the literature that deals with the concept of reflective judgment. King and Kitchener (1994) and Wood (1983) have written extensively about the reflective judgment model, and several studies in adolescent and college-age students have validated their approach (Love and Guthrie 1999; Kitchener et al. 1993). They define reflective judgment as "reasoning about the basis for knowing in relation to ill-structured problem solving" (Wood, 1983). These ill-structured problems have no "right answer," and even qualified experts can be expected to show some disagreement about them.

Briefly, King and Kitchener (1994) suggest that there are stages of development in individuals' abilities to reason reflectively. During "prereflective thinking," knowing is limited to single concrete instances, and individuals believe that there are right and wrong answers. Students at this stage may not find ill-structured problems perplexing, because they do not acknowledge that knowledge itself may be uncertain. They assume that a correct answer does (or will) exist, and their knowledge largely comes from authority figures or from their own observations. In the stage of "quasi-reflective thinking," students recognize elements of uncertainty, and do see some situations as problematic. However, developing and justifying a position are not distinguished from merely asserting an opinion. In the highest level, that of "reflective thinking," students can come to defensible conclusions about complex problems. They acknowledge the uncertainty of knowing but believe a judgment can be constructed by integrating available evidence and opinions on different sides of an issue.

Reasoning in these studies has largely been assessed using the Reflective Judgment Interview (RJI), which asks subjects to form judgments about several ill-structured problems and to talk about the assumptions that underlie their decisions (Wood 1997). The RJI is labor intensive and must be hand-scored by at least two certified raters. It has been studied extensively in college students and has been found to be reliable in its ability to track groups and to assess responses to curricular changes and other educational experiences. Interestingly, higher level students (e.g., advanced undergraduate and graduate level vs. high school) show more variability in their reasoning between dilemmas, perhaps indicating that different dilemmas may force students to reason at different stages. As Coles suggests, and in contrast to the models of moral reasoning, it is not believed that individuals are at a single point on a scale, or at a single stage in all contexts (Coles 2002; Kitchener et al. 1993). In fact, Fischer (1980) suggests that there are two levels at which individuals operate: an optimal level, which is the highest level at which a person can make judgments, and a functional level, which is where people typically operate. It has been argued that no skill exists independent of the environment, and an individual's competence— or ability to reason reflectively—will vary depending on the context in which it is assessed. They further suggest that, with contextual support and practice, people can achieve higher stages of reasoning.

Several other methods of assessing reflective judgment have also been tested. For example, in the Reasoning Around Current Issues (RCI) test, which has been tested on almost 10,000 college students, subjects are asked to discriminate between paired essays written in response to five controversial issues and to determine which is reasoned at a higher level (P. K. Wood, K. S. Kitchener, and L. Jensen, personal communication, 2003). In a second phase, they are asked to read 10 statements that represent different levels of sophistication in reasoning according to reflective judgment theory. They are asked to rate each statement in terms of how closely it resembles their own thinking about the issue. These tests are much simpler to score and have been able to demonstrate differences between undergraduate and graduate students of different levels, even when corrected for general academic aptitude.

In one of these studies, a group of entering medical students was assessed, and they scored somewhere between undergraduate and advanced graduate students (P. K. Wood, K. S. Kitchener, and L. Jensen, personal communication, 2003). To our knowledge, apart from this result, the assessment of reflective judgment has not been tested in health professions education, but there are some similarities to what we are finding in our analysis of students' reasoning strategies. For example, we also found differences in students' reasoning strategies between dilemmas; in fact, this variability precluded us from analyzing the data by student—instead, we grouped students together and analyzed them as a group, from the perspective of the unique scenarios (Ginsburg et al. 2003a). Despite this, we also found that some students appeared, overall, to be reasoning at higher levels, for example, by acknowledging that some dilemmas exist for which there is no right answer and that different principles and implications must be taken into account when deciding how to act. It might be worthwhile to study the use of the RCI test in medical students to see if could be a reliable and valid measure of their abilities to reason around these sorts of ill-structured dilemmas and could assess responses to curricular interventions.

What Processes Are Required to Adopt This Approach?

In contrast with other methods presented in this book, the analysis of professional reasoning is in its infancy. Although not yet ready for widespread application in practical settings, it provides unique insight into a critical aspect of professionalism that is not revealed through other means. In this chapter, we have attempted to outline and elucidate the theories that underlie our approach to using reflection and rhetoric as methods to understand students' decision making in professionally challenging situations. In order to adapt these approaches for purposes of evaluating professionalism in medical students or residents, further research is required in the following areas.

First, it would be important to confirm the generalizability of the dominant motives and reasoning patterns in other medical school populations, for example, determining if differences exist between schools with different curricula (e.g., traditional vs. problem-based learning); also, our studies have largely been conducted in Canada, and it would be important to determine if cultural differences exist between medical schools in Canada, the United States, and internationally. Second, the methods outlined above have tended to involve labor-intensive approaches, for example using videotaped scenarios, semistructured interviews, and qualitative analysis of transcripts. The feasibility of using this sort of approach would be greatly increased if pencil-and-paper or computer-based formats could be shown to yield similarly rich responses from the subjects being studied. Furthermore, the issue of scoring such assessments has not yet been addressed. Any framework developed should be simple and easy to apply and would have to be able to discriminate between students with respect to levels of reasoning and critical insight into individuals' motives. Another area that needs to be explored relates to the stability of an individual's reasoning strategies across different situations. As discussed above, it seems that at higher levels of reasoning there may be less correlation between situations than at lower levels, meaning the context itself is a crucial factor to consider when assessing reasoning abilities. Our own studies with medical students seems to support this theory, but further research is required to determine the optimal number and range (e.g., degree of difficulty or uncertainty) of cases to use in order to create a reliable and valid method of assessment. Finally, these approaches may be able to give us accurate insights into individuals' attitudes, rhetorical reasoning, and motives, but further study would be required to determine the ability of this sort of evaluation to authentically predict professional behavior in practice. Some of these issues are currently being explored in ongoing research studies in our labs.

Note

1. From its classical tools, such as Aristotle's appeals to ethos, pathos, and logos (Aristotle 1984), to its more recent heuristics such as Toulmin's model of claims and warrants (Toulmin 1964) and Burke's dramatistic Pentad (Burke 1945), rhetoric offers powerful means for exploring the relation between language, knowledge, and action.

References

Aristotle. Rhetoric. Roberts RW, trans. In: The rhetoric and poetics of Aristotle. New York: Modern Library, 1984; 12–19.

Brady DW, Corbie-Smith G, Branch WT Jr. What's important to you? The use of narratives to promote self-reflection and to understand the experiences of medical residents. Ann. Intern. Med. 2002; 137: 220–223.

Brownell AKW, Cote L. Senior residents' views on the meaning of professionalism and how they learn about it. Acad. Med. 2001; 76: 734–737.

Burke K. A grammar of motives. New York: Prentice-Hall, 1945.

Burke K. Language as symbolic action: essays on life, literature, and method. Berkley, CA: University of California Press, 1966.

Burke K. A rhetoric of motives. Berkley, CA: University of California Press, 1969.

Clack GB, Head JO. Gender differences in medical graduates' assessment of their personal attributes. Med. Educ. 1999; 33: 101–105.

Clever SL, Edwards KA, Feudtner C, Braddock CH. Ethics and communication: does students' comfort addressing ethical issues vary by specialty team? J. Gen. Intern. Med. 2001; 16: 560–566.

Coe RM. Process, form, and substance: a rhetoric for advanced writers, 2nd ed. Englewood Cliffs, NJ: Prentice Hall, 1990.

Coles C. Developing professional judgment. J. Cont. Educ. Health Prof. 2002; 22: 3–10.

Feudtner C, Christakis DA, Christakis NA. Do clinical clerks suffer ethical erosion? Students' perceptions of their ethical environment and personal development. Acad. Med. 1994; 69: 670–679.

Fischer KW. A theory of cognitive development: the control and construction of hierarchies of skills. Psychol. Rev. 1980; 87: 477–531.

Flaherty JA. Attitudinal development in medical education. In: Rezler A, ed. The interpersonal dimension in medical education. New York: Springer, 1985; 147–182.

Ginsburg S, Kachan N, Lingard L. Before the white coat: perceptions of professionalism in the pre-clerkship. Med. Educ. 2005; 39: 12–19.

Ginsburg S, Regehr G, Lingard L. The disavowed curriculum: understanding students' reasoning in professionally challenging situations. J. Gen. Intern. Med. 2003a; 18: 1015–1022.

Ginsburg S, Regehr G, Lingard L. To be and not to be: the paradox of the emerging professional stance. Med. Educ. 2003b; 37: 350–357.

Ginsburg S, Regehr G, Lingard L. Basing the evaluation of professionalism on observable behaviours: a cautionary tale. Acad. Med. 2004; 10(suppl): S1–S4.

Ginsburg S, Regehr G, Stern DT, Lingard L. The anatomy of the professional lapse: bridging the gap between traditional frameworks and students' perceptions. Acad. Med. 2002; 77: 516–522.

Ginsburg S, Stern DT. The professionalism movement: behaviors are the key to progress. Am. J. Bioethics 2004; 2: 14–15.

King PM, Kitchener KS. Developing reflective judgment. San Francisco: Jossey-Bass, 1994.

Kitchener KS, Lynch CL, Fischer KW, Wood PK. Developmental range of reflective judgment: the effect of contextual support and practice on developmental stage. Dev. Psychol. 1993; 29: 893–906.

Lavine E, Regehr G, Garwood K, Ginsburg S. The role of attribution to clerk factors and contextual factors in supervisors' perceptions of clerks' behaviors. Teach. Learn. Med. 2004; 16(4): 317–322.

Lingard L, Garwood K, Szauter K, Stern DT. The rhetoric of rationalization: how students grapple with professional dilemmas. Acad. Med. 2001; 76: s45–s47.

Lingard L, Haber RJ. Teaching and learning communication in medicine: a rhetorical approach. Acad. Med. 1999; 74: 507–510.

Love PG, Guthrie VL. King and Kitchener's reflective judgment model. N. Dir. Stud. Serv. 1999; 88: 41–51.

Niemi PM. Medical students' professional identity: self-reflection during the preclinical years. Med. Educ. 1997; 31: 408–415.

Niemi PM, Vainiomaki PT, Murto-Kangas M. "My future as a physician"–professional representations and their background among first-day medical students. Teach. Learn. Med. 2003; 15: 31–39.

Patenaude J, Niyonsenga T, Fafard D. Changes in students' moral development during medical school: a cohort study. Can. Med. Assoc. J. 2003; 168: 840–844.

Pelligrino ED, Thomasma DC. The virtues in medical practice. New York: Oxford University Press, 1993.

Rennie SC, Crosby JR. Students' perceptions of whistle blowing: implications for self-regulation. A questionnaire and focus group survey [comment]. Med. Educ. 2002; 36: 173–179.

Rest JR, Narvaez D. Background: Theory and research. In: Rest JR, Narvaez D, eds. Moral development in the professions: psychology and applied ethics. Hillsdale, NJ: Erlbaum Associates, 1994; 1–26.

Rezler A. Attitude changes during medical school: a review of the literature. J. Med. Educ. 1974; 49: 1023–1029.

Richards IA, Ogden CK. The meaning of meaning: a study of the influence of language upon thought and the science of symbolism. New York: Harcourt, Brace, & World, 1923.

Rowley BD, Baldwin DC Jr, Bay RC, Karpman RR. Professionalism and professional values in orthopaedics. Clin. Orthop. Rel. Res. 2000; 378: 90–96.

Rudy DW, Elam CL, Griffith CH. Developing a stage-appropriate professionalism curriculum. Acad. Med. 2001; 76: 503–504.

Satterwhite RC, Satterwhite WM, Enarson C. An ethical paradox: the effect of unethical conduct on medical students' values. J. Med. Ethics 2000; 26: 462–465.

Schon D. The reflective practitioner: how professionals think in action. London: Basic Books, 1983.

Testerman JK, Morton KR, Loo LK, Worthley JS, Lamberton HH. The natural history of cynicism in physicians. Acad. Med. 1996; 10: S43–S45.

Toulmin S. The uses of argument. Cambridge: Cambridge University Press, 1964.

Wolf TM, Balson PM, Faucet JM, Randall HM. A restrospective study of attitude change during medical education. Med. Educ. 1989; 23: 19–23.

Wood PK. Inquiring systems and problem structure: implications for cognitive development. Human Development 1983; 26: 249–265.

Wood PK. A secondary analysis of claims regarding the reflective judgment interview: internal consistency, sequentiality and intra-individual differences in ill-structured problem solving. In: Smart J, ed. Higher education: handbook of theory and research. Bronx, NY: Agathon, 1997; 243–312.

12

The Use of Portfolios to Assess Professionalism

Kelly Fryer-Edwards, Linda E. Pinsky, and Lynne Robins

Addressing Professionalism Through Portfolio Use

On *Scrubs*, a popular TV sit-com about medical residents, there is a scene in which a patient seeks reassurance from an intern. "Are you a good doctor?" she asks. "Too soon to tell," he replies in an eager and earnest manner. The intern faces a dilemma faced by most medicine trainees. His goal is to become a good doctor, but his medical school experience has been limited to course grades and fairly general evaluations with which to assess his progress. His eagerness to become a good doctor may even interfere with his professional development because personal insecurity compounded by institutional pressures may encourage him to pretend he knows things he has not yet learned and to hide his deficiency from others. The medical student's teachers may be unable to distinguish what he already knows and what he still needs to learn. He realizes that he is supposed to be a "lifelong learner," but trained in neither thorough and honest self-assessment nor goal setting, he responds by thinking he should just do more nontargeted learning such as reading a textbook from cover to cover.

Scenarios such as these illustrate the need for comprehensive systems of assessment that can be used to both foster the learner's development of professional skills and provide meaningful assessment and remediation. As discussed throughout this volume, professionalism involves building foundational elements, reflecting on aspirations, and demonstrating application of principles in practice. A professional portfolio is an example of a tool that can address these features of interest to teachers of professionalism.

In this chapter, we offer a working definition of portfolios, discuss how portfolios are uniquely suited to assessing professionalism, review pertinent literature on portfolio use within academic medicine, provide a case study of portfolio use in residency, outline key elements of successful portfolio programs, and suggest tips for implementing a portfolio program. Throughout, we distinguish between using portfolios as a basis for formative evaluations and using them for summative evaluations. Existing theory, literature, and experience show that portfolios serve equally well to foster professional development as well as to showcase a learner's developing attitudes, skills, behaviors, and values.

What Is a Portfolio?

A portfolio is a purposeful collection of evidence gathered by individuals in their roles as learners, recording and reflecting on a learner's progress and achievement in selected domains. Portfolios involve more than merely keeping a file of achievements; portfolios themselves become tools for reflection.

The idea of portfolios is not new to professional education. Visual artists historically have used portfolios as a way of reflecting on and displaying their learning. The portfolio allows artists to reflect on their work, to set goals, to continually revise those goals based on their work, and to directly observe their own progress over time (Jones 1994; Parboosingh 1996). The task of developing a portfolio is not complicated, but it is complex. Artists identify gaps in their present skills and target future areas in which they would like to work. They must cultivate a critical eye as to which of their pieces of work will best display their achievements; they must be aware of relevant criteria in their discipline that will influence others to judge their work favorably. They must review their work and select examples that will demonstrate the depth and range of their work. In so doing, they come to know their skills and limitations intimately. In developing their portfolios, artists develop a sense of who they are as artists.

Visual artists have the advantage of having a tangible product on which to reflect; by viewing their work, they can see their progress. In medicine, we lack that kind of tangible product to view, but we may learn from the field of teacher education where teachers-in-training have adapted the portfolio approach to make the activity of teaching visible. Teaching, like medicine, is a multifaceted activity that cannot be captured fully through exam scores alone (Black et al. 1994). Clinician-educator faculty have begun to create teaching portfolios composed of various pieces of evidence of their teaching (e.g. syllabi, student evaluations, statements of teaching philosophy, and reflections upon lessons learned) so they are able to view, reflect upon, and demonstrate their professional growth and achievements (Beecher et al. 1997; Simpson et al. 1997). Like the artists, teachers select the evidence to include in the teaching portfolio by reflecting on their growth as teachers over time, and where learning and excellence have occurred. Using the portfolio, teachers can see strengths as well as limitations or gaps that need work in the coming year.

Portfolios constitute an integrated system of learner-directed evaluation that is well suited for formative and summative assessments of complex and multifaceted skills and competencies, including professionalism. They highlight the identification of learning needs, the details of learning experiences, and a demonstration of the new skills learned. The formative and summative functions are distinguished by delineating two types of portfolios: the working and performance portfolios respectively. The working portfolio provides a sense of progress and process, while the performance portfolio displays final products. Developing both aspects of the portfolio is critical for success. The portfolio itself can take many forms, from web-based files to three-ring binders, and may consist of many items, including verbal and written forms, videotaping, and critical incident narratives (see table 12-1 for sample entries). Innovative medicine programs around the world are currently using portfolios to demonstrate professional competencies at every stage of development, from medical students to continuing medical education (CME) programs (Ben-David et al. 2001; Challis 1999; Mathers et al. 1999).

Table 12-1   Sample Portfolio Items for Medical Education

Professionalism goals
Learning plan
Standardized and real patient evaluations
Videotape segments
Self-evaluation forms
Peer feedback
Reflective exercises
Formative faculty feedback from small groups or mentoring
Faculty evaluation forms

The Role of Reflection in Professional Development

Experiential learning is a major part of the process of becoming a physician. Reflection translates the experience of clinical practice into learning; that is, the crucial intellectual task is to transform a description of the experience into understanding the learning derived from that experience (Kolb 1984; Smith and Irby 1997). As John Dewey succinctly expressed it, "We learn by doing and realizing what we did." The pace of medicine and medical education exemplified by the adage "see one, do one, teach one" rarely allows for the reflective time needed to bring the experiences one is having to the level of learning (Westberg and Jason 1994, 2001). However, increasingly educators are bringing attention to the tight connection between professional competency and reflection (Epstein 1999; Irby 1992; Pinsky and Irby 1997; Pinsky et al. 1998).

Work on reflective practitioners categorizes reflection into three time periods: anticipatory reflection, reflection-in-action, and reflection-on-action (Schon 1983). Anticipatory reflection involves preparation prior to the event including organizing and preparing material, selecting strategies or diagnostic and treatment approaches, and considering how to tailor care to the specific patient. Initial goal setting helps to identify areas for further learning and develop measures of the effectiveness of the approach. Reflection-in-action refers to the process of thinking or problem solving while directly engaged in the activity. It includes moment-to-moment monitoring of action and making immediate adjustments to developments in the situation. It may include recognizing the need to use of point-of-care evidence-based resources. Deliberative reflection takes place after the activity and represents reflection-on-action that then leads to planning and action. Portfolios can be the catalyst for prompting this iterative process of renewed goal setting and can foster the skills of reflection-in-action over time.

Educational Principles and Practices

Insights are common, although not uncontroversial, among educators that learners are more effective at learning when they are self-directed, goal oriented, and problem or practice directed and the learning has immediate applications for the skills or knowledge learned (Knowles 1984, 1988; Norman 1999; Brown 2001). Social learning theory indicates that experiential learning, as well as observation and modeling, is necessary in order to adopt new behaviors or skills (Bandura 1970; Vygotsky 1978). The developmental perspective suggests that learning is maximized when new knowledge is linked to activated prior knowledge in a manner that allows for individual scaffolding of the material. The formation of these links, or scaffolding, requires deliberate time set aside for this process. Learning is best served when the learner is actively involved in constructing personal meaning, because the learning can become internalized rather than remaining at a surface level, demonstrated for external evaluation purposes only (Kinzie 2005).

Learning that is goal oriented, learner centered, and experiential is one part of the picture needed for effective learning to occur. Research by Kolb (1984) and by Smith and Irby (1997) looking specifically at learning in ambulatory medicine shows that experiential learning is a cyclical process including concrete personal experiences, reflection, abstraction, generalizations, and testing implications of the learning (see figure 12-1). Central to this process is the hypothesis that reflection translates the experience of clinical practice into learning. The crucial intellectual task of creating a portfolio is thus to transform a description of the experience into understanding the learning derived from that experience.

Educators promote the portfolio as an effective vehicle for promoting "deep" learning of the type that enables learners to perform capably and professionally in varied environments (Snadden and Thomas 1998). Deep learning is made possible by coupling experiences and learning activities that facilitate learners' efforts to interpret those experiences. Assisting learners to reflect on and interpret events helps them to bring to awareness the principles, ideas, and concepts that underlie their interpretations.

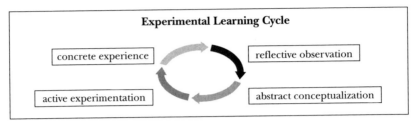

Figure 12-1   Experimental Learning Cycle as Adapted from Kolb.

Portfolio Use in Medicine

Educators in the United Kingdom have been leaders in portfolio development for medical professionals (Snadden et al. 1999; McMullan et al. 2003). Portfolios have been implemented at every level of medical training and practice, from medical school to CME. In an early pilot, the Postgraduate Education Allowance (PGEA) in Britain experimented with portfolios as a flexible, targeted means of meeting CME requirements (Challis et al. 1997; du Boulay 2000; Mathers et al. 1999). In this study, physicians were individually responsible for identifying their own learning objectives and outlining how they were going to achieve and document those objectives. The physicians each met with a mentor to review appropriate objectives and realistic means for achieving them. Structured reflection was built into the process and was seen as a strength, explicitly moving away from the passive approach that educators take in most traditional lecture-based CME courses.

In the PGEA experience, not surprisingly, the shortcomings identified were time and mentor availability. However, the deep learning and personal mastery the participants achieved was felt to be well worth the effort. In addition, accrediting bodies had something of substance to review in assessing the practitioners' continuing education. Far more than a signature on an attendance sheet for CME credits (the current model), portfolios provide a window into the physician's professional development.

Taking on the challenge of demonstrating reliability with portfolio-based assessments, O'Sullivan and colleagues ran a demonstration project in a psychiatry residency education program at the primary affiliate of a state university medical school (O'Sullivan et al. 2002; Cogbill et al. 2005). The residency requested a "showcase" portfolio where residents exhibited their best work to demonstrate competency. In this model, a resident selects from cases or experiences that best represent specific psychiatric skills. The resident writes a brief reflective self-assessment describing why the case demonstrates competency and explaining how the accompanying documentation supports this view. Trained raters scored the portfolios. The researchers demonstrated that five portfolio entries were necessary to achieve a reliable assessment of the learner (O'Sullivan et al. 2002; Feldt and Brennan 1989; Reckase 1995). Furthermore, if raters were trained in the individual assessment tools, only two raters were required for each entry of the portfolio. Because the portfolio is composed in part of other assessment tools (e.g., videotape review, peer feedback, reflection statements), the validity and reliability of those individual instruments apply to the whole.

Ben-David et al. (2001) used portfolios at the University of Dundee School of Medicine to assess medical students' achievement related to 12 learning outcomes in an outcomes-based curriculum. Outcomes related to professionalism specifically included self-awareness (demonstrated through reflective practice), self-learning (demonstrated through an ability to self-assess), and self-care (demonstrated through an awareness of the internal and external factors that influence professional development, career choice, and commitment). Students were required to assemble portfolios that contain evidence of their achievement of all 12 learning outcomes and to defend their selections in an oral exam procedure. The portfolios were reviewed by independent examiners using standardized criteria and were an integral component of students' final exams. Graduation was dependent upon receipt of a passing grade. Requiring students to reflect on their learning and make decisions about how to best demonstrate their achievements is one element in the process that sets portfolio assessment apart from other assessment tools.

Lending further legitimacy to the use of portfolios as an assessment tool in medical education is the recent inclusion of portfolios among the review of possible assessment tools recommended by the Accreditation Council for Graduate Medical Education (ACGME). For residency programs meeting the core requirements as defined by the ACGME, portfolios provide an option for both an intervention and assessment, both in a format that achieves documentation requirements. Even high-stakes evaluations are moving into this territory. The American Board of Internal Medicine was one of the first to explore portfolios. To date, the ABIM offers use of peer and patient evaluations of physician professionalism as an optional route to recertification. The American Board of Family Practice (ABFP) is beginning a compilation of practice-based and prescriptive testing as well as patient and peer evaluations for recertification and evidence of maintenance of certification. The ABFP has plans to require resident portfolios to qualify for certification.

Portfolios and Professionalism

Some authors have criticized the recent push to enhance professionalism curricula as being motivated solely by an interest in meeting ACGME requirements rather than involving any substantive changes to learners' experiences (Wear and Kuczinski 2004). Others have noted the concepts that comprise professionalism remain too lofty or abstract to implement into meaningful behavior changes or assessment measures (Wear and Nixon 2002). Despite these valid concerns, portfolios are a tool with the potential to make teaching and learning professionalism authentic and grounded in the experiences of both teachers and learners.

Professionalism implies both competence, or mastery of appropriate knowledge, skills, and attitudes; and capability, or the ability to adapt to change, generate new knowledge, and continue to improve (Fraser and Greenlagh 2001). Professionalism is built on a foundation of clinical and communicative competence, including both the aspiration to a set of principles and the ability to apply these principles wisely in the context of clinical care (Arnold and Stern, this volume). Professionalism is seen as a skill that is developmental, impermanent, and context dependent, requiring a commitment to lifelong learning, self-assessment, and excellence. Multiple-choice questions and performance-based assessments are useful tools for assessing the foundational knowledge and skills of professionalism, respectively. Additional methods are needed to ascertain the learners' applications of these attributes in clinical work and their ability to choose among conflicting values in complex clinical situations and to routinely apply this knowledge in different contexts.

Portfolios are well suited to this task, documenting the experiential learning process that promotes (or inhibits) learners' attempts at bringing their professional behaviors in line with those to which they aspire. Elements in a portfolio can capture learners' achievements under realistic circumstances and record them using authentic evidence and tangible products (Snadden et al. 1999). Further, a portfolio program can help learners identify, understand, and grapple with issues of professionalism that occur in the routine course of their practice and training but are seldom identified or discussed.

Portfolios in Practice: The PERL Program

The PERL (Portfolio of Evaluation for Reflection on Learning) program at the University of Washington constitutes an integrated system of learner-directed reflection and evaluation. The internal medicine continuity clinic in which the PERL program was piloted has approximately 45 residents and 15 faculty preceptors. Residents are paired with faculty with mentoring groups of three or four residents. PERL was designed to foster and evaluate essential professional skills. The program is learner directed, integrated, comprehensive, and adaptive to learner needs. Frequently used components are featured in tables 12-1 and 12-2. PERL is presented here as a model for portfolio implementation.

Fundamental Elements of Effective Portfolios

Portfolio implementation will differ from site to site according to programmatic needs and faculty preferences. Experience from educational assessment has highlighted key features of successful portfolio assessment programs (Gredler 1996; Fenwick and Parsons 2000). In a recent report, we synthesized recommendations from the

Table 12-2   Items in PERL Portfolio for Residents

Primary goals worksheet
Goal tracking worksheet
Critical-incident–type narratives
Mini-CEX structured observations
CD-ROM compilation of resident's videotaped encounters with accompanying goal setting and self-evaluation
Evidence Based Medicine clinical question presentations
Preclinic conference self-evaluation
Preclinic conference teaching evaluation
Colleague feedback worksheet
Self-summary of learning
Trimester self-assessment
Summary of resident/attending meeting
Overall departmental evaluations

education literature into five fundamental elements of successful portfolios based on the PERL program experience (see table 12-3). We discuss each of these fundamental elements to describe the spirit in which portfolios should be introduced; we then discuss the more pragmatic tips for implementation.

Establish Separate Guidelines for Working (Self-Reflection) and Performance (Evaluated) Portfolios

An effective portfolio separates the two functions it serves clearly. To encourage honest self-assessment, the program is divided into separate working and performance portfolios, the former to reflect on progress to self-designed goals (with guidance from a mentor) and the latter to highlight achievements via a portfolio display. The formative portion, or working portfolio, is composed of any and all evidence and reflective work that the learner thinks may be relevant to building and demonstrating his or her professional development. The working portfolio may include assigned activities, may require items be submitted for review, and may include returned feedback or comments from peers and faculty. Mentor feedback about the portfolio at this stage is intended to be formative, in that it assists the learner to develop selected aspects of professionalism.

Summative feedback occurs when the learner makes an assessment about which pieces of evidence from the working portfolio should be put forward to create a cumulative picture of his or her professional development thus far. This final product is referred to as the performance portfolio. Important reflective and self-assessment work is done when the learner makes decisions about what work to put forward in this final product.

A program could make a range of decisions about how frequently to request such a product (e.g. quarterly, at the end of a year or the end of a 6-week rotation). The critical issue for successful im-

Table 12-3   Elements of Successful Portfolio Programs (Pinsky and Fryer-Edwards 2004)

Establish separate guidelines for working (self-reflection) and
    performance (evaluated) portfolios
Promote a supportive climate for learning and feedback
Advance the development of self-assessment and mentoring skills
Chart progress over time through observation and iterative goal setting
Support learners' development through structured autonomy

plementation is that the learner is clear about the different purposes of the two portfolios. The learner must feel safe and open enough to reap the developmental benefits of a working portfolio while cultivating the assessment skills to make appropriate selections for the performance portfolio.

Promote a Supportive Climate for Learning and Feedback
A safe and encouraging learning climate must be actively developed. One way to do this is to conceptualize the clinic as a learning community where faculty and residents interact as colleagues with differing in levels of experience and knowledge. The PERL program found this framing essential for creating the necessary learner safety, which is then enhanced by teaching communication skills and making feedback routine within the community.

Regular and repeated training in giving and soliciting feedback is recommended for both residents and faculty. Scheduled and impromptu feedback must be a cultural expectation that not only improves the participant's skills but also changes their attitudes toward receiving it. Feedback training is especially effective when it provides opportunities for practice and concrete examples of how to phrase feedback. Collegiality is reinforced by faculty routinely asking for feedback on their attending skills from residents. Using the same feedback forms for faculty and resident evaluations of residents (preclinic conference teaching evaluation and colleague feedback worksheet) also demonstrates evaluative symmetry (see chapter 1) and reflects collegiality.

Advance the Development of Self-Assessment and Mentoring Skills
Effective self-assessment skills are integral to being a good doctor. These can be learned and, indeed, need to be learned (Gruppen et al. 2000). Learners and mentors both require training in self-assessment skills. These skills are then calibrated by comparison with external feedback and evaluation.

Self-assessment involves areas of knowledge, skills, and attitude, which can be developed through experiential learning, feedback, and reflection. It is fostered by a cultural climate where learners and mentors are valued for their honesty and ability to identify and reveal weaknesses and strengths. This can be challenging in medicine, where traditionally learners (and faculty) are rewarded for not admitting weaknesses. To change the institutional or departmental climate, mentors need to role model this behavior by demonstrating both insight and honesty. It proved helpful to have faculty when participating in discussions such as "time management in clinic" not only to discuss tips for achieving timeliness but also to honestly share with others the ways they fall short of their goals and how they are working to improve.

Reflection is a key component of self-assessment. However, "being reflective" had to be demystified for residents. In PERL, this was done by guiding residents through reflective exercises such as considering "What is hard about being a resident?" and "What things have you tried to do to make your life better that have worked?" One must explain to residents that reflection can be this simple, and then lead them through more sophisticated consideration with reflections on "What do you think about a time you made a mistake in patient care?" or "Who was your most meaningful patient this month/year and why?" (critical-incident–type narratives, table 12-2).

Using portfolios with medical students can be challenging because they do not traditionally have as much clinical contact as do residents, nor do they often have the opportunity to work closely with faculty mentors (with some notable exceptions; Baernstein et al. n.p.; Goldstein et al. 2005). That said, similar work can be done to cultivate self-assessment skills and to promote reflection. Questions can be posed periodically to promote medical students' reflection on issues related to professionalism, for example, "What does it mean to you to be a physician?" "What do you think the obligations or expectations of a physician should be?" "What do you feel you have lost and gained since you have started medical school?" "What is the hardest part about interviewing patients right now for you? What is the best part?"

Chart Progress Over Time Through Observation and Iterative Goal Setting
The reflective questions discussed above can be revisited to promote insights into professional growth. Asking students or residents to revisit their expectations and sense of who they are as physicians can be important in identifying emerging and damaging cynicism. Continuing to ask about emerging skills, charting progress, and setting new goals promotes awareness of growth. To promote this type of reflection, learners were reoriented from a competitive stance that asks "Who is the best doctor?" to a developmental one that asks "How can I be the best doctor I can be?" Trainees are coached to view their work as a learning process; portfolio entries serve to highlight their professional development over time (e.g., table 12-2, primary goals worksheet).

Questions posed to residents included "What are your goals?" "How will you get there?" and "How will you know when you are there?" Individual residents will have different levels of skills in goal setting, from "My goal is to read more so I can learn more" to "I want to know more about common symptoms seen in outpatient medicine. I am keeping a log of every patient I see or we discuss in chart review that I don't know about and read specifically about that. I then will track future patients and assess if I am now adequately familiar with that condition." Residents must divide goals into measurable units to assess progress. Rather than "As the senior resident, I want to be a better teacher to my team," they can devise a plan such as "I am going to try a different approach each week and survey the interns and students about which worked best for them," or perhaps assess teaching evaluations or observe rate of knowledge improvement by the team using different approaches.

Discussing goal setting as a group (e.g., during clinic conferences) helped raise the level of goal setting skills in all of participants. Questions from mentors or peers prompt reflection and more meaningful goal setting, for example, "Who are residents you respect? What do you respect about them? Are those things you do well or wish to improve? Let's brainstorm on how you would do that. Is it something you can learn from reading or would it help more to talk with them or observe them?" Holding an annual resident retreat for the PERL program devoted to goal setting conveyed the importance of this skill. Developmental mapping is facilitated by having goal setting framed as an iterative process in which anticipatory reflection forms preactivity goals ("what I hope to get out of this videotaping") and reflection on action goals are the stimulus for the next set of goals ("what I am going to work on now is . . ."; Pinsky and Wipf 2000).

Support Learners' Development Through Structured Autonomy
Through discussions with their mentor, residents deepen their understanding and broaden the range of knowledge they derive from reflection on their portfolios (e.g., 12-2, trimester self-assessment). Resident professional development is fostered by providing illuminative prescriptive entry items in portfolios, building in mentored meetings both during and outside of clinic time, and remaining learner centered while working toward individual goals and growth.

The faculty mentors are involved with both formative feedback and summative evaluation. Ende (1983) distinguishes between feedback and evaluation by defining feedback as conveying information and evaluation as conveying judgment. Both approaches are used with portfolio assessment. When giving feedback, faculty convey information that facilitates the resident's ability to self-evaluate and come to his or her own conclusions about what might need to change or improve. Centering this responsibility in the learners helps assure they will choose a solution that will make sense to them, increasing the likelihood of adoption. These skills of self-assessment can be applied to the lifelong learning that is necessary in becoming a good physician. The attending does have a responsibility to assure a standard of care is being met by residents, and judgment can be required to help a resident recognize certain skills that are needed, or to prioritize some goals over others. A common situation is one in which standards are being met, but only minimally, and the attending can help the resident strive for improvement. The overarching message of the portfolio process is that although "passing" may have been the goal for some students in medical school classes, striving for excellence should be the goal of a successful medical career. Instilling the values and practices of excellence are part of the focus of mentored dialogues as well as incumbent on the culture of the residency program itself.

Tips for Implementing a Portfolio Program

While elements of a portfolio will vary from one educational context to another, portfolio assessment literature (Challis 1999) and the PERL experience suggest some practical steps to employ when implementing portfolio programs (see table 12-4).

Determine Portfolio Elements

Documenting or reflecting on almost any meaningful experience the resident has can be used as a portfolio entry. It is important to be

Table 12-4   Practical Tips for Successful Portfolio Implementation

Determine portfolio elements
Establish a mentoring system
Ensure faculty buy-in
Anticipate learner resistance
Incorporate portfolios into existing learning activities
Plan outcomes and evaluation strategies

creative and flexible in thinking about concrete examples that illustrate the less tangible knowledge, skills, or attitudes you are attempting to cultivate and capture.

Establish a Mentoring System

Because portfolios rely on the structured autonomy model of assessment, with faculty mentors providing feedback and facilitation, one must first identify faculty who will serve as guides to the learning process. Establishing a mentoring system begins with soliciting interested faculty who will make a commitment to serve in this role. It allows the work load to be shared rather than born solely by the director. A potential limitation of shared responsibility for assessment is that the process becomes diffuse and open to variability in measurement. Faculty development becomes critical, along with the development of consistent assessment tools, shared vocabularies, a review structure, and common practices. To use portfolios as an evaluative tool, the faculty must agree on benchmarks of competency for each level of training and coordinate their assessments to assure interrater reliability.

Just as it takes time and training to become a good teacher, faculty often need development specifically aimed at skills for mentorship. These include some basic skills, including skills in providing feedback in an effective manner and assisting learners in setting appropriate goals for themselves. Also needed is a more philosophical shift of perspective regarding the kind of teaching or guidance that is required of them as faculty in a mentoring role. When using portfolios, the faculty mentor serves less as a traditional teacher, and more as a facilitator or coach. It is helpful to address faculty concerns about mentoring through discussion of time needed and compensation for this time, and their cognitive dissonance with the traditional image of the mentor as a "known and chosen sage" and the more diverse "AMA" role in this system as an (assigned) advisor, mentor, and advocate.

Ensure Faculty Buy-In

Faculty should be recruited early in the planning process both to ensure the best possible product and to engage their participation. The program should be framed as a pilot and initial ideas can be presented in a "works-in-progress" format, with an invitation for faculty to comment and participate in strategic planning. It is helpful to engage faculty ideas on the benefits and challenges of the portfolio system, from their own, residents, and system perspectives and to brainstorm on their resolution. PERL used a slide presentation featuring Picasso's evolving self-portraits to allow the faculty to experience how the process of reflecting on one's work can be used to create new personal goals that ultimately result in professional growth.

Use of standard "change agent" techniques such as identifying local champions, "preaching to the choir" to build a critical mass of support, and offering training to address faculty fears optimize the probability of success. Time spent during an already attended meeting was used for PERL faculty education on mentoring, reflection, goal setting, and feedback skills, so the faculty felt prepared and competent. Explicit recognition that the use of portfolios requires new skills and a cultural transformation in the role of the teacher facilitates acceptance of the change.

Anticipate Learner Resistance

As with any educational intervention, the more a learner can see the merit in the activity, the more wholeheartedly he or she will participate. The pay-off from portfolios comes with time, as learners experience the benefits of goal setting, feedback, and reflection. To assuage concerns that the learners will immediately dismiss portfolio-related activities as "busy work" in an already busy schedule, introduce the components individually and slowly into existing activities to minimize resistance to what learners might perceive as additional work. Use of this stealth introduction gives enough time for the learners to experience the value of portfolio activities before they are formally named as a portfolio system. PERL used discussion of the vignette from *Scrubs* that began this chapter to engage residents while introducing them to the purpose of the portfolio.

Concretely, portfolio work begins with learners completing a worksheet outlining their goals at the start of each designated period. In dialogue with a mentor, learners identify the means by which they can achieve their goals, and also suggestions for achieving those goals. The work with a faculty mentor is critical, because setting appropriate and specific goals is challenging and often takes practice. The work of identifying experiences that will help them achieve the goals, and some tangible evidence they can name to know they have achieved the goal, can lead to further goal refinement and new levels of specificity. The learners then use the worksheet periodically to track their progress toward their goals and have a designated time, usually at the end of a specific time period, when they revisit the goals with their faculty mentor. In the PERL program, building these activities into the preclinic conference schedule helped to encourage resident and faculty participation, because time was set aside to complete and discuss the worksheets, rather than having them become extra paperwork done in time found elsewhere.

Learner acceptance can be helped by starting early in an educational program. In our experience, it takes some time initially to engage the senior residents in this new approach, but over time it becomes an established practice. If portfolios are seen as simply part of the program and begun in internship year, as opposed to something that is added during the third year of residency, habits can be cultivated and learners can experience success with the portfolio and come to endorse it in their later years.

Incorporate Portfolios Into Existing Learning Activities
Embedding portfolio activities into existing teaching and learning time slots can help to increase faculty buy-in and minimize learner resistance. Generating the activities that comprise a portfolio, doing the work of goal setting, and the reflective practices required take time. However, many activities are likely already in place and can simply be formalized as parts of a portfolio. As mentioned above, setting aside time for activities such as goal setting in a preclinic conference can help the learners develop skills of reflection and goal setting, as well as enhance the opportunity to see the clinical impact of the work.

Plan Outcomes and Evaluation Strategies
Anytime a major change in the learning environment is implemented, one should be thinking about putting into place a process evaluation and a system for tracking longitudinal outcomes. If a residency or school was interested in the impact of a portfolio program, certain measures should be captured before and after implementation. Possible areas for measurement include learning climate (measuring both learner and faculty attitudes), learners' self-assessment skills, learners' goal setting skills, learner autonomy, learners' clinical skills, faculty attitudes toward mentoring, and job placement data. For PERL, the failure to proactively plan an evaluation system and thus the lack of baseline data on resident and faculty experience of the preexisting evaluation system limited postintroduction analysis to subjective estimates of the effects of the change. One should not underestimate the importance of developing an evaluation plan

proactively and collecting baseline data in order to compare items of interest before and after portfolio adoption.

Postimplementation, one would want to ask learners and faculty about the utility of the portfolio, for example, "Is it worth the time it takes to get the process going and keep it going?" Further assessments can be used to determine if the faculty see improvements in learners' performance.

Discussion

Faculty Concerns

The time demands increase for faculty, just as they increase for learners, and as such, it will help to have faculty buy into the process. One way to achieve this is to review current curricular efforts, including assessment strategies, and to consider how portfolios can fit in with existing work. A well-planned portfolio effort may serve to consolidate several disparate faculty activities into one. For example, if clinical faculty members conduct videotape reviews, give feedback on bedside presentations, distribute literature review assignments, critique patient write-ups, and elicit informal feedback from staff about learners, all of these activities could be collected by the learner and submitted at once.

Support staff to assist in the distribution and collection of portfolio activity sheets, videotaping, scheduling of trimester self-assessment meetings, and so forth, lessens the burden on faculty. For both faculty and support staff time, consideration should be given to reasonable compensation, either financial or in creating time in their present activities.

Further management issues must be considered. The portfolio can be paper based or electronic, depending on the resources available to the program. For paper-based portfolios, decisions need to be made regarding ongoing storage of the portfolio, either at the institution (which requires space and a secure filing system) or with the learner (with an increased risk of material being lost).

Learner Concerns

In PERL, the control of the portfolio rests with the learner. This may be problematic for some, but we believe that learner control of the portfolio is key to its success. Faculty should have access to only those portions of the portfolio for which the learner grants permission. This restriction can feel frustrating to faculty or administrators who would like to have easy access to all data to assure standards are being met. Other programs have made the decision to have central control of portfolios for administrative reasons. For the purposes of the PERL program, it was important that the learner felt safe enough to reflect openly in the portfolio and to bare mistakes and flaws as readily as successes. Within a good mentoring relationship, all formative pieces may certainly be shared. Distinguishing clearly between the formative and summative purposes of the portfolio will also help.

Conclusion

The dynamic and flexible qualities of a portfolio system are well suited for the assessment of the multifaceted and complex nature of professionalism. In the case of the portfolio assessment tool, the work of assessment itself cultivates skills and features that are essential elements of professionalism, such as reflection and self-assessment. The developmental and longitudinal nature of the portfolio allows students and faculty alike to observe progress over time. The time invested in such a comprehensive system pays off in meaningful professional development.

References

Bandura A. Social Learning Theory. Englewood Cliffs, NJ: Prentice Hall, 1970.

Beecher A, et al. Use of the Educator's Portfolio to Stimulate Reflective Practice Among Medical Educators. Teach Learn Med 1997; 9(1): 56–59.

Ben-David MF, Davis MH, Harden RM, et al. Portfolios as a Method of Student Assessment. Med Teach 2001; 23(6): 535–551.

Black L, Daiker DA, Sommers J, Stygall G, eds. New Directions in Portfolio Assessment: Reflective Practice, Critical Theory, and Large-Scale Scoring. Portsmouth, NH: Boynton/Cook Publishers, Inc., 1994.

Brown JO. Know Thyself: The Impact of Portfolio Development on Adult Learning. Adult Educ Q 2001; 52(3): 228–245.

Challis M. Portfolio-Based Learning and Assessment in Medical Education. Med Teach 1999; 21: 370–386.

Challis M, Mathers N, Howe A, Field N. Portfolio-Based Learning: Continuing Medical Education for General Practitioners—A Mid-point Evaluation. Med Educ 1997; 31: 22–26.

Cogbill KK, O'Sullivan PS, Clardy J. Residents' Perceptions of Effectiveness of Twelve Evaluation Methods for Measuring Competency. Acad Psychiatry 2005; 29(1): 76–81.

du Boulay C. From CME to CPD: Getting Better and Getting Better? Individual Learning Portfolios May Bridge Gap Between Learning and Accountability. BMJ 2000; 320(12): 393–394.

Ende J. Feedback in Clinical Medical Education. JAMA 1983; 250: 777–781.

Epstein RM. Mindful practice. JAMA 1999; 282(9): 833–839.

Feldt LS, Brennan RL. Reliablity. In: Educational Measurement (Linn RL, ed.). 3rd ed. New York: American Council on Education, 1989; 105–146.

Fenwick TJ, Parsons J. The Art of Evaluation: A Handbook for Educators and Trainers. Toronto: Thompson Educational Publishing, 2000.

Goldstein EA, Maclaren CF, Smith S, Mengert TJ, Maestas RR, Foy HM, Wenrich MD, Ramsey PG. Promoting Fundamental Clinical Skills: A Competency-Based College Approach at the University of Washington. Acad Med 2005; 80(5): 423–433.

Gredler ME. Program Evaluation. Englewood Cliffs, NJ: Prentice-Hall, 1996.

Gruppen LD, White C, Fitzgerald JT, Grum CM, Woolliscroft JO. Medical Students' Self-Assessments and Their Allocations of Learning Time. Acad Med 2000; 75(4): 374–379.

Irby DM. How Attending Physicians Make Instructional Decisions When Conducting Teaching Rounds. Acad Med 1992; 67: 630–637.

Jones JE. Portfolio Assessment as a Strategy for Self-Direction in Learning. New Dir Adult Cont Educ 1994; 64(winter): 23–29.

Kinzie MB. Instructional Design Strategies for Health Behavior Change. Patient Educ Couns 2005; 56(1): 3–15.

Kolb D. Experiential Learning. Englewood Cliffs, NJ: Prentice Hall, 1984.

Mathers N, Challis M, Howe A, Field N. Portfolios in Continuing Medical Education—Effective and Efficient? Med Educ 1999; 33: 521–530.

McMullan M, Endacott R, Gray MA, Jasper M, Miller CM, Scholes J, Webb C. Portfolios and Assessment of Competence: A Review of the Literature. J Adv Nurs 2003; 41(3): 283–294.

Norman GR. The Adult Learner: A Mythical Species. Acad Med 1999; 74: 886–889.

Parboosingh J. Learning Portfolios: Potential to Assist Health Professionals With Self-Directed Learning. J Cont Educ Health Prof 1996; 16: 75–81.

Pinsky LE, Fryer-Edwards K. Diving for PERLS. J Gen Intern Med 2004; 19(5 pt 2): 582–587.

Pinsky LE, Irby DM. If At First You Don't Succeed: Using Failure to Improve Teaching. Acad Med 1997; 72(11): 973–976.

Pinsky LE, Monson D, Irby DM. How Excellent Teachers Are Made: Reflecting on Success to Improve Teaching. Adv Health Sci Educ 1998; 3: 207–215.

Pinsky LE, Wipf JE. A Picture Is Worth a Thousand Words: Practical Use of Videotape in Teaching. J Gen Intern Med 2000; 15(11): 805–810.

Schon DA. The Reflective Practitioner: How Professionals Think in Action. New York: Basic Books, 1983.

Simpson D, Beecher AC, Lindemann JC, Morzinski JA. The Educator's Portfolio. 4th ed. Milwaukee: Medical College of Wisconsin, 1998.

Smith C, Irby DM. The Roles of Experience and Reflection in Ambulatory Care Education. Acad Med 1997; 72(1): 32–35.

Snadden D, Thomas M. The Use of Portfolio Learning in Medical Education. Med Teach 1998; 20: 192–208.

Snadden D, Thomas M, Challis M. The Use of Portf   >-Based Learning in Medical Education. AMEE Medical Education Guide No. 11 (rev.). Dundee, Scotland: Centre for Medical Education, 1999.

Westberg J, Jason H. Fostering Learners' Reflection and Self-assessment. Fam Med 1994; 26: 278–282.

Westberg J, Jason H. Fostering Reflection and Providing Feedback: Helping Others Learn From Experiences. New York: Springer, 2001.

13

Admission to Medical School: Selecting Applicants With the Potential for Professionalism

Norma E. Wagoner

Selecting applicants to medical school has been a longstanding endeavor with numerous attempts to make it scientific. Efforts to create a selection process that seeks to choose students who possess the qualities we desire in future physicians has led to a wealth of literature, innumerable discussions, and considerable controversy over valid and reliable selection criteria. Medical school admissions committees have long relied on cognitive measures in their selection. Academic leaders, proponents of humanism and professionalism, and the general public, however, have been advocating for physicians who possess not only cognitive skills but also professional characteristics that include good communication abilities, compassion, respect, empathy, and altruism. Their advocacy has prompted medical schools to search for a means of selecting candidates with the attributes that predispose them to become competent, caring physicians. Over the past several years, they have placed greater emphasis on codifying and employing noncognitive criteria to ensure the admission of more students with the potential for professionalism.

Efficiency and fairness have always been the goal of selecting students. While admissions committees can rather easily attain efficiency in the selection process, achieving fairness has proven more elusive, particularly when it comes to selecting applicants with desired preprofessionalism behaviors. Although admissions committee members generally agree on the importance of admitting such applicants, it is difficult to obtain a consensus as to exactly which premedical behaviors are associated with specific aspects of professionalism. Opinions on a range of variables differ widely, with each committee member likely to weigh one favored variable over another, leading to less-than-optimally articulated criteria.

If it were easier to evaluate the behaviors of medical school graduates who possess the highest levels of professionalism, then it might be possible to use these behaviors more effectively to select entering students. "This lack of evaluation is not due to a lack of consensus on what constitutes professionalism—in fact, every major national commission set up to identify the traits of tomorrow's physicians emerges with a similar list of professional characteristics" (Stern et al. 2005, p. 76). Instead, this lack of assessment reflects a dearth of reliable and valid measurement instruments, and incomplete systems with which to track students from admissions to graduation and beyond. Other chapters in this book describe new tools and systems of professionalism assessment, and those discussions are not repeated here. This chapter focuses on the admissions process and the use of data sources to select students who will develop the kinds of professional behaviors that faculty, patients, and the society as a whole expect.

This chapter reviews the major cognitive and noncognitive measures in use by medical schools and reports on relevant research studies that sought to weigh the effectiveness of both measures in detecting preprofessional behaviors. Recommendations in this chapter are based both on research findings and my own 26 years of experience in various aspects of the admissions process. The chapter also offers an interpretation of an ideal admissions process that has as its goal increasing the number of entering students who have the greatest potential for professionalism.

Context of Admissions

Factors both internal and external to medical schools complicate the task of selecting humanistic students.

External Factors

Reputation

The applicant pool that a school garners is due in large measure to the school's reputation, including its rank among all medical schools. The reputation of certain schools enables them to attract academically top-rated students. Knowing that a sufficiently large cadre of these students will apply, these schools can be much more selective in screening applicants into the interview pool, thereby allowing them to focus on professionalism rather than grades. Schools that do not enjoy the same status have to compete harder to attract top academic students and therefore often make their selections regardless of whether applicants possess a broader set of desired characteristics.

U.S. News & World Report *Ranking*

The medical school ranking published yearly in the *U.S. News and World Report* has as one of its parameters the aggregate grades and Medical College Admissions Test (MCAT) scores of entering students. Results released in this publication tend to exert tremendous pressure on schools to recruit students with the highest cognitive scores. Deans and faculty pay close attention to this list. Some deans target a specific ranking for their schools to achieve and exert pressure on admissions committees to meet that goal, limiting their latitude to focus on professionalism.

Assessment of Students' Potential

Admissions committees have a difficult time assessing candidates with less than perfect academic records, such as those who had a slow start in college or who initially lacked focus and maturity. Undergraduate students in both categories often eventually do find direction, become highly motivated, and do very well in their final years of college. However, their grade-point averages (GPAs) fall short of the medical school's desired performance level. Another group of candidates that committee members have difficulty evaluating are those with poor undergraduate records who ultimately attain master's or PhD degrees in science. Also challenging are assessments of those who have acquired 50 or more hours of postbaccalaureate work at the honors level after an initial academic record that is less than stellar. Similar problems arise with a poor showing on the first MCAT, which raises questions as to whether an improved set of scores on a

second test is more valid. While most admissions committees understand that true passion, driven by altruism, can overcome a slightly
lower GPA or MCAT score and catapult a student to success, the student may not be accepted because of the effect a lowered cumulative undergraduate GPA or MCAT would have on a school's overall
ranking in *U.S. News and World Report*.

State Financial Support

Nearly all states compensate their medical schools to some degree
for educating state residents. In states with a number of public medical schools with an imperative to fill the class with state residents,
competition for applicants can become exceptionally keen. Schools
invest in ongoing public relations efforts to portray their school's
greatest strengths in order to attract the "best students." The admissions committee makes every effort to ensure that each new class
has an academic and personal profile comparable or better than the
previous class. If the applicant pool diminishes in size, filling the
class, rather than seeking humanistic students, becomes the goal.

Applicant Pool Fluctuation

From 1997 to 2003, the applicant pool declined 22% but the
2003–2004 applicant pool increased 3.4% over the 2002–2003 cohort, largely due to a 7% rise in the number of women applicants
(AAMC Newsroom 2003). In years that schools receive an excess
number of applications, admissions committees raise the bar in
choosing students who meet their desired criteria. During lean times,
when competition for the "best" becomes keen, the need to fill the
class surpasses other considerations, and some students may be admitted who would not have been in a more competitive environment.
That means that the committee is unable to hold desired characteristics, including aspects of professionalism, as a high priority.

Accreditation Requirement

The Liaison Committee on Medical Education (LCME 2004) has specific standards for the admissions process:

1. "Each medical school must develop criteria and procedures
   for the selection of students that are readily available to potential applicants and collegiate advisors" (p. 24).
2. "The final responsibility for selecting students to be admitted for medical study must reside with a duly constituted
   faculty committee" (p. 24).

3. "Each medical school must have a pool of applicants sufficiently large and possessing national level qualifications to
   fill its entering class" (p. 24).
4. "Medical schools must select students who possess the intelligence, integrity, and personal and emotional characteristics necessary for them to become effective physicians"
   (p. 25).

Given these requirements, if the applicant:place ratio becomes small
enough to worry the admissions committee members, they will likely
put less emphasis on noncognitive measures of professional attributes rather than reduce class size.

Desired Diversity
Another LCME accreditation standard that focuses on schools'
achieving a desired diversity in their student population reads as follows: "Each medical school should have policies and practices ensuring the gender, racial, cultural and economic diversity of its students" (LCME 2004, p. 25). For many years prior to the June 23,
2003, Supreme Court decision limiting the use of race and ethnicity in selecting students to achieve diversity, medical schools selected
students from among four designated underrepresented minority
groups (Powell 1978). With the Court's decision, schools must be
very careful in their attempts to achieve diversity for fear of litigious
action. However, the decision also states that schools must devise and
follow "narrowly tailored" policies designed to serve the compelling
interest in diversity that can withstand legal scrutiny. Accordingly,
the Association of American Medical Colleges (AAMC) has provided
schools with the following definition of "narrowly tailored": quotas
and separate admissions tracks are forbidden, schools must consider
individually each applicant, race-neutral and ethnicity-neutral alternatives that could enhance diversity should be explored in good faith,
and institutions should periodically review the need for race or
ethnicity-conscious measures (AAMC Executive Committee 2004).
To some extent, the Court's decision supports the use of noncognitive criteria through its requirement to provide "individualized consideration of each applicant."

Internal Factors

According to McManus (1998) in his retrospective study on admissions, a degree of similarity occurs among the criteria used by med-

ical schools across the United States: academic ability (cognitive measures), insight into medicine, extracurricular activities and interests, personality, motivation, and linguistic and communication skills.

Targeted GPA and MCAT Averages
Most medical schools seek to maintain or exceed targeted GPA and MCAT averages. Given that the applicant pool in most medical schools normally exceeds the number of entering places, committees feel compelled to first consider the highest academic performers, even if their files disclose no overt evidence of preprofessionalism behaviors.

Because of the need to be exacting in class size, schools keep careful statistics on the number of acceptances required to fill a class and how far down the wait list they will likely go. Having to maintain targeted GPA and MCAT averages means that the school must consider cognitive scores first and foremost as the class fills. If schools could gear the weighting system to focus on professionalism without the pressure of maintaining cognitive averages that are published yearly, forcing overt competition among schools, most would opt to select the brightest *and* most professional students. Unfortunately, these attributes may not always be in the same package.

Institutional Mission
Many schools have institutional missions, such as recruiting students for primary care, or serving the underserved or rural areas of a state. Research-oriented institutions often seek to educate physician scientists and researchers as future academic physicians. Admissions committees are well aware of their institutional missions and may put more of a priority on finding the types of students likely to help fulfill it, rather than on those most likely to behave professionally.

Self-Interest
Because medical school faculty members who serve on the admissions committee are asked to consider criteria and establish policies for the admissions process, they can significantly influence the characteristics of the students being sought. Sometimes, these faculty have been accused of wanting to "replicate themselves," and if they do not consider the traits of outstanding professionalism the most important to replicate, these traits may not be emphasized in the admissions process.

Recruiting Faculty

In general, faculty members view the admissions process as highly important yet burdensome and expensive and many feel they can not afford to commit the time involved in selecting students. In the best interest of the process, schools should recruit only those faculty members with the demonstrated ability to serve as outstanding mentors and role models, a keen interest in young people, excellent intuition about others and the willingness to become fully educated in the best methods of selecting students. However, this is not an easy task.

Admission Committee Member Influences

Elam et al. (2002) at the University of Kentucky studied their committee members' deliberations from a 2-year admissions cycle (1999–2000 and 2000–2001). They analyzed voting patterns to determine the change between their initial review of the applicant's file and their final decision. Analysis revealed that approximately 20% of the members changed their votes after committee deliberation. The authors found that knowledgeable and experienced committee members could influence newer members to change their votes, typically from "hold" to "accept" or "hold" to "reject," based on an expanded interpretation of a student's MCAT performance, medical experiences, or grades. The authors noted that committee members expressed much more ease in "assessing cognitive data than in trying to decipher which applicants demonstrated altruism" (Elam et al. 2002, p. 102).

Frequently Used Cognitive and Noncognitive Admissions Criteria

Cognitive Measures

As mentioned above, medical school admissions committees have tended to rely heavily (some almost exclusively) on various cognitive measures to determine an applicant's qualifications and likelihood of success, despite research studies showing that relying on cognitive data alone does not yield the intended results. Primary selection factors traditionally center on science GPA and/or cumulative GPA and MCAT scores. A review by Ferguson et al. (bjm.com 2002) identified 62 peer-reviewed articles on the relevance of previous academic performance to success in medical school. The authors used hierarchical linear modeling to analyze data found in two broad areas of achievement in medical training (undergraduate [all 4 years of medical school] and postgraduate [internship year]). They found that 23% of variance in medical school performance could be explained by previous academic performance. For the internship year, on average, previous academic performance accounted for less than 3% of variance, and with the corrected coefficient, 6% of variance. The overall results of their study indicate that previous academic performance is a limited predictor of clinical success during medical school and offers even less validity in predicting excellence in clinical performance in the internship year.

Hojat et al. (2002) found empathy scores are associated with ratings of clinical competence and gender but not with performance on objective examinations such as scores in the biological sciences (BS), physical sciences (PS), and verbal reasoning (VR) sections of the MCAT, first- and second-year GPAs, and scores in the United States Medical Licensing Examination step 1. They noted the difficulty in defining and measuring empathy, since empathy has been described as a concept involved in cognitive as well as affective or emotional domains.

GPA/Academic Performance
The differential between the intellectual strengths required for successful performance during the preclerkship and clerkship years of medical school offers researchers a rich opportunity for comparison. A study by Rhoads et al. (1974) highlights some of these differences: "[O]nly half the students who excelled in basic science courses did so in clinical courses, while 70% of those who excelled in clinical courses did not do so in basic sciences" (p. 1119). This leads to the conclusion that while cognitive scores have some degree of predictive validity for success in the basic science years, selecting for cognitive strengths alone will not meet the goal of attracting students with professionalism attributes, particularly those attributes that are sought during the clinical years.

With grade inflation in college on the rise, admissions committees have yet another challenge in interpreting and placing value on grades as a predictive measure. In their 1997 study, Rigol and Kimmel (1997) found that "grade inflation now appears at all levels of education" (p. 6). A syndicated press article (Bombardieri 2004) noted that Harvard dealt with the concern that 91% of students were graduating with an honors designation, and Princeton was considering action because 45% of students were now achieving "A" grades. However, grade inflation may have some benefits, causing committee members to ask what else about the applicants they should be considering and turning to important professionalism characteristics to aid their selection.

MCAT Scores

Committee members give almost as much weight to MCAT results as academic achievement, even though these scores may not predict a candidate's true potential. Sedlacek et al. (1998), in a review of standardized tests at the college entrance level, remarked, "Standardized tests do not measure motivation, study habits, personal or professional goals, and other factors that can affect academic performance and persistence to graduation" (p. 5). The MCAT scores fall into a score scale ranging from 1 to 15 in each of three major areas: verbal reasoning (VR), physical sciences (PS), and biological sciences (BS). The fourth area is a writing sample, scored using letters of the alphabet ranging from L to T. Most admissions committees average all the MCAT scores (VR, PS, and BS) and measure that against a predetermined performance threshold that accepted applicants must meet. There is little in the literature to suggest the predictive validity of MCAT scores with respect to professionalism. Only Kulatunga-Moruzi and Norman (2002a) have shown statistical correlations between the VR score and communication skills.

Limitation on Exclusive Use of Cognitive Scores in Selecting Candidates

Cognitive scores do not assess creativity. When medical schools describe their entering students as the "the brightest and the best," they are generally referring to those who acquired the high grades and MCATs that enabled them to be selected. Committee members also apply the terms "intelligent," "gifted," and "talented" to their students, all of which suggest an ability to perform at an exceptional level in one or more areas. Even if we assume that these scores do represent intelligence, they do not ensure that the candidate also possesses desired humanistic behaviors.

For example, numerical ratings do not necessarily indicate whether a candidate possesses the quality of creativity, an attribute that has been shown to be a critical asset in becoming a humanistic physician. Individuals are deemed creative when they have the ability to solve or interpret a problem or create a significant or novel product (Powis 1994). Sternberg (1985) describes three types of in-

telligence: *componential* (ability to interpret information in a hierarchical and taxonomic fashion [good standardized test takers]), *experiential* (ability to interpret information in a changing context), and
contextual (ability to adapt to a changing environment). Using Sternberg's classification, Sedlacek (2004) found that the admissions
processes of most medical schools placed heavy emphasis on choosing students with strong componential intelligence, bypassing students with a high degree of experiential or contextual intelligence.
In a later study, Sternberg and Lubart (1996) concluded that
creativity comprises a key element of experiential intelligence. Interpretations of this work indicate that someone who possesses
"intelligence" responds to a circumstance appropriately *and with
motivation*, applying knowledge and skill when it is a relevant contribution (Sternberg's "practical intelligence"). Research by David A.
Powis convinced him that creativity has the greatest predictive validity in determining medical students' success (Powis 1994). Greenlaugh (2001) states, "[G]ood clinical hunches and competent moral
judgment are not simply picked out of the sky. They arise from the
same creative imagination that allows the scientist to generate worthwhile hypotheses" (p. 819). Cognitive scores alone do not allow an
admissions committee to determine whether an applicant possesses
the creativity to be successful.

Cognitive scores do not reflect motivation. Although motivation can
be defined in various ways, it reflects an individual's inner drive to
achieve a goal based on personal values and beliefs. Such values may
include a desire to influence others, to share one's knowledge, or to
dedicate oneself to serving others, all of which hinge on elements of
altruism, empathy, compassion, and communication. A particularly
critical motivational factor that falls outside the realm of cognitive
variables, and that should be assessed in much greater depth, is a
student's true interest in medicine. In the admissions interview, the
question, "Why do you want to become a physician?" will likely elicit
a rehearsed response, rather than reveal true motivation. Any number of students with high scores fail in medical school because they
lack the inner drive to become physicians. This occurs for a variety
of reasons—their real interests may lie elsewhere (but they followed
their parents' wishes by pursuing medicine), they may have entered
the field with a limited understanding of a physician's responsibility,
they may not have realized how hard they would have to work for so
many years, or they may have discovered that becoming a physician

can preclude other values they held dear (e.g., having equal time for family and friends). Without the personal satisfaction derived from following inner motivation, students find it exceedingly difficult to look beyond their own needs and desires to devote themselves to caring for others. To the extent that an individual's value system focuses on empathic relations, altruism, and commitment to service, being able to live these values is central to being both humanistic and professional in medicine.

Cognitive scores do not assess biases. With our rapidly changing patient population and new LCME standards, it has become imperative to capture data in the admissions process that provide insight into whether students understand their own cultural and gender biases and appreciate diverse cultures and belief systems. An increasingly diverse applicant pool compounds the challenge. Since many of the applicants' families have only recently immigrated to this country, assessing personal growth, character qualities, values, and beliefs is a monumental undertaking that cannot be accomplished exclusively through the use of cognitive measures.

Noncognitive Measures

The emphasis on recruiting students with the potential to achieve high levels of professionalism has led academic leaders to assign greater weight to noncognitive criteria in the admissions process. Historically, admissions committees have attempted to predict the capacity for professionalism from four sources: letters of evaluation or recommendation, personal statements on the American Medical College Application Service (AMCAS) application, supplemental application forms, and interviews.

Letters of Evaluation or Recommendation
In order to complete an application to most medical schools, students must submit letters from their college's premedical committee or from several science professors or other faculty with whom they have worked and who can describe important character qualities.

Personal Statement on the AMCAS Application
Each student must complete a uniform computer-based national application that has as one of its component parts, a "personal state-

ment" section, wherein the student can write on any topic (AMCAS). Most committees search personal statements for both positive comments and "red flags" that may indicate questionable or potentially negative aspects of a student's background. When made available to the interviewer, the personal statement serves as a potential resource for discussion. Committees are especially alert to the disclosure of personal or academic situations generally associated with attrition from medical school. On the positive side, if students choose to provide insightful, personal comments about their experiences and growth, they may add value to the final review of their candidacy.

Supplemental Application

Admissions committees sometimes require students to answer a series of questions in a supplemental application designed to develop insights into the students' level of altruism, empathic skills, and personal values and beliefs. Many medical schools also use their supplemental applications to determine why a student has chosen to apply to that particular school. Responses on supplemental forms offer the admissions committee more information about various aspects of the applicants' personalities, including whether they have demonstrated the desired humanistic behaviors. Questions might include those aimed at determining a candidate's level of responsibility in other-person–directed activities, leadership activities, and organization/time management. Questions may also seek responses that reveal the individual's challenging life experiences and coping ability, as well as values and beliefs that have guided daily living. Committee members use the student responses to acquire new information, to corroborate information in the letters, or as a prompt for further discussion during interviews.

Interviews

Although interviews are time-consuming and expensive, they can produce valuable information, and medical schools have long relied on them to ascertain important personal traits. In a 1990 survey, Mitchell (1990) found that 99% of medical schools used some form of interview as part of their selection process. Another survey, in 1992, corroborated Mitchell's findings, concluding that 99% of U.S. medical schools interviewed applicants (Nayer 1992).

Data Gathered During the Campus Visit

In addition to the formal interview(s), several opportunities exist to assess prospective students when they come to campus. These include a chance to meet enrolled students through an overnight host program or during interviews. Schools keep admissions staff members on the front line to answer applicants' questions. These informal exchanges serve as important recruitment tools for schools, although they have the added value of providing the admissions committee with an ability to detect unusual behavioral changes between the more relaxed informal environment and the interview.

Limitations of Noncognitive Measures

No current studies appear to exist that *first* define critical professionalism traits, then systematically assess relevant noncognitive admissions data to determine their reliability and validity. However, Kulatunga-Moruzi and Norman (2002a) did publish study results on the predictive validity of data gleaned from the McMaster Medical School admissions process, which uses a series of admissions tools that enable the committee to give greatest weight to noncognitive criteria. As testament to their seriousness about noncognitive weighting, the school does not require the MCAT, nor does it require specific course prerequisites. Kulatunga-Moruzi and Norman undertook this study after the Medical Council of Canada's Licensing Examination (LMCC, part II) began to include reliable and valid multistation objective structured clinical examinations (OSCEs) designed to measure communication and problem exploration. McMaster's admissions tools assess both these areas, providing an excellent opportunity to assess the reliability and validity of these variables against selected LMCC results. In a regression analysis, the researchers found that their noncognitive admissions tools did not predict success in either communication or problem exploration, and that traditional cognitive measures—science and cumulative undergraduate—GPA—have the most utility in predicting future academic and licensing exam performance. The authors noted that regression analyses research unfortunately yields low correlations between the predictor and the outcome variables. They stated that the "low correlation can be interpreted in two opposing ways: that the admissions measures have poor predictive validity simply because the correlations are low, or paradoxically, that the predictors are working as intended, selecting a homogenous cohort at the very top of the ability range with low correlation reflecting the lack of variability among the very best" (Kulatunga-Moruzi and Norman et al. 2002b, p. 44).

Since none of the McMaster noncognitive admissions measures proved useful in predicting performance on the LMCC part II communication and problem exploration skills component, Kulatunga-Moruzi and Norman (2002a) chose to examine other cognitive variables and focused on the VR score of the MCAT. (Even though Mc-Master does not require MCAT scores, applicants tend to have them because they are applying to other Canadian medical schools that do.) This particular regression analysis yielded a final R value of 0.50, which accounted for 25% of variance. Given the statistical significance of this finding, the authors concluded that the VR score of the MCAT is a valid predictor of communication skills as assessed on the LMCC part II.

Arnold (2002) questions whether some or all elements of professionalism are present in premedical students or whether these develop in different stages of their medical careers. Baldwin (2003) postulates that professionalism "includes and builds upon a core of epigenetic, evolving, interrelated and interactive elements—humanism, morality and spirituality—all of which have their own developmental sequences" (p. 8). Baldwin believes that teaching in the pre-clerkship years should place emphasis on issues of morality and humanism, with focus on peer relationships, conflicting roles, and the moral dilemmas that students deal with on a daily basis. He believes that the teaching of professionalism should come later—when medical students have become physicians and can understand the greater complexities that constitute professionalism (Baldwin 2003). If further research concludes that applicants should be held accountable for specific preprofessional behaviors, a national task force would need to factor this into the development and assessment of a revised AMCAS personal statement that incorporates the concept of a supplemental application (see An Ideal Admissions Process, below). Should research show that professionalism occurs in developmental stages as suggested by Baldwin, it would be unfair to assess traits that emerge only with greater clinical experience.

Letters of recommendation or letters of evaluation. Ferguson et al.'s (2002) comprehensive review of the literature on factors associated with success in medical school revealed no data showing that letters of recommendation had any predictive value in identifying students' subsequent academic or clinical achievements. He noted that this finding was consistent with the conclusions of other studies on the value of references in other occupations.

One of the major difficulties with either individual letters or those from a premedical committee is that the writer may not be aware of the students' academic ability or personal qualities. Some premedical program personnel work with hundreds of students and simply don't come to know them on a personal level. Their letters tend to be standardized, containing factual information about courses taken and grades received. On the other hand, faculty in small colleges or universities may have much greater knowledge of their students and will include commentary on student behaviors in their letters, thus classifying these as letters of evaluation. Admissions committee members quickly become familiar with those schools that have letter writers who provide accurate, reliable information about their candidates, and consequently, they place more weight on these in the final decision-making process.

Over the years, many undergraduate programs with premedical students have made efforts to codify important and desired areas of information in their letters. Yet a true understanding of a candidate's personal qualities—those important to recognizing whether someone possesses the capabilities to become an exemplary professional—will not be available to an advisor with limited time and resources.

Personal statements on the AMCAS application. In an article entitled "Assessing Personal Qualities in Medical School Admissions," Albanese et al. (2003) state, "A literature search yielded no citation of its [the personal statement] being used or evaluated to assess personal characteristics of the applicant. This would seem to be an untapped resource" (p. 318).

Stern and colleagues reported on a detailed qualitative analysis of the predictive power of admissions essays as a tool for identifying professional behavior in the clinical years. Coding for common themes across an entire medical school class, they found no relationship in bivariate analyses between the presence of any theme and future professional behaviors as identified in the third year of medical school. The authors identified significant predictors only in domains where students had opportunities to demonstrate conscientious behavior or humility in self-assessment during the first 2 years after entrance to medical school (Stern et al. 2005).

A few research studies examining the use and value of personal statements furnished little evidence that they help predict early, preclinical success (Roth et al. 1996). Although it is the one consistent noncognitive source for all applicants, personal statements provide inconsistent information, since neither AMCAS nor the medical schools dictate their content. Thus, this document fails to provide reliable or valid data in the selection process. Another difficulty with the personal statement is that there is no guarantee that the candidate actually wrote it. Students have numerous opportunities to receive assistance in writing through the Internet, test-preparation organizations, and health professions advisors, as well as from parents, family, and friends.

Supplemental application. During the fall of 2003, on the listserv for the Group on Student Affairs of the AAMC, admissions' deans questioned the benefit of retaining supplemental applications. While some felt they were losing applicants who chose not to apply to schools that required an additional form, others felt the required form helped eliminate candidates unwilling to make an extra effort. Although responses on supplemental applications provide valuable data, the questions are not standardized and applicant responses vary widely, rendering them unreliable and invalid as an admissions tool.

The interview. Several interesting research studies examined whether data gleaned from the interview process helped predict which candidates would become competent, humanistic clinicians. Albanese et al (2003) noted that many studies have sought evidence for the value of the interview and that the results show that the reliability and validity of interview data "have been equivocal."

Even if an admissions committee has identified important assessment criteria, most interviewers have significant latitude in defining "most important traits," making their efforts of low reliability. Interviews tend to be loosely or moderately structured, with interviewers generally receiving minimal training in interview techniques. Interview formats can be highly variable: one or two interviews per applicant on a one-on-one basis, panel interviews with multiple faculty members and a single applicant, one or two faculty members interviewing a panel of students, student interviews, administrative interviews, open-file interviews, and closed file interviews. Given this variability, coupled with interviewer latitude, the Albanese et al. (2003) finding that interview data is "equivocal" is not surprising.

In her 1990 study, Mitchell determined through survey analysis that only 47% of the medical schools engaging in interviews collected valid assessment data. Edwards et al (1990) concluded from their research that interviewer bias posed one of the major problems with interviews, leading to low validity and reliability. They contend that "bias can arise from a number of sources, including but not limited to rater tendencies, stereotyping, and interviewer background" (p. 170). Harasym et al. (1996) concluded that interviewer variability accounts for 56% of the total variance in interview ratings.

Kelman and Canger (1994) conducted two studies to assess the value of the applicant interview in identifying the important attributes of communication, problem-solving ability, and social responsibility/dedication to professional service. In the first study, the authors discovered no extant relationship between earlier interview scores and later clinicians' assessments of the same characteristics. In their second study, they assessed the characteristics of two entering classes, one of students who had been interviewed and one of students who had not. Using selected characteristics, the authors found that faculty members were unable to distinguish between the two student cohorts. According to these authors, the most frequently cited interviewer errors that prevent reliability and validity include

> over-weighting the first impression (snap judgment), over-generalizing from one trait to another (the halo effect), order effect (being first or last in a series of biases due to an interviewee who made a strongly positive or strongly negative impression), losing control of the interview, naive views about the relationships between traits (e.g., persons with red hair are emotionally volatile) and biases due to stereotypes about gender, race, national origin, sexual preference or handicap. (Kelman and Canger 1994, p. 2)

An interesting aspect of interviewer bias is the effect of an applicant's "personality" on decisions. In researching the question "Do interviewers seem to make judgments about applicant personality?" Jelley et al. (2003) considered (1) the extent to which medical admissions interviewers evaluated specific personality traits in the interview, (2) the impact of perceptions of personality on individual admissions decisions, and (3) the interrater reliability of personality perceptions. Using a semistructured interview process, the authors asked a three-person panel to complete a research-generated personality-rating instrument concurrent with the normal admissions interview. Three hundred forty-five interviews were completed. The authors hypothesized that certain personality traits did, in fact, affect the interview panel members' final weighting either positively or negatively. Data disclosed that the following personality traits are likely to have a positive effect on a candidate's overall score: achievement, cognitive structure (perfectionism, accuracy), dominance, endurance, nurturance, and order. Conversely, Jelley et al. (2003) found that traits of excessive abasement, impulsivity, and aggression carried negative weight. From their data, the authors determined that significant correlations exist between personality ratings and interview scores.

Data gathered during the interview process. Albanese et al. (2003) suggest that "much can be gained from the non-interview portion of the campus visit" (p. 319), and that medical schools adopt the 360-degree evaluation model now being used by the Accreditation Council for Graduate Medical Education and the American Board of Medical Specialties. One of the difficulties with the 360-degree approach, however, is the lack of consistency among those with whom the candidates interact when they come for interviews. The admissions process tends to span 7 months, and within that period, applicants meet a wide range of individuals, including highly critical and noncritical medical students, admissions front desk personnel who may change over time, and various overnight hosts. Given the number and type of reviews furnished unsystematically by numerous individuals, the information provided may be biased and unfair.

Summary of Cognitive Versus Noncognitive Measures

Both grades and MCAT scores will always play a key role in any selection process since they prove critical in predicting competency and retention. However, these variables measure neither motivation nor the ability to achieve important professionalism traits, and relying exclusively on them may have adverse effects. These can include student attrition, with commensurate cost implications to the school, and, more important, rejecting deserving candidates who would have been excellent students and fine physicians. Another significant consequence has been that in the last decade, as high GPA and MCAT scores have become the standard for medical school selection, college students have invested the majority of their time in academics, to the detriment of engaging in experiences that offer opportunities to learn about themselves and their values. Many students enter medical schools without having tested their ability to handle responsibility, without knowing the depth of their coping skills from engaging in challenging experiences outside their comfort zone, and without having participated in sustained activities that enable them to understand the personal sacrifices that true commitment to others requires.

Today's medical student bodies have become highly diverse, not only racially and ethnically, but also in terms of life experiences and career motivation. Sedlacek (2004) argues that diverse individuals have different experiences and different ways of demonstrating their attributes and abilities. Thus, he concludes, it will be difficult to develop a single cognitive or noncognitive measure or test item that would prove equally valid for all. Rather, he states,

> we should concentrate on results (students with the greatest degree of professionalism) rather than intentions, such that we could conclude that it is important to do a good job of selecting for each group (majority, minority, nontraditional, etc.), not that we need to use the same measures for all to accomplish that goal. (p. 33)

An Ideal Admissions Process

In a perfect world, medical schools would orchestrate the admissions process in a sophisticated, effective manner dedicated to recruiting and selecting competent, humanistic students with the greatest potential for sustaining high levels of professionalism throughout their lives. With this worthy goal in mind, an ideal admissions process would begin well before a candidate submits an application and continue beyond that candidate's matriculation. Many of the elements described here can also be used appropriately in residency and practice settings.

Prior to Admission

Revise the AMCAS personal statement to include questions aimed at attaining both contextual, and experiential information about student experiences, values, and beliefs. Questions should reflect research findings on the developmental stages of professionalism. In order to allow for variation in institutional goals and missions, 8–10 questions should be developed for general use, and individual schools should choose the six most suitable for their needs. These answers would provide the basis for in-depth questions during the interview. Content areas could include (1) challenges to students' values and beliefs as they encounter experiences outside their comfort zone (detail the experience and talk about exploration of values and beliefs); (2) challenging life experiences that required creative thinking to develop solutions (detail each situation and describe why the solution was considered creative); (3) a self-reflection piece that provides insight into a student's demonstrated conscientiousness; (4) an example of an experience in which communication proved difficult and an analysis of how the situation might have been handled differently; (5) a description of the means by which the student learned about commitment to medicine, providing the reader insight into the knowledge and understanding gleaned from the experience; (6) moral and ethical dilemmas that arose out of interpersonal relationships—how they were handled and what lessons were learned; (7) leadership positions that taught a lesson; and (8) the University of Michigan's item, "an experience in which cultural diversity—or lack thereof—made a difference" (Schmidt 2003). Modifying the AMCAS personal statement in this way would negate the need for individual school supplemental applications.

Devise a system by which to score the AMCAS personal statement and train AAMC reviewers to use it, much as the AAMC has trained reviewers to score the writing skills section of the MCAT examination. This admissions tool would serve as an important noncognitive filter to eliminate students whose low scores reflect the fact that they have not had the relevant experiences.

Standardize the interview process by developing a model that medical schools can adopt, preferably one that uses multiple mini-interviews as described in the research findings of Eva et al. (2004) below. This would necessarily involve devising a means by which medical schools can train standardized interviewers to perform the interviews and assess the findings, developing case studies to be used in interviews, and devising a behaviorally anchored evaluation instrument that builds on the AMCAS personal statement and focuses on important aspects of professionalism, communication, and interpersonal skills. Standardized case studies are necessary both to ensure their quality and, as Eva et al. (2004) point out, to include enough variability that each applicant has a "first-time" experience in answering questions.

Actions to Be Taken by Prematriculation Advisors

Provide applicants with the questions found on the AMCAS personal statement. Advisors would work with students to identify appropriate experiences that would address the questions on the AMCAS personal statement. The advisor would develop a portfolio for each premedical student, and the student would craft a piece reflecting on personal growth and insights gained as each experience is completed. The advisor would meet regularly to discuss the student's portfolio entries. From ongoing discussions with the student throughout the college years, the advisor would be able to glean information on such areas as (1) how well the student works as a part of the team, (2) the student's level of maturity and judgment, and (3) the student's overall orientation to service. The close relationship between advisor and student, along with accumulated data, will enable the advisor to construct a quality letter of evaluation that more accurately reflects a student's level of empathy, conscientiousness, creativity, and motivation. Such information would greatly aid admissions committees in identifying candidates who have the greatest strengths in areas of professionalism, communication, and interpersonal skills (Note: in 2004 J. R. Suriano submitted a grant proposal to the Arnold P. Gold Foundation for a pilot project based on this model).

Actions to Be Taken by Individual Medical Schools

Establish admissions policies that take into account issues of diversity as well as professionalism. As it relates to diversity, such policies should heed the recommendation of the AAMC Executive Committee (2004) that "medical schools should base their admissions policies on an explicit articulation of legitimate aspirations: to achieve the educational benefits of a diverse student body, including enhancing the cultural competency of all the physicians it educates and improving access to care for underserved populations" (p. 2). Enrolling a diverse student population in our medical schools will ultimately ensure greater ability to create sound patient–physician relationships, resulting in professional care to individuals in all segments of society (AAMC Executive Committee 2004).

Develop an applicant weighting system to determine whether a student meets an academic threshold. Using data accrued from previous graduates, including composite GPA and MCAT scores, establish the threshold necessary for success in the medical school's program. Kulatunga-Moruzi and Norman (2002a) demonstrated that the VR section of the MCAT was a reliable and valid predictor of the communications segment of the LMCC part II. After 2005, U.S. medical schools could enjoin with the National Board of Medical Examiners following the first administration of the U.S. Medical Licensing Examination step 2 clinical skills examination, and perform a similar analysis to that of Kulatunga-Moruzi and Norman (2002a) on the communications section. To the extent that VR proves a reliable and valid predictor of communications, this score could receive increased emphasis in developing the academic threshold. The school's weighting system should also factor in experiences, college attended, difficulty of the major, excellence in advanced course work in the major, and the rigor of the academic workload. Other items that should be included are extenuating circumstances such as illness, death in the family, and the need to work to fund one's own education.

Publish cognitive and noncognitive data depicting information of previous successful applicants. The key to fairness in the admissions process lies in furnishing applicants with published data against which their ratings will be compared. In these more litigious times, access to greater specificity about the admissions process would benefit everyone involved. Thus, the critical first step is for medical schools to fully disclose its desire for students who have demonstrated through their experiences and personal behaviors those traits central to humanism and professionalism. Currently, too many candidates guess at the formula they believe most likely to gain them acceptance, with a majority convinced that grades and MCAT scores are the only aspects of their application that truly matter (and schools have tended to reinforce this). Thus, applicants invest extensive time and effort into producing a perfect numerical record, while forgoing life-enriching experiences. Disclosing the school's selection criteria would encourage potential applicants to concentrate on other important areas of development.

St. George's Hospital Medical School in the United Kingdom provides an example through its disclosure document, "Medical School Admissions Policy: Arrangements to Prevent Unfair Discrimination." The section entitled Admissions Process in Detail contains a subsection entitled Non-academic Personal Qualities, which delineates those qualities that the school seeks in its students in three major areas: communication and motor skills, personal attitudes and attributes, and personality. Each area contains questions that applicants must answer on-line, giving examples or evidence to illustrate or support their answers. In addition, the questionnaire seeks information about the applicant's insight into a medical career, reasons for wanting to be a doctor, and perspectives on personal limitations (St. George's Hospital Medical School 2003).

It will take considerable effort on the part of medical schools to determine the attributes and experiences they consider critical in their students and to make available printed and on-line material that outline these in detail. The information must clearly point out the attributes of professionalism that the school considers critical in its students. The information should also describe the variety of experiences in which the school expects its students to engage before entering medical school, particularly those that support interest in research, primary care, rural medicine, teaching, community service, and serving the underserved, such that they can successfully respond to questions on the AMCAS personal statement. Emphasis will be given to the important humanistic behaviors being sought and to the baseline academic performance needed for admission.

Restructure the interview process to encompass the standardized interviewer approach as suggested below.

The Admissions Process at the Individual Medical School

Initial screening of applicant through cognitive measures. The admissions committee would review each applicant using the school's previously developed weighting system. The admissions dean would review the file of each applicant who fails to pass this screen to ensure fairness to the candidate.

Initial screening through noncognitive measures. AMCAS personal statement: In this ideal admissions process, all medical schools would accept the modification of supplemental questions, and AAMC trained reviewers would score this segment of the AMCAS application.

Letters of evaluation or recommendation: Because premedical advisors have worked one on one with students throughout their college years, their letters would contain information about the nature of the student's experience, the degree of achievement, insight gained, and personal growth as well as about important attributes of professionalism that center on integrity, respect, empathy and compassion. Given that there will still be variability, schools will need to develop a scoring system for letters that factors into their final selection.

Interviews: Kevin Eva and colleagues at McMaster capitalized on the research findings of Kulantunga-Mourzi and Norman to construct an admissions system focusing on the interview process. They developed multiple mini-interviews modeled after OSCE type stations. Eva et al. (2004) describe the concept of multiple mini-interviews, which they claim are neither "objective" nor "clinical" but build on the concept of the multistation OSCE presently used by nearly all medical schools in North America. They chose four domains for station development: critical thinking, ethical decision making, communication skills, and knowledge of the health care system. Recognizing that interviews are plagued by context specificity, the authors designed 10 short stations that present scenarios requiring applicants to discuss a health-related issue, interact with someone from their standardized patient group to discern strengths in interpersonal skills, and answer standard interview questions. They rated the reliability of the multiple mini-interviews at 0.65, based on their tests of two student populations at McMaster (Eva et al. 2004).

In an ideal admissions process, standardized interviewers would become the norm, rather than having faculty or admissions committee members interview applicants on an ad hoc basis. A training process would enable institutional faculty to qualify to serve the institution's needs. In keeping with the study by Eva et al. (2004), students would go through some sort of admissions OSCE. Many of the stations would make use of standardized case studies. Some of the stations could use video technology to depict moral and ethical dilemmas, followed by questions from the standardized interviewer. Other stations would offer an opportunity for interviewers to directly observe and rate interpersonal skills and communication styles through constructed cases in which the candidate participates. If the work of Eva and others proves particularly useful, one might even argue for a national admissions OSCE, rather than multiple individual school-level examinations as part of the application process.

Given that most medical schools use the interview day as a time for recruitment, setting aside an additional hour beyond the time required for the standardized interviewer process could create an opportunity for enrolled students and faculty to provide specific information about the school and to answer questions.

Key to the success of the standardized interviewer process is the buy-in of the school, adequacy of high-quality case studies, and a sufficient cadre of trained faculty available to manage those chosen for interviews.

Rating applicants: Using the nationally designed, behaviorally anchored evaluation tool, interviewers would rate each applicant and compile scores that would be added to those obtained from the AMCAS personal statement and letters of evaluation. The admissions committee would then weigh all the relevant cognitive and noncognitive scores and make its final selection.

Subsequent to the admission process. Create a portfolio for each entering student: The student's advisor or the Dean of Student Affairs would create a portfolio that contains all the information collected from the admissions process, the AMCAS personal statement and the score given, the standardized interview reports and scores, and any relevant notes that would help the school develop a baseline for the student's level of professionalism.

Meet with the entering student: Initially the dean/advisor would meet with the student to review the baseline data in the student portfolio and to develop a plan for professional growth. The dean/advisor would continue to meet regularly with the student throughout the four years of medical school to proffer academic and personal counseling geared toward facilitating the development of professionalism attributes. From the outset, the dean/advisors should help students understand that there are no "perfect" medical students and that being one is not the goal. Rather, the plan involves ensuring systematic professional development, which includes holding students to specific professional standards. Students should be advised that they can meet these standards through course work, community service, and other means devised by the school.

Use OSCEs to assess various competencies after years 1, 2, and 3: Scores and comments derived from these OSCEs should be used to assess clinical skill development and to determine how well the student is progressing in terms of professionalism, communication, and interpersonal skills.

Maintain the student portfolio: Information derived from the OSCEs would be included in the student portfolio, as would records of extracurricular activities that facilitate personal and intellectual growth. Also included in the portfolio would be notations on research, leadership, or community service experiences, along with the student's written comments describing the learning experience and insights gained. When the student reaches the fourth year, the documents in the student portfolio would be forwarded to the Dean of Student Affairs, who would use the data to write the Dean's Letter (now known as the Medical Student Performance Evaluation).

Challenges to Making the Ideal Admissions Process Work

Making significant changes in the admissions process will require, first, a consensus among medical schools that such changes are needed and second, that the possibility for such change exist. The following issues represent challenges to reaching consensus:

1. Gaining national acceptance for change and enlisting all schools in the process of change;
2. Agreeing on the value of assigning weight to noncognitive experiences in the selection process;
3. Establishing a range of acceptable GPA and MCAT scores for matriculating students, that is, identifying a floor below which a student will not be accepted;
4. Willingness of each school to publish data on acceptable GPA and MCAT ranges and a statement of important professionalism traits desired in entering students;
5. Agreeing on a modification of the requirements of the AMCAS personal statement to specifically identify areas the student must address;
6. Agreeing on the content areas to be included on the AMCAS personal statement;
7. Developing the AMCAS personal statement in a manner that does not give entrepreneurial individuals/companies an opportunity to devise answers for students at a price;
8. Developing a cadre of trained standardized interviewers;
9. Developing a wide array of case studies for interviews so that students cannot prepare for specific cases described by previous applicants;
10. Establishing research studies on information derived from case studies;
11. Getting premedical advisors to change their approaches to working with students and agree to the more time-consuming, one-on-one relationship needed to help students construct their student portfolios;
12. Getting deans/advisors in medical schools to set aside the time to meet regularly with students.

With the dedication of medical educators, these challenges can be met. Changes in the admissions process would afford a number of benefits, in addition to the primary one of selecting students with outstanding attributes of professionalism. In light of this established goal, admissions committees would be empowered to give greater weight to assessing important noncognitive attributes, a critically important step. The consistency of approach in the process would, over time, increase the opportunities for research to identify valid and reliable criteria for making selections. Data gathered during the admissions process will offer an excellent understanding of where students stand developmentally, enabling schools to more effectively tailor their curricula to meet their needs.

Since the majority of medical students eventually graduate and are then faced with new and increasing requirements related to accreditation, licensure, certification, and recertification, it behooves medical schools to assist them in attaining the highest standards of professionalism. This commendable mission begins with the admissions process. All schools should make a concerted effort to move from the current process to one that emphasizes the selection of students with the potential to become the outstanding professionals that the schools and the public want and expect.

References

AAMC Executive Committee. Status of the new AAMC definition of "underrepresented in medicine." Association of American Medical Colleges, March 19, 2004.

AAMC Newsroom. Applicants to U. S. medical schools increase [press release]. Association of American Medical Colleges. Available at: http://www.aamc.org/newroom/pressrel/2003/031104.htm. Accessed November 5, 2003.

Albanese M, Snow MH, Skochelak SE, Huggett KN, Farrell PM. Assessing personal qualities in medical school admissions. Academic Medicine, 2003; 78: 313–321.

AMCAS. American Medical College Application Service. Washington, DC: Association of American Medical Colleges, 2004: 353.

Arnold L. Assessing professional behavior: yesterday, today and tomorrow. Academic Medicine, 2002; 77: 502–513.

Baldwin DC Jr. Toward a theory of professional development: framing humanism at the core of good doctoring and good pedagogy. Presented at the Arnold P. Gold Foundation Overcoming the Barriers to Sustaining Humanism in Medicine Symposium VI, New York, January 2003.

Bombardieri M. Princeton plan seeks to ease grade inflation. Boston Globe. April 8, 2004.

Edwards JC, Johnson EK, Molidor JB. The interview in the admissions process. Academic Medicine, 1990; 65: 167–177.

Elam CL, Stratton TD, Scott KL, Wilson JF, Lieber A. Review, deliberation and voting: a study of selection decisions in medical school admissions committee. Teaching and Learning in Medicine, 2002; 14(2): 98–103.

Eva K, Rosenfeld J, Reiter H, Norman G. An admissions OSCE: the multiple mini-interview. Medical Education, 2004; 38(3); 314–326.

Ferguson E, James D, Madeley L. Factors associated with success in medical school: systematic review of the literature. British Medical Journal, 2002; 324 (7343): 952–957. Available at: http://www.pubmedcentral.nih.gov/articlerender.fcgi?artid=102330. Accessed September 20, 2003.

Greenlaugh T. Storytelling should be targeted where it is known to have greatest added value. Medical Education, 2001; 35: 818–819.

Harasym PH, Woloschuk W, Mandin H, Brudin-Mather R. Reliability and validity of interviewers' judgments of medical school candidates. Academic Medicine, 1996; 71(suppl): 540–542.

Hojat M, Gonnella JS, Mangione S, et al. Empathy in medical students as related to academic performance, clinical competence, and gender. Medical Education, 2002; 36: 522–527.

Jelley R, Parkes M, Rothstein M. Personality perceptions of medical school applicants. Medical Education Online [serial on line], 2002; 7: 11. Available at: http://www.med-ed-online.org/res00038.htm. Accessed September 20, 2003.

Kelman E, Canger S. Validity of interviews for admissions evaluation. Journal of Veterinary Medical Education 1994; 21: 2 Available at: http://scholar.lib.vt.edu/ejournals/JVME/V21–2/kelman.html. Accessed September 25, 2003.

Kulatunga-Moruzi C, Norman G. Validity of admissions measures in predicting performance outcomes: the contribution of cognitive and noncognitive dimensions. Teaching and Learning in Medicine, 2002a; 14(1): 34–42.

Kulatunga-Moruzi C, Norman G. Validity of admissions measures in predicting performance outcomes: a comparison of those who were and were not accepted at McMaster. Teaching and Learning in Medicine, 2002b; 14(1): 43–48.

LCME. 2004. Functions and structure of medical school: standards for accreditation of medical programs leading to the M.D. degree. Washington, DC: Liaison Committee on Medical Education.

McManus IC. Factors affecting the likelihood of applicants being offered a place in medical schools in the United Kingdom in 1996 and 1997: a retrospective study. British Medical Journal, 1998; 317: 1111–1116.

Mitchell K J. Traditional predictors of performance in medical school. Academic Medicine, 1990; 65: 149–158.

Nayer M. Admission criteria for entrance for physiotherapy schools: how to choose among many applicants. Physiotherapy Canada, 1992; 44: 41–46.

Powell L. 1978. Bakke, 438 V.S. at 312–313n.48.

Powis DA. Selecting medical students. Medical Education, 1994; 28: 443–69.

Rhoads JM, Gallemore JL, Gianturco DT, Osterhout S. Motivation, medical admissions and student performance. Journal of Medical Education, 1974; 49: 1119–1127.

Rigol G, Kimmel E. A picture of admissions in the United States. New York: College Entrance Examination Board. Unpublished manuscript. 1997.

Roth PL, BeVier CA, Schippmann JS. Meta-analyzing the relationship between grades and job performance. Journal of Applied Psychology, 1996; 81: 548–556.

Schmidt P. U. of Michigan will use application essays to help enroll diverse undergraduate class. Chronicle of Higher Education, August 29, 2003. Available at: http://chronicle.com/weekly/vol50/02/02a02801.htm.

Sedlacek WE. Multiple choices for standardized tests, 1998. AGB Priorities 1998; 10: 1–15. Available at: http://www.agb.org/_content/priority/past/v10n1/covnd97.htm.

Sedlacek WE. Why we should use non-cognitive variables with graduate and professional students. The Advisor: The Journal of the National Association of Advisors for the Health Professions 2004; 24(2): 32–39.

St. George's Hospital Medical School. Medical school admissions policy: arrangements to prevent unfair discrimination. Available at: http://www.nottingham.ac.uk/medical-school/school/admissions_policy.html. Accessed October 7, 2003.

Stern DT, Frohna AZ, Gruppen LD. The prospective prediction of professional behavior. Medical Education, 2005; 39(1): 75–82.

Sternberg R. Beyond IQ. London: Cambridge University Press, 1985.

Sternberg R, Lubart TI. Investing in creativity. American Psychologist, 1996; 51: 667–688.

14

Assessing Professionalism for Accreditation

Deirdre C. Lynch, David C. Leach, and Patricia M. Surdyk

If medicine and education are moral enterprises (Eisner 2003), it follows that medical education has a substantial responsibility to help learners and teachers do the right thing (Leach 2001). Accrediting organizations play an important role in determining what the "right things" are. Assessing professionalism for accreditation means that educational programs are judged on their ability to foster professionalism. Implementation of this initiative, however, is still relatively new. Thus, this chapter addresses an important initial consideration: how to organize professionalism assessments to meet educational program goals.

Accreditation is a process for articulating standards and determining whether programs or institutions meet them. In the United States, the Accreditation Council for Graduate Medical Education (ACGME) is the accrediting body for allopathic residency training programs that prepare physicians for independent practice after they have graduated from medical school. Medical schools are accredited by the Liaison Committee on Medical Education. This model contrasts with that of Canada, where medical schools and residency programs are accredited by the same organization, the Royal College of Physicians and Surgeons of Canada. Accreditation differs from certification, which is the process for determining whether an individual meets discipline-specific requirements (ACGME 2003). To be certified in a specific specialty in the United States, an individual physician must meet established requirements set by the board for that specialty.

The ACGME provides the mechanism by which the medical profession self-regulates graduate medical education (GME). Physicians, selected by their peers, determine whether residency training programs meet established educational standards. The ACGME accredits 7,878 residency programs in the United States, with about 99,000 residents (ACGME 2003b). It has three points of leverage: residency programs must be accredited to obtain government funds, residents must have attended an accredited residency program to apply for board certification, and physicians seeking state licensure must have completed training in an accredited residency program (Leach 2001).

In parallel with the outcomes movement in patient care, the ACGME began to move accreditation away from a focus on processes and structures to focus on educational outcomes. Examining a program's actual accomplishments changes the accreditation question "Can you educate?" to "What is the evidence that you have educated?" (Swing 2003). Consequently, in 1999, the ACGME board of directors approved a plan that would require GME programs to teach and assess residents in six general competencies (in addition to other requirements): professionalism, patient care, interpersonal and communication skills, medical knowledge, practice-based learning and improvement, and systems-based practice (ACGME 1999). The competencies should be integrated into practice; they are not meant solely as discrete behaviors. Professionalism, for instance, can be observed with practice-based learning and improvement when residents reflect on their performance and ask themselves, "How could I have done it better?" It can be associated with systems-based practice when residents seek and collaborate with community-based resources to aid and maintain patient health or with interpersonal and communication skills and with patient care when residents are respectful in their interactions with others. Professionalism is therefore central to the development of new physicians.

GME is a rich arena for examining professionalism because it evokes the ability to meet the relationship-centered expectations required to practice medicine competently (Kuczewski et al. 2003; Surdyk et al. 2003). Medicine is a cooperative endeavor; relationships unite the practice of medicine and the construct of professionalism. GME can be understood in terms of these relationships (Leach and Stevens 2001) wherein residents must learn with whom to interact and how to interact with them in order to complete the tasks of residency. Key relationships for residents include those with patients, peers, supervising physicians, medical students, and other health care workers (Surdyk et al. 2003).

GME has three goals: Its immediate goal is to aid resident learning, its intermediate goal is to improve the process of patient care, and its long-term goal is to have a positive impact on patient outcomes. The purpose of this chapter is to describe an organizing framework for integrating these goals in the assessment of professionalism.

Designing a System to Assess Professionalism

Planning a system to assess professionalism requires answers to six questions.

Why Assess Professionalism?

There are at least two reasons to assess professionalism. The first reason is to gauge learners' abilities and the second reason is to aid curriculum or program improvement. With regard to learners, two critical questions must be addressed: (1) should professionalism be assessed to determine whether learners meet a given standard (i.e., summative assessment), or (2) should it be assessed to determine learner's strengths and weaknesses to aid subsequent teaching and learning (i.e., formative assessment)? Formative assessment is predicated on the belief that learners can change, and some evidence indicates that components of professionalism can be improved. With targeted, defined interventions, the research suggests it is possible to change specific professional attitudes and beliefs (e.g., Hayes et al. 1999; Tang et al. 2002), reasoning (e.g., Godkin and Savageau 2001; Self and Olivarez 1996), and behaviors (e.g., Beckman et al. 1990; Phelan et al. 1993). From the perspective of accreditation, professionalism should be both formatively and summatively assessed. These two systems of assessment can potentially achieve both the immediate goal of aiding resident learning (formative) and the longer term goals of improving patient care and patient outcomes (summative). In both cases, learners should be apprised of the purpose and criteria of assessment early in the education process.

What Should Be Assessed?

The process of deciding what to assess begins with broad questions about content and outcome domains and advances to specific questions about the most important expectations. This is part of the process of establishing content validity of assessment, and these decisions can be aided by examining the relevant literature, asking experts to identify key expectations, and making sure that what is assessed parallels the educational goals and objectives. It is not feasible to assess all aspects of professionalism in all contexts; thus, it is necessary to select a sample of what will be assessed. The sample should consist of the most important and representative expectations for a given specialty and developmental level. Culhane-Pera and Reif (2003), for instance, have determined that advanced family medicine residents should be able to "incorporate patients' desires into medical care" (skill) and "accept responsibility to understand cultural issues in health and illness" (attitude).

A relationship-centered perspective on professionalism provides a framework for identifying the content of professionalism curricula. Examples of professionalism within each type of relationship include (1) patient–physician: being careful and thorough when performing physical examination, considering patients' cultural preferences during treatment planning, disclosing all relevant information about health status and treatment effects; (2) society–physician: collaborating with governmental agencies to reduce health care costs, participating in initiatives to improve health care safety, providing services to poor patients; (3) health care system–physician: involving other health care providers when appropriate, interacting respectfully with other health care providers, participating in cross-department improvement activities; (4) physician–physician: teaching medical students and residents, consulting with expert peers when needed, lobbying for professional group membership needs that do not compromise societal needs; (5) physician–self: self-reflecting on performance, identifying areas that need improvement, balancing personal and professional activities. In the case of professionalism, outcomes in the affective, cognitive, behavioral, and environmental domains are interrelated. Thus, each of these levels should be captured at some point, possibly sequentially, by assessment. Since medical education ultimately strives to affect patient care indicators, the ideal assessment system would also include assessments that capture this level (table 14-1).

How Should Professionalism Be Assessed?

The fundamental technical requirements of assessment are that it yields valid and reliable (credible) data. The practical requirement is that it must be feasible. The credibility of high-stakes, summative assessments such as certifying examinations depend greatly on the technical characteristics of a single instrument, which is used to assess the same individual relatively infrequently. Alternatively, residency education provides other approaches to enhancing data cred-

Table 14-1 An Organizing Framework to Assess Professionalism

Outcome category	Type of outcome	General assessment method	Example assessment
Learning	Affective	Resident questionnaire	Schwartz Values Scale (Eliason and Schubot 1995)
	Cognitive	Cognitive test	Barry Challenges to Professionalism Questionnaire (Barry et al. 2000)
	Behavioral	Focused observation	Ethics OSCE (Singer et al. 1996
Practice	Patient care processes	360-degree, focused observation	Musick 360-Degree Assessment (Musick et al. 2003), Modified Amsterdam Attitude and Communication Scale (DeHaes et al. 2001)
	Other relationships	360-degree	Musick 360-Degree Assessment (Musick et al. 2003)
Results	Environment	Resident survey	Scale to Measure Professional Attitudes and Behaviors in Medical Education (Arnold et al. 1998)
	Patient care outcomes	Patient survey	Wake Forest Physician Trust Scale (Hall et al. 2002)

ibility. During residency, it is possible to use various assessment methods, to assess over time, and to access various assessors. Tapping into these parameters helps to provide a more complete picture of resident abilities, thus enhancing data credibility.

Regarding multiple methods, each assessment method has strengths and weaknesses. Rating forms, although considered relatively easy to use, can be biased by raters' gneral impressions of learners (Gray 1996). The Ethics Objective Structured Clinical Examination (Ethics OSCE) may mitigate the latter weakness but requires several cases, and hence testing time, to obtain stable estimates of learner performance (Singer et al. 1996). Consequently, using more than one assessment method helps to compensate for the weaknesses associated with any single approach, thus enhancing data validity. Because professionalism is a complex construct, it is unlikely that a single assessment will adequately measure it. Using a combination of assessments, however, such as a cognitive test together with direct observation is more desirable. Finally, using multiple methods improves validity due to the enhanced scope and depth of information obtained, which provides more information about learners' abilities.

Who Conducts the Assessment?

Different types of assessors should be involved. Research indicates that different assessors offer different perspectives, thus enhancing the breadth and thus validity of assessment (Wooliscroft et al. 1994). Multiple assessors enhance reliability (Swanson 1987). Studies indicate that it is feasible for nonphysician co-workers, for instance, to assess residents (Butterfield and Mazzaferri 1991; Musick et al. 2003). As with the administration of any effective assessment, assessors should also be interested in education and be willing to participate in training required to improve assessment or be experienced assessors.

When Should the Assessments Be Given?

To be congruent with a formative approach and to enhance data credibility, assessment should begin early (Lowe at el. 2001), be conducted frequently, be implemented long-term, and provide learners with opportunities to change (Van Luijk et al. 2000). Summative assessment occurs at key transition points during training, including program completion.

Where Should Assessment Take Place?

Ideally, assessment should be conducted at various sites to identify context specific issues that influence learner professionalism. The context specificity of professionalism assessment is a fundamental challenge to measurement, as outlined in chapter 1. Measuring professional behaviors as close as possible to real-life contexts can aid data validity.

Assessing Professionalism in GME: An Organizing Framework and Example Assessments

As mentioned above, GME has three goals: Its immediate goal is to aid resident learning, its intermediate goal is to improve the process of patient care, and its long-term goal is to have a positive impact on patient outcomes. Paralleling these goals are three outcome categories: learning, practice, and results (Miller 1990; Kirkpatrick 1998). Learning can be gauged by examining postteaching changes in the affective, cognitive, and behavioral domains. Practice can be gauged by examining performance in applied settings such as the hospital. Results can be gauged by examining practice impact (table 14–1). Below we describe how an individual program could address all three goals of GME for the competency of professionalism using existing instruments. (Please note the general assessment methods and example assessments in table 14–1 are intended to stimulate thinking on this topic and are not mandated by the ACGME.)

Learning

Affective outcomes encompass personal values, opinions, and beliefs about, or attitudes toward, pertinent issues; these are collectively referred to as meaning schema. When it comes to assessing professionalism, why does information about affective outcomes matter? The rationale for behavior can be partially explained by an individual's meaning schema (McClelland 1985). In other words, some aspects of professionalism are related to personal values. Exemplary family physicians, for example, consider honesty to be the most important personal value and social power the least important (Eliason and Schubot 1995). Instruments have been designed to assess affective outcomes for components of professionalism such as ethics or personal characteristics. Examples of these include the Coverdale Attitudes Toward Doctor's Social and Sexual Contact with Patients Questionnaire (Coverdale and Turbott 1997) and the Baldwin Cheating Questionnaire (Baldwin et al. 1996), which contains items such as "in the long run cheating doesn't really hurt anyone."

The purpose of such instruments in a system designed to measure professionalism may be threefold. The first is to gauge learners' meaning schema to tailor relevant course content. For example, if an instructor discovered that residents had positive attitudes toward dating patients, then teaching content could be developed to address the topic of professional relationships with patients. Second, these assessments may be used as a teaching tool to help learners identify and reflect on their own attitudes and values so that they may subsequently engage in discussions about these issues and their relationship to medical professionalism. A third reason to use assessments that measure affective outcomes involves determining whether participation in interventions designed to improve professionalism change learners' meaning schema.

Cognitive outcomes focus on knowledge or reasoning about professionalism. Identifying the behaviors involved in professional lapses may delineate what happened but do not always reveal why the lapses occurred. Thus, information about cognitive rationales behind professional behavior or lapses thereof can help to inform instructional strategies. An example might involve a resident leaving an emergency to write patient notes because he did not know his presence was required. Instruments designed to assess the cognitive aspects of professionalism include the Barry Challenges to Professionalism Questionnaire (Barry et al. 2000) and the Wenger Orthopaedic Surgeons Ethics Questionnaire (Wenger and Lieberman 1998). Both address contemporary issues in medicine, such as resolving conflicts of interest, dealing with incompetent colleagues, and communicating honestly with patients. Although these cognitive tests have been used for research purposes with residents and practicing physicians, they can easily be applied to education to help gauge learners' knowledge about professional issues and to stimulate discussion. Another way to assess cognitive aspects of professionalism is to conduct focus group sessions with learners. The advantage of this approach, which requires group participants to generate professionalism issues, is that it can reveal learners' perceptions of the meaning of professionalism and how it is apparent in their daily activities (Ginsburg et al. 2002).

Behavioral outcomes encompass actions that can be directly observed by others. Professional behavior has been assessed via simulations such as encounters with standardized patients (Prislin et al. 2001) and the Ethics OSCE (Singer et al. 1996). Due to strong interest in assessing professional behavior in applied settings versus simulations, however, the behavioral assessment of professionalism is addressed further below.

Practice

Practice can be ascertained by examining performance in applied settings. Thoroughness as a characteristic of professionalism, for example, can be assessed by observing the completeness of residents' physical examination of patients; respect as another characteristic can be assessed by observing resident interactions with patients. Generally, two broad approaches are used to assess professional behaviors in applied settings. One approach involves assessment based on impressions of a learner derived from interacting with or observing him or her over a given period of time. At the end of the time period, assessors document their impressions by rating items on a performance rating scale or, less commonly, by writing notes. This approach is often exemplified in the end-of-rotation evaluation forms typically completed by supervising physicians. Until relatively recently, if included at all, professionalism was denoted in such forms by one or two global items such as, "acts professionally" or "meets responsibilities." More recently, however, some end-of-rotation evaluation forms expand from a single global professionalism item to a few items or include descriptive anchors for points along the scale on which a single professionalism item is measured. Although these steps advance assessment of professionalism, a more notable improvement is the use of 360-degree assessments where various health care professionals assess learner professionalism (e.g., Musick et al. 2003). An example of early work in this area is Butterfield's Nurse Evaluation of Medical Housestaff Form designed to aid nurse evaluation of resident professionalism (Butterfield and Mazzaferri 1991).

In the second approach to the behavioral assessment of professionalism in applied settings, learners are directly observed and assessed during specific tasks or focused activities that typically involve a patient encounter. Observations are recorded on checklists or performance rating forms either during or soon after the encounter. The Amsterdam Attitudes and Communication Scale is an example of this approach (DeHaes et al. 2001). It was designed to assess professionalism and communication skills; thus, professionalism is measured by six of nine items.

Results

Results refer to the impact of professionalism in applied settings. With regard to professionalism, two categories of results, namely, environmental outcomes and patient care outcomes, are important. Environmental outcomes pertain to the context in which teaching and learning occurs. This type of information addresses the behavior of learners, their peers, teachers, supervisors, co-workers, and relevant others. Other important environmental information includes policies, rules, expectations, traditions, routines, and reporting relationships. Why does an environmental index of professionalism matter? The educational environment, whether through formal or informal curricula, appears to influence learner attitudes and behavior (Brownell and Cote 2001; Feudtner et al. 1994; Stern 1996). Furthermore, research suggests that business and cultural environments influence professionalism among practicing physicians (Freeman et al. 1999; Hoffmaster et al. 1991). Consequently, assessments that gauge professionalism in the environment may also provide insight into the professionalism of individuals. At least two questionnaires have been designed to measure professionalism in the educational environment as reported by residents: the Baldwin Survey of Resident Reports of Unethical and Unprofessional Conduct (Baldwin et al. 1998) and the Scale to Measure Professional Attitudes and Behaviors in Medical Education (Arnold et al. 1998).

Patient care outcomes refer to the impact of health care, such as improving health or satisfying patient expectations. Professionalism is related to results in the following areas: patient compliance, satisfaction, trust, selecting and changing physicians, and legal action (Hall et al. 2002; Hickson et al. 2002; Hauck et al. 1990). Regarding professionalism, feedback from patients appears to be the most frequently used assessment method. Feedback may be obtained by survey or by patient complaint records. Although the latter can provide useful information, complaints typically pertain to a small subset of health care providers, thus precluding feedback about all physicians. The American Board of Internal Medicine (ABIM) Patient Satisfaction Questionnaire was designed to assess physicians' communication skills and professionalism. With only 10 items, it is relatively easy to administer. Like many patient surveys, however, it tends to yield negatively skewed data; thus, feedback from many patients is required to obtain stable estimates of performance. Tamblyn et al. (1994) found, for instance, that 25–30 patient surveys were needed per resident. On the other hand, the Wake Forest Physician Trust Scale (WFPTS) appears to yield less skewed data; thus, it may require fewer samples (Hall et al. 2002). Also a 10-item scale, the WFPTS contains such items as "[Your doctor] will do whatever it takes to get you all the care you need"; therefore, it is more oriented toward professionalism areas than is the ABIM questionnaire, which mostly addresses communication skills. Construct validity of the WFPTS was inferred from positive correlations between trust (as measured by the WFPTS) and satisfaction, willingness to recommend to friends, and length of time with physician. Criterion validity was inferred from a positive relationship between WFPTS ratings and those from another validated instrument that measured trust. Interitem reliability of data yielded from the WFPTS is high at 0.93 and test–retest reliability is acceptable at 0.75. In sum, the WFPTS appears to be both a credible and feasible questionnaire for obtaining patient feedback about physician professionalism.

Conclusion

Professionalism is not new to medicine. In the past, however, it was referred to in terms of noncognitive abilities, ethics, and personal qualities. Furthermore, it was typically considered desirable but not necessary material for explicit teaching and assessment. Now, as one of the six general competencies for the ACGME, programs are expected to foster professionalism and graduating physicians should be able to demonstrate professionalism. Gauging and detecting changes in professionalism are impossible without measurement, but measurement is challenging because professionalism (unlike procedural skill sets, which consist of discrete steps) is a complex construct. A first step to address this challenge is to use a systems approach to measurement. Important systems variables encompass purpose and use, methods, personnel, timing and frequency, and setting. An organizing framework and example assessments are presented here to advance a previous prototype for assessing professionalism in GME (ACGME 2002) and to stimulate more thinking about this topic.

Although we describe broad steps for incorporating the competency of professionalism into accreditation, the ACGME views implementation as a complex process (Bertalaffy 1969) where effective strategies will likely emerge and evolve over time. Because it focuses on programs (vs. individuals), accreditation offers a unique and useful perspective on assessing professionalism. GME programs consist of sets of relationships—the substance of professionalism. Good programs, therefore, are likely to foster professionalism among residents, faculty, and other key players. Credible data about individuals' professionalism should be used to improve the program, which in turn will do a better job of fostering professionalism. Progress will also occur when the links between professionalism and patient care indicators become apparent. In the long term, focusing on professionalism will lead to models of excellent approaches to teaching, assessing, and integrating professionalism into medical education and care so that ultimately there will be "good learning for good health care."

References

ACGME. General competencies. ACGME Outcome Project, Accreditation Council for Graduate Medical Education. 1999. Available at: www.acgme.org/outcome/comp/CompFull.asp. Accessed October 15, 2003.

ACGME. List of Accredited Programs and Sponsoring Institutions. In: About the ACGME. Accreditation Council for Graduate Medical Education. 2003b. Available at: www.acgme.org/adspublic/. Accessed October 15, 2003.

ACGME. Outcome Project Think Tank. ACGME Outcome Project. 2002. Available at: http://www.acgme.org/outcome/project/thinktank.asp. Accessed October 15, 2003.

ACGME. Essentials of Accredited Residencies in Graduate Medical Education. In: GME Useful Information. Accreditation Council for Graduate Medical Education. 2003a. Available at: http://www.acgme.org/adspublic/. Accessed October 15, 2003.

Arnold, E., L. Blank, K. Race, and N. Cipparrone. Can professionalism be measured? The development of a scale for use in the medical environment. Acad Med. 1998;73:119–121.

Baldwin, D. C. Jr., S. R. Daugherty, B. D. Rowley, and M. D. Schwarz. Cheating in medical school: a survey of second-year students at 31 schools. Acad Med. 1996;71:267–273.

Baldwin, D. C., S. R. Daugherty, and B. D. Rowley. Unethical and unprofessional conduct observed by residents during their first year of training. Acad Med. 1998;73:1195–1200.

Barry, D., E. Cyran, and R. J. Anderson. Common issues in medical professionalism: room to grow. Am J Med. 2000;108:136–142.

Beckman, H., R. Frankel, J. Kihm, G. Julesza, and M. Geheb. Measurement and improvement of humanistic skills in first-year trainees. J Gen Intern Med. 1990;5:42–45.

Bertalaffy, L. General systems theory. New York: George Braziller, 1969.

Brownell, A. K. W., and L. Cote. Senior residents' views on the meaning of professionalism and how they learn about it. Acad Med. 2001;76:734–737.

Butterfield, P. S., and E. L. Mazzaferri. A new rating for use by nurses in assessing residents' humanistic behavior. J Gen Intern Med. 1991; 6:155–161.

Coverdale, J., and S. Turbott. Teaching medical students about the appropriateness of social and sexual contact between doctors and their patients: evaluation of a programme. Med Educ. 1997;31(5):335–340.

Culhane-Pera, K.A., and C. Reif. Ramsey's five levels of cultural competence: conceptualizing Bennett's model into curricular objectives for multicultural medical education. Ann Behav Sci Med Educ. 2003;9:106–113.

DeHaes, J., F. Oort, P. Oosterveld, and O. ten Cate. Assessment of medical students' communicative behaviour and attitudes: estimating the reliability of the use of the Amsterdam Attitudes and Communication Scale through generalisability coefficients. Patient Educ Counsel. 2001; 45(1):35–42.

Eisner, E. The educator and professionalism: knowing how to look. Paper presented at the ACGME and ABMS conference Fostering Professionalism: Challenges and Opportunities; September 19, 2003; Chicago.

Eliason, B. C., and D. B. Schubot. Personal values of exemplary family physicians: implications for professional satisfaction in family medicine. J Fam Prac. 1995;41:251–256.

Feudtner, C., D. Christakis, and N. Christakis. Do clinical clerks suffer ethical erosion? Students' perceptions of their ethical environment and personal development. Acad Med. 1994;69(8):670–679.

Freeman, V. G., S. S. Rathore, K. P. Weinfurt, K. A. Schulman, and D. P. Sulmasy. Lying for patients: physician deception of third-party payers. Arch Intern Med. 1999;159:2263–2270.

Ginsburg, S., G. Regehr, D. Stern, and L. Lingard. The anatomy of the professional lapse: bridging the gap between traditional frameworks and students' perceptions. Acad Med. 2002;77:516–522.

Godkin, M., and J. Savageau. The effect of a global multiculturalism track on cultural competence of preclinical medical students. Fam Med. 2001; 33(3):178–186.

Gray, J. D. Global rating scales in residency education. Acad Med. 1996; 71(10 suppl):S55–S63.

Hall, M.A., B. Zheng, E. Dugan, F. Camacho, K. E. Kidd, A. Mishra, and R. Balkrishnan. Measuring patients; trust in their primary care providers. Med Care Res Rev. 2002;59:293–318.

Hauck, F.R., S. J. Zyzanski, S. A. Alemagno, and J. H. Medalie. Patient perceptions of humanism in physicians: effects on positive health behaviors. Fam Med. 1990;22:447–452.

Hayes, R. P., A. Stoudemire, K. Kinlaw, M. Dell, and A. Loomis. Changing attitudes about end-of-life decision making of medical students during third-year clinical clerkships. Psychosomatics. 1999;40:205–209.

Hickson G. B., C. F. Federspiel, J. W. Pichert, C. S. Miller, J. Gauld-Jaeger, and P. Bost. Patient complaints and malpractice risk. JAMA. 2002;287: 2951–2957.

Hoffmaster, C. B., M. A. Stewart, and R. J. Christie. Ethical decision making by family doctors in Canada, Britain, and the United States. Soc Sci Med. 1991;33:647–653.

Kirkpatrick D. L. Evaluating training programs. 2d ed. San Francisco: Berrett-Koehler, 1998.

Kuczewski, M., E. Bading, M. Langbein, and B. Henry. Fostering professionalism: the Loyola model. Camb Q Healthcare Ethics 2003;12: 161–1666.

Leach, D. C. Changing education to improve patient care. Qual Health Care. 2001;10(suppl 2):54–58.

Leach D. C., and D. P. Stevens. Substance, form, and knowing the difference. Front Health Serv Manage. 2001;18:35–37.

Lowe, M., I. Kerridge, M. Bore, D. Munro, and D. Powis. Is it possible to assess the "ethics" of medical school applicants? J Med Ethics 2001; 27:404–408.

McClelland, D C. How motives, skills, and values determine what people do. Am Psychol. 1985;40:812–825.

Miller, G. E. The assessment of clinical skills/competence/performance. Acad Med. 1990;65(9 suppl):S63–S67.

Musick, D. W., S. M. McDowell, N. Clark, and R. Salcido. Pilot study of a 360-degree assessment instrument for physical medicine and rehabilitation programs. Am J Phys Med Rehabil. 2003;82:394–402.

Phelan, S., S. Obenshain, and W. R. Galey. Evaluation of non-cognitive professional traits of medical students. Acad Med. 1993;68:799–803.

Prislin, M. D., D. Lie, J. Shapiro, J. Boker, and S. Radecki. Using standardized patients to assess medical students' professionalism. Acad Med. 2001; 76(10 suppl):S90–S92.

Self, D. J., and M. Olivarez. Retention of moral reasoning skills over the four years of medical education. Teach Learn Med. 1996;8:195–199.

Singer, P., A. Robb, R. Cohen, G. Norman, and J. Turnbull. Performance-based assessment of clinical ethics using an objective structured clinical examination. Acad Med. 1996;71(5):495–498.

Stern, D. T. Values on call: a method for assessing the teaching of professionalism. Acad Med. 1996;71(10 suppl):S37–S39.

Surdyk, P. M., D. C. Lynch, and D. C. Leach. Professionalism: identifying current themes. Curr Opin Anaesth. 2003;16:597–602.

Swanson, D. B. A measurement framework for performance based tests. In: Further developments in assessing clinical competence: proceedings of conference held in Ottawa, Ontario, June 27–30, 1987 (I. Hart and R. Harden, eds.; pp. 13–45). Montreal: Can-Heal Publications, Inc., 1987.

Swing, S. R. The Outcome Project: an introduction. In: ACGME Outcome Project. Accreditation Council for Graduate Medical Education. 2003.

Available at: http://www.acgme.org/outcome/project/OutIntro.htm. Accessed October 3, 2003.

Tamblyn, R., S. Benaroya, L. Snell, P. McLeod, B. Schnarch, and M. Abrahamowicz. The feasibility and value of using patient satisfaction ratings to evaluate internal medicine residents. J Gen Intern Med. 1994; 9:146–152.

Tang, T. S., J. C. Fantone, M. E. Bozynski, and B. S. Adams. Implementation and evaluation of an undergraduate sociocultural medicine program. Acad Med. 2002;77:578–585.

Van Luijk, S., J. Smeets, J. Smits, I. Wolfhagen, and M. Perquin. Assessing professional behaviour and the role of academic advice at the Maastricht Medical School. Med Teach. 2000;22(2):168–172.

Wenger, N., and J. Lieberman. An assessment of orthopaedic surgeons' knowledge of medical ethics. J Bone Joint Surg. 1998;80(2):198–206.

Wooliscroft, J., J. D. Howell, B. P. Patel, and D. B. Swanson. Resident-patient interactions: the humanistic qualities of internal medicine residents assessed by patients, attending physicians, program supervisors, and nurses. Acad Med. 1994;69(3):216–224.

15

Measuring Professionalism: A Commentary

Fred Hafferty

This volume establishes a new benchmark within ongoing efforts to define, assess, and ultimately construct learning environments to promote medical professionalism across medicine's educational trajectory. What began in the mid-1980s as medicine's response to the mercurial rise of corporate medicine has evolved into a rather formidable organizational movement. Debates as to meanings and measures, curricula, and competencies have been vigorous and visible—a healthy sign. What is not healthy is the very real possibility that educational authorities will anoint a particular measure or methodology as "the one" and thus (even indirectly) announce that the "professionalism problem" has been solved. This would be a grave mistake (*American Journal of Bioethics* 2004). While no one questions (as a general principle) the need to develop ever more sophisticated assessment tools and strategies, great care must be taken within this empirical quest not to reduce professionalism to a "static thing"—a conceptual mass at rest. At its most elemental level, professionalism is an *action system,* sharing some of the properties of quantum physics. Like particles that do not exist in the absence of movement, professionalism is best viewed as residing within a system of social action. As such, professionalism must not be approached (or configured) as something that can exist external to or independent of context. In turn, the social and interactive nature of professionalism demands that the medical education community (which includes faculty, students, administrators, and practicing clinicians) has a fiduciary responsibility to keep the professionalism "debate" ever alive and ever vibrant.

Socialization: The Engine of Professionalism

The formal identification of professionalism as a "core competency" (chapter 14) brings new challenges to medical training. Early studies of medical school by Robert K. Merton and colleagues (*The Student-Physician*, 1957) and Howard Becker and colleagues (*Boys in White*, 1961) devoted considerable attention to physician socialization. In fact, these two studies were designed, in large part, to test core sociological theories about socialization, with the Merton study adopting a traditional socialization perspective (e.g., the internalization of core medical values) while Becker found training to be more situational and temporary in its impact (Hafferty 2000). Over the ensuing decades, however, the concept of socialization, like that of professionalism, began to lose its critical cache. "Professionalism" became an adjective (e.g., a "professional effort"), as well as a general social claim to technical expertise and/or product quality (e.g., professional-strength toilet bowl cleaner). Socialization, meanwhile, became a synonym for "training."

Defining professionalism as a competency puts brakes on this backsliding—at least, it should. Framing professionalism as a competence turns a critical gaze toward how it is supposed to be attained and how the process of attainment is supposed to be accessible to the individual via self-reflection (chapters 11 and 12), to peers via peer review (chapter 10), and to external evaluators for the purpose of certifying that competency (chapter 14). It also forces us to re-examine and then make explicit whether we consider professionalism to be an object of socialization-as-internalization (the "Merton" camp) or to be a part of an overall strategy of situational adaption (the "Becker" camp). Such specification needs to happen prior to the development of measurement tools, because the tools themselves will reflect this underlying distinction (whether we want them to or not). Being more analytically critical about professionalism and socialization comes with the added benefit of making explicit something that has long (too long) been considered a natural by-product of medical training. In other words, one becomes "professional" by virtue of qualifying for the M.D. degree. Defining professionalism as a competency, however, makes everything more explicit—at least in principle. However, there remains considerable danger (and self-deception) if we label professionalism as a competency and yet continue to treat it as axiomatic. As I argue below, if we set our standards such that virtually everyone (except for medicine's ubiquitous "one or two bad apples") attains that status, then this will distort the notion of competency. Attainment must be problematic,—not automatic. Furthermore, maintenance of this competency must be treated as contingent—not complementary.

Ultimately, medicine must avoid the self-serving inconsistency of claiming to establish professionalism as an internalized and deep competency (chapter 12) while willing to settle for graduates who manifest it only as at a surface phenomenon. Such fence sitting, of course, calls into question just how core professionalism is to the nature and identity of medicine. A professionalism that is deep must exist at the level of identity. Surface professionalism, on the other hand, is nothing more than doing one's job in a "professional manner." Surface professionalism sidesteps issues of identity and treats professionalism as something physicians can put on and take off like one's stethoscope. Professionalism as a deep competency might generate the same behavior, but the behavior in question is more real/authentic because the behavior is consequentially linked to the social actor's underlying identity (as a professional) rather than to how the job was carried out (in a professional manner). Although sociologists would frown at the use of "authentic" in this context, it does help to make the point of whether we want professionalism to be a "who" or a "what." Do we want physicians who are "professional," or will we settle for physicians who can act in a "professional" manner (the what)?"

This brings us to the issue of how best to measure professionalism. By tying much of the assessment of professionalism to observable behaviors, this book leaves substantially underaddressed the deep-surface distinction, along with the socialization-as-internalization versus socialization-as-situational-adaptation distinction. Nonetheless, a few of the chapters do highlight the internalized, identity-based and therefore deep version of professionalism (chapters 7, 11, and 12) despite the challenges of validating these internal and very personal changes in what it means to be a professional person.

Measurement Issues

Authenticity and Professionalism

Medical students are socialized across a variety of curricula (e.g., the formal, informal, and hidden curriculums) to be acutely sensitive to "what faculty want and this fact demands that we pay particular attention to the presence of power and social hierarchies within the structure of medical education. Issues of legitimacy aside, medical students spend an inordinate amount of time "scoping out" their learning environments to determine who they are (statuswise), what they will be held responsible for, and who has the power to hold their noses to the pedagogical grindstone. They want to know what will be on the next test, just as they seek to establish what kinds of questions their attending physicians will ask during the transient, time-limited, and evanescent interactions with patients, faculty, and peers that comprise clerkship and residency education (Christakis and Feudtner 1997).

As exemplified by *Boys in White* (Becker et al. 1961), the theoretical perspective of symbolic interactionism (chapter 10) has played an important role in understanding the process and impact of medical training. Using symbolic interactionism theory, we can see how medical students are engaged in a constant process of "impression management" (Goffman 1959, 1967) as they struggle to control and ultimately routinize their physical, social, and emotional environments (Christakis and Feudtner 1997; Bucher and Stelling 1977). The hierarchical nature of medical training adds both intensity and poignancy to students' efforts to garner the approval of their superiors and to avoid loosing face (Clouder 2003; Haas and Shaffir 1977) as they seek to acquire a cloak of competence (Haas and Shaffir 1982). Regardless of their personal insights and self-reflective abilities, all medical students are acutely aware that faculty evaluate behavior not simply as evidence of skills or as reflections of knowledge but also as indicators of manifested attitudes. In other words, students expect faculty to treat conduct, such as industriousness or altruism, as windows into students' inner qualities. As such, I wonder what will happen when medical educators inform students, via measures of professionalism, that inner states do not matter and that only behaviors "count."

Furthermore, there is a thin line (sociologically speaking) between issues of impression management and gaming. Whether it be in the form of cheating (with a negative connotation) or coping skills (with its more positive connotation), these behaviors have particular relevance for professionalism and its measurement. The problem of providing socially acceptable answers plagues instruments that rely on self-reporting or multiple-choice formats because respondents (in our case, medical students) quickly learn—within the ambiguities that mark medical knowledge—to differentiate between answers that are technically correct versus answers that faculty want. This is a reality of medical training. To avoid this bias in assessment, one must either move to more realistic contexts (e.g., faculty and peer performance appraisals) or create situations in which students feel free to provide honest responses rather than those that are socially acceptable (e.g., formative reflection, portfolios, peer assessment).

More fundamental to the formation of a professional character is whether impression management is "unprofessional"—at least within the context of professional education. The question is a difficult one to answer, in part because what is and what is not considered appropriate behavior within the culture of medicine can be so variable (e.g., note the different rates of professional lapses reported for obstetrics-gynecology and surgery in chapter 9). Like much of social life, "it depends." Medical students, for example, seek to provide themselves with moral space or buffers by defining issues of normative behavior as "situational"—rather than universal. Whether cheating (e.g., using crib notes) is considered inappropriate by medical students depends on such things as "importance of the class" or whether a test is considered "fair." In short, the exact same behavior may be seen by students as reprehensible in one context (an important pharmacology exam) while justified in another (a "Mickey Mouse biostats class"). All of this "situating" leaves us with a rather important question. At what point does finessing one's way through a clerkship cross that invisible line and become "unprofessional" rather than the frequently referenced (and implicitly justified) presence of "coping skills" or "adaptive behaviors"?

A further question speaks to the concept (and process) of professional socialization. Are medical students *obligated* to cooperate with the socialization process in the quest to create a professional self? The image of cohorts of medical students marching lock-step to the normative chant of their professors has a certain disquieting and Fascist ring to it. Nonetheless, because being (or becoming) a professional is considered foundational within organized medicine, we must ask how much leeway students have within their subculture regarding impression management practices. If professionalism is good—and the overall thrust of this book assumes this to be the case—then it would appear that medical students are at least somewhat obligated not only to acquire the knowledge and skills of their professional calling but also to internalize its core values.

Conversely, perhaps it is enough only to *appear* professional, at least so that patients, staff, and other co-workers believe that someone is carrying out their work in a concerned and concerted manner. After all, why should it be crucial (all within the context of "being professional") that one behave with an underlying motivation and self-identity that is professional in nature? Time and again, the message in this book is to assess behavior. However, professional identity is at best an indirect aspect of behavior, and most certainly a different dimension. It will be interesting, over time, to see whether organized medical education will stop with behaviorally based measures or whether it will move aggressively to tap these other dimensions. Of even greater interest will be whether medical education will move beyond assessing individuals and formal-structural units such as departments or clinical services to constructing (and assessing) overall learning environments where the use of impression management techniques (by both students and physicians) would be considered (by all) to be unnecessary, improper, and normatively devalued.

On Language and Professionalism

Assessing professionalism is a difficult and morally "touchy" issue. The upsides of being labeled a professional, or the downsides of being considered lacking in this respect, carry great moral weight within medicine. Whatever the underlying psychometric properties of our measurement tools, special care must be directed toward the terms and concepts we employ in those assessments. In short, we need to play special attention to our language of failure and our vocabulary of success. Furthermore, because any measure will (hopefully) discriminate (technically speaking) among students, we must be willing to wrestle with the presence of both professionalism "stars" and "slouches"—namely, those students who score markedly higher or lower than their classmates as a whole. Ultimately, we need a language of assessment that captures the presence of these outliers.

With all of this in mind, the prevailing terminology used in this book to indicate the absence of professionalism is notable. For the most part, it is an absence represented by the term "lapse," a characterization that appears in other publications, as well (Arnold 2002; Ginsburg et al. 2000, 2002; Lingard et al. 2001; Whitcomb 2002). While I do not wish to imply that there is a perfect lexicon, a professionalism of "lapses" is troubling in three key respects. First, a professionalism that operates within a language (and standard) of lapses is a far different professionalism than one rooted in a language of transgressions, errors, or violations. "Lapse" connotes a particular relationship between the social actor and his or her actions. It is a language of distance, as if the act in question is not only unusual but also uncharacteristic of that person's character and motives. It connotes a slip, a gaffe, or an oversight rather than a mistake. Furthermore, a lapse (as a slip or gaffe) is not something that occurs with malice or forethought.

Second, medicine already has a language of mistakes and shortcomings (and accompanying rationalizations) by which physicians manage troubling events (Lingard et al. 2001; Bosk 1979). How, then, does "lapse" jibe with the underlying standards implied by the well-recognized term "critical incident" (Branch et al. 1993, 1997)? Can something as benign and innocently sounding as a lapse (e.g., a flub or foible) really be considered a critical incident? Furthermore, what do we do about the fact that one physician's "lapse" is another's "mistake" or "transgression"? A case in point is the implicit underreporting of lapses described in chapter 9 and in George (1997) and Self et al. (1992).

A third problematic aspect of lapse involves the subdefinitions that are built into this term. The usual connotation of lapse is that of one "slipping away from," but from what? The implicit message is a slippage from an already established and functioning platform of professionalism. However, if professionalism truly is developmental, how do we have lapses among neophyte trainees—individuals whose professional stature is more embryonic than formed?

Norm-Referenced Versus Criteria-Referenced Standards

The fact that professionalism can be approached from within two standards, norm referenced and criteria referenced (chapter 6), provides us with yet another opportunity to step back and ask how we want to think about professionalism. Should professionalism be evaluated from within the context of a reference group (e.g., peers), or should it be assessed via standards generated by, for example, an expert panel? My own preference is for criteria-based assessment. We are, after all, quite early in the professionalism assessment business. The fact that most medical students enter medical school with little understanding of why medicine is a profession and/or why physicians are professionals (try asking this during a medical school interview and see what kind of answers you get) suggest that criteria-based assessment provides faculty and students with more opportunities to identify (and identify with) core elements of professionalism, than the more informal standards or definitions that might circulate within a given reference group. The fact that students qua students function within their own subculture, along with the parallel fact that most "instruction" about professionalism still takes place within the hidden and informal curricula, practically assures us that student and peer-generated conceptions of professionalism will be different from (and perhaps even antagonistic to) those definitions held by faculty and/or advanced by administration. As long as the language of professionalism has some cache within the occupational culture of medicine, and as long as the term "professional" is used within and around medical work, students are learning about professionalism—a lack of formal instruction notwithstanding. The lessons learned might not be exemplary, and the definitions may be far from authoritative, but students still will internalize lessons—incorrect definitions and all. As one example, and recalling a definition offered in chapter 6, I am fairly certain that current medical students, residents, and faculty do not view professionalism as "a reciprocal covenant of expected and learned behaviors among students, faculty, and institutions" (with the emphasis here being professionalism as a "reciprocal covenant"). Norm-referenced measurement may be more helpful once standards have been established and anchored within group culture, but not before.

A similar rationale can be extended to a debate referenced in chapter 6 between focusing our efforts on assessing professionalism at the extremes of our population (the "stars" and "slouches") versus seeking to scale professionalism so that we can track, over time, the professionalism of all individuals or cohorts. My own position is that we know too little about the trajectory of professionalism across the course of medical training to reject the insights that are gained by tracking both performance and change. At the same time, organizations have legitimate concerns with social control regarding professionalism, particularly those whose low scores suggest the need for remedial action or a sanctioning response.

The Sensitivity and Specificity of Professionalism: Context Matters

Once we decide what we want to measure and the terms we wish to employ, how will we know when we have assessment tools capable of establishing the presence or absence of these social entities with a reasonable degree of certainty? In other words, and borrowing from the language of clinical decision making, how do we establish the "sensitivity" and "specificity" of our new assessment tools? What will we use for our gold standard (for calibration purposes)? Finally, what will we call the absence and presence of "disease"? In our case, and for remainder of the present discussion, "disease" will be the absence of professionalism (1—false negative rate), while the "absence of disease" is the presence of professionalism (1—false positive rate).

However, reflecting clinical medicine, we are not interested in the probability of a positive test given the presence of disease ($P[T+/D+]$, or sensitivity) or the probability of a negative test given the absence of disease ($P[D-/T-]$, or specificity). Instead, we want to know the antithesis, the probability of disease (or its absence) given a positive (or negative) test result. In short, we want to know the predictive value of our assessment tools. However, predictive value requires one additional piece of information to complete our assessment. We need to know the prior probability of disease (or how likely is it, prior to running our test, that our "patient" has, or does not have, the condition in question?).

This last piece of information is of critical importance because we know that the ability of a diagnostic test to "rule in" and/or "rule out" disease is *extremely* dependent on the prior probability (the prevalence) of disease in the relevant population (Motulsky 1995). How, then, do we propose to develop measurement tools to diagnose something (professionalism and/or its absence) within a culture where almost everyone is considered a "star"? If our prevalence is accurately reflected by the phrase "one or two bad apples," then what we have is a rather low prior probability of unprofessionalism—something, let us say, below 2%. Based on this standard, we would expect the vast majority of our "test" results (~98%) to be negative—indicating (in our case) the presence of professionalism. Under such conditions (and still operating from within a biostatistical perspective), such a rate also tells us that we need to be far more concerned about false-positive test results (the remaining 2%) than with false-negative outcomes. In other words, within a population that is awash with "stars," we would want to reduce our false-positive rate as much as possible (thereby assuring us that a positive test result really means what it says). In short, we should be far more concerned about falsely identifying a "slouch" as a "star" than about falsely labeling a star as a slouch.

The above discussion only skims the surface of this somewhat unconventional approach to thinking about professionalism and its assessment. One key point (captured within the concept of prior probability) is that diagnostic tests are not "situation neutral." The "worthiness" of any professionalism test (recalling that many contributors to this text advise against developing a unidimensional professionalism rating scale) rests within the general circumstances and context of the assessment. It rests upon the "environmental factors" within which the test will be applied—which includes the prior probability or prevalence of the "condition" in question. In short, there is no such thing as a "context-free" test for professionalism.

Finally, I want to use the above discussion to lobby once again for measurement tools that can discriminate within a given group or population where the modal finding truly is considered (normatively speaking) as "average" and where the distribution around that mode properly captures and identifies outliers that reflect the necessarily present subpopulations of "hyper" and "hypo" professionalism.

Professionalism and the Hidden Curriculum

Educators no longer believe that all (or even a majority) of the learning that takes place during medical training occurs within the confines of what we now term the "formal curriculum." While labels may differ (e.g., explicit vs. tacit, formal vs. informal, stated vs. unstated, real vs. shadow), there are good pedagogic reasons to reject any claim that the authoritative voices of administration and faculty command a singular and privileged place at the curricular table. At minimum, there are at least three distinct domains of medical learning (however labeled): the formal (the officially stated curriculum as it exists in course catalogues and course objectives), the informal (built around the idiosyncratic and happenstance lessons that are learned within the social interactions that weave their way through and around the educational and work settings of clinical medicine), and the hidden curriculum (lessons that emanate from the very structure, process, and content of the educational endeavor, including the "organizational culture" of that particular medical school or residency program; Hafferty and Franks 1994; Hafferty 1999). A fourth concept, with its own academic pedigree, is the "null curriculum" (messages that emanate from what was not taught or said and thus things that become unofficially labeled as "irrelevant," "unimportant," or "not essential"; Burack et al. 1999; Eisner 1985; Stern 1998).

Any meaningful recognition that professionalism transcends the mere issues of technical knowledge and skills *must* be accompanied by the acknowledgment that traditional medical education has, for the most part, relegated the teaching of professionalism to its other-than-formal curricula (Stern 1998). One reason for this rather myopic view of medical learning resides in the aforementioned (and longstanding) belief within organized medicine that physicians become professionals not by virtue of any targeted instruction but simply by virtue of having completed the training process. "Good" basic science teachers took care of the knowledge part, while "good" clinical faculty added relevant skills and knowledge—the end result being a "professional person." This is not to insist that medical education has ever totally ignored issues of pedagogy and professionalism. Medical educators have long and steadfastly acknowledged the importance of such things as role models in the educational process (Linzer and Beckman 1997; Skeff and Mutha 1998; Paukert 2001; Wright et al. 1998). Nonetheless, and up to the present time, the anointing/attribution of the physician as a "professional person" has been more a matter of faith than evidence. Few training programs have taken the necessary steps to formally ensure that what was being conveyed within these relationships was consistent with broader statements about educational goals and professional ideals.

A second problem with these rather optimistic and distancing scenarios that professionalism is something that "just happens" is that data from the shop floor of medical education has consistently portrayed medical training as a rather inhospitable place. Studies in the 1950s by Eron (1955, 1958) documented a shift from idealism to cynicism among medical students—a transformation process in evidence that continues or remains (Goldie 2004; Morris 2000; Testerman et al. 1996). Studies in the 1960s and 1970s (Becker et al. 1961) documented a medical student subculture that was largely invisible to, and off limits for, faculty. Studies in the 1990s began to document the negative impact of the educational process on such things as moral reasoning (Self et al. 1998, 2003) along with the pervasive presence of medical student abuse (Baldwin et al. 1998; Uhari et al.

1994). Physician autobiographies echoed these studies. Such depictions of medical education range from the early and pseudonymous *Intern* by Doctor X (1965) and Samuel Shem's classic *House of God* (1978), through engaging accounts by physicians such as William Nolen (1970) and Robert Marion (1990, 1993, 1998), to highly detailed and analytical tomes from physician-anthropologist Melvin Konner (1987) and Atul Gawande's artfully written *Complications* (2002). Taken as a whole, the image reflected in these sources is "good students—bad schools" (or bad learning environments). Medical school was more damaging than developmental. Students were depicted as learning, almost continuously, but the lessons learned often were not the ones being heralded in course descriptions, in medical school mission statements, or being reported to licensing and certification authorities.

So, what can we do? How are we to measure the impact of all these curricula on the professional development of students? Recognizing that a thorough answer far exceeds the space allotted, a few general guidelines must suffice. First, we need to better understand the lessons being conveyed within the informal and hidden curricula. Although the learning that takes place within the informal curriculum cannot be eliminated (almost by definition), it must be acknowledged as a legitimate source of learning and, when necessary, countered. Meanwhile, change at the level of organizational culture, while admittedly difficult, must be taken on as well—beginning with the acknowledgment that individual medical schools operate as organizational microsystems, each as a discrete and identifiable moral community. Second, all efforts to measure professionalism must acknowledge the multidimensionality of student learning. Assessing only what takes place within the formal curriculum is insufficient. Worse yet, such assessments send messages to medical students (and society) that intent (e.g., *teaching*) matters more than outcomes or consequences (e.g., *student learning*). This is a very stilted (and self-protective) view of education—and a rather sorry lesson (via the hidden and/or informal curriculum) for students to learn about professional responsibilities. Surveys of the organizational professionalism (chapter 6) and peer assessment (chapter 10) provide windows into these more informal settings.

Third, and related, formal steps taken to counter aspects of the informal and hidden curricula must be issue, context, and stage specific. Supersaturating the formal curriculum with perfect pedagogical principles will not, in and of itself, counter the concurrent and negative lessons being conveyed within the informal and hidden curricula. While it is theoretically possible for the hidden and informal curricula to contain "good" messages and to reinforce positive lessons within the formal curriculum (and the formal curriculum does contain many good elements), the fact remains that subcultures are not created to praise Caesar. They are formed in response to, or out of perceived problems within, the dominant culture (or learning environment).

Fourth, all social groups need to celebrate their heroes and denounce their villains. In other words, all social groups require deviance. Supportive social and institutional structures and the positive reinforcement of professional behaviors are all important, but groups also must establish their normative and moral boundaries. "Anything goes," along with adjudication on a literal case-by-case basis, conveys none of the social order that groups require to function effectively over time. For the purposes of this chapter, the concept of deviance captures both positive and negative departures from the norm. The presence of both heroes and villains represents a particular challenge to medical education. Allowing a student caught cheating or a faculty caught falsifying patient records to slip quietly away in the night may satisfy those immediately involved (e.g., the individual student or faculty, and along with various administrators), but it does nothing to inform the greater community as to the outer limits of acceptable behavior, and that these limits are being enforced. In short, we need to avoid creating Lake Wobegon colleges of medicine—where everyone is above average and special because we say it is so and because we like to believe this to be the case (Hafferty 2001). In her autobiographical account of undergraduate training, Perri Klass, describing her first few days of medical school, captures this attributional tomfoolery: "What they tell you, of course, is that . . . some of you will be superb . . . and the rest of you will be merely excellent" (Klass 1987). Garrison Keillor's mythical Lake Wobegon may sound endearing, supportive, and eternally affirmative, but in reality, a community stripped of anything other than "above average" members is highly dysfunctional. Educational strategies such as formative assessment based on critical incident reports (chapter 9), exercises based on personal reflection (chapter 11), and portfolio assessment (chapter 12) can all serve a role, but not if the interpretation, formation, and sanctioning of group norms take place behind closed doors.

Fifth, faculty (basic science, clinical, full time, and "auxiliary") must be on the same page regarding the core competencies identified by their medical school and/or residency program. Standards and their enforcement cannot be carried out on an ad hoc or teacher-by-student basis. Schools must move beyond the current era of educational anarchy, where the number of ways to "best" create "professional" learning environments is set by the number of schools and/or residency programs under consideration. Thus, there are not 125 "best" ways to deliver professionalism at the undergraduate medical education level, nor are there 7,878 ways to do so at the residency level. At the same time, having a singular "best" is creatively stifling and stunts the aforementioned need to maintain a dynamic model of professionalism. The goal of developing "best practices," as noted in chapter 14 on accreditation and professionalism is a positive step. Perhaps something in the middle, with 10 or 20 at the undergraduate level and 100 or so residency models across the various specialties, would allow for both excellence and a continued striving for ever better learning tools.

Professionalism and Altruism

Altruism is the "missing hero" of this book. What once stood as core and definitional has begun to disappear from the professionalism lexicon. Traditional references to, and definitions of, professionalism almost always identify altruism as a/the core principle. When the American Board of Internal Medicine (ABIM) launched "Project Professionalism" in the late 1980s, altruism was clearly and unequivocally identified as *the* core element of professionalism. Similarly, the Association of American Medical Colleges (AAMC) Medical School Objectives Project (AAMC 1998) identified four core medical student competencies (altruism, knowledge, skill, and dutifulness), with the AAMC considering altruism's placement at the head of the quartet to be both intentional and message bearing. By the time the ABIM Foundation, the American College of Physicians–American Society of Internal Medicine (ACP–ASIM) Foundation, and the European Federation of Internal Medicine delivered its Physician's Charter (Members of the Medical Professionalism Project 2002), however, the temper of things had begun to shift. Altruism, as a term and ideal, had begun to fade. In its place stood "primacy of the patient" (as the first of three primary principles identified in the charter). The term "altruism" does appear in this document, but in a supporting role. Altruism has a notable appearance in this present volume (chapter 2, figure 2-1) as one of the four "core principles"/"Corinthians" standing in support of a capstone of professionalism—and yet the term is virtually invisible for the remainder of this book.

There are other movements taking place within medical education and medical practice that chronicle altruism's fall from professional grace. Rowley and colleagues (2000) found that orthopedic physicians ranked altruism 19th of 20 professional qualities in terms of importance to professionalism. In a recent class exercise, first-year students barely 2 weeks into their medical school experience produced similar results by ranking altruism 24th of 25 professional qualities, trailing only by "charity" (Hafferty 2004). The rise of "lifestyle specialties" (Schwartz 1989) and the push for a "balance" between one's professional and personal responsibilities (with personal and professional usually framed as antagonists) point to still other domains of contention and conflict (Croasdale 2003; Dorsey et al. 2003; Schwartz et al. 1990; Henningsen 2002). Over a 6-year period, entering students at one medical school consistently identified altruism as the professional value they most worried about in terms of its potential to negatively affect on their lives (Hafferty 2002, 2004). Rather than an ideal and object of occupational reverence, these students saw altruism as something that would "tie you to your work," with altruistic physicians the ones most likely to be "taken advantage of" by their "manipulative patients." In a similar vein, these same students feared that medicine's power elite (senior residents or faculty) would use altruism as a lever to get them to do more work or to take on unwanted (and, for the students, unwarranted) responsibilities (Hafferty 2002, 2004). In summary, while altruism has not yet been declared passé, the newest generation of medical students, residents, and emerging physicians are wary of what has long been considered a hallmark of the profession. *Altruism has become suspect.* It is something that manipulative patients and senior physicians alike use to exploit the naiveté and powerlessness of students. Far from empowering, it seems that altruism makes physicians weak and vulnerable.

Can there be real professionalism without altruism? I am not sure. On the one hand, I can easily imagine medicine continuing to employ the term, but in an eviscerated form, devoid of traditional connotations. At the same time, there must be some way of exposing students to issues of obligation and responsibility without igniting student fears that they are entering a career of victimhood.

The medical literature, meanwhile, has been curiously silent on this altruism/professionalism conundrum. Searches for "altruism" within medical literature databases capture a number of articles—virtually all of which focus on transplantation and the altruism of . . . donors (Brown-Saltzman et al. 2004). The theme of provider selflessness in turn is inconspicuously absent. Ironically, there are normative expectations regarding altruism within medical education, but they are almost singularly directed at patients—and with students as the demanding party. For medical students, patients are harlequins. They are both the recipients of medical care and "learning tools" (Baldwin et al. 1998; Gawande 2002; Christakis et al. 1993; George 1998). This clash of interests and identities surfaces most palpably among third- and fourth-year clerkship students, and first-year residents, all of whom can do little for, but learn much from patients. Within this overall context, it is students, eager for the opportunity to practice and master, can become angry (even indignant: "Who do they think they are?") when patients refuse to be "procedured." There are myths that circulate among medical students asserting the "fact" that patients in teaching hospitals get better care *because of* the extra eyes and redundancies that are built into the educational system. Studies supporting this rhetoric do not exist. Teaching hospitals may deliver better care (Allison et al. 2000; Rosenthal et al. 1997), but this "better" has not been linked in any causal way to a relationship between "number of times examined by students" and "quality of care."

The topic of the patient as a learning tool is both fascinating and complex, and so I will emphasize here that while society does benefit from having a well-trained physician corps (with students using this rationalization for why patients are "obligated" to acquiesce), the immediate patient does not directly benefit from having a lesser-trained person perform procedures on them. This is why patient consent under these circumstances truly is selfless (DeAngelis et al. 2004). When patients say "yes," the beneficiaries are students and not the acquiescing patient. In summary, when we look to medicine for signs of altruism, we find it most routinely with patients, not doctors.

Professionalism and Commercialism

When managed care and corporate medicine began its expansionary drive in the 1980s (both having a prior existence, but in a more sanguine form), the response by organized medicine was swift and unequivocal. Medical leaders identified "commercialism" as medicine's axis of evil and denounced the conflicts of interest that were enticing physicians (Angell 1993, 2000; Kassirer 1994, 1995, 1997a, 1997b, 1998; Kassirer and Angell 1997; Lundberg 1985, 1990, 1997, 2001; Relman 1980, 1987, 1991, 1993, 1997; Relman and Lundberg 1998). Military metaphors, long a staple in the oral and written culture of medicine, were aggressively deployed. Organized medicine declared itself to be at "war"—an "epic clash" between the cultures of commercialism and professionalism (McArthur and Moore 1997).

Twenty years later, these fears have proved to be prophetic. One does not have to travel far beyond the pages of the *New York Times*, the *Wall Street Journal*, *USA Today*, or business periodicals such as *Forbes*, *Fortune*, or *BusinessWeek* to discover just how commercial medicine has become and just how entrepreneurial physicians and medical researchers can be. And yet commercialism, like altruism, has an almost invisible presence in this book.

The overall issue of how best to represent and locate commercialism within any assessment of professionalism is a difficult yet unavoidable issue. One difficulty is tied to organized medicine's traditional ambivalence about conflicts-of-interest issues. Organized medicine publicly has denounced certain conflicts (e.g., self-referral) while remaining essentially silent (the qualification is purposeful) on others (e.g., selling patients to commercial clinical trial companies). This "ambivalence" is further compounded (for students and practitioners alike) when organized medicine fails to take formal, adjudicative steps against physicians who engate in clear-cut examples of conflict. The aforementioned sale of patients to clinical trials companies is a case in point. There are more than 40,000 clinical trials taking place in this country, today, requiring tens of thousands of patient-subjects overall (Winslow et al. 2000). Community physicians are an important source for these patients, and drug companies and private contract research organizations pay these clinicians handsomely for these patients—upward of $40,000 per patient for rare conditions (Eichenwald et al. 1999a, 1999b, 1999c; Klein 2003; *New York Times* 1999). A lecture on conflicts of interest will mean little if students (via the informal and hidden curriculums) routinely encounter physician–role models who earnestly tell them about the "consulting fees" they earn "in the service of science"—with fees that "just happen," in certain instances, to dwarf their clinical practice income.

There are broader issues afoot as well. If selling one's patients to a for-profit corporation is fundamentally antithetical to professionalism (and I posit here that it is), how is it that so many physicians engage in this practice and do so with impunity? (See Pound [2000], in addition to the above references, for examples of how widespread this practice has become.) This is not an issue that is best addressed at the level of curriculum. This is an issue where organized medicine must be willing and able to act in a proactive and decisive manner. Labeling such practices as "unprofessional" is not enough. Organized medicine also must sanction the offending physicians as well. What we have, instead, is an ethically awkward state of affairs where it appears that organized medicine views the recruitment and sale of patients as an acceptable practice. Once again we have an example of "mixed messages" where a lecture about commercialism and the dangers of conflicts of interest is effectively neutralized by antiprofessional influences within medicine's informal and hidden curricula.

Finally, we need to recognize that the problem of commercialism is more than "just" an out-of-sight, out-of-mind issue. Today, physicians who transform biomedical discoveries into marketable products, and then bring those products to Wall Street, are the new heroes of academic medicine. Faculty are urged (with salary and pay raises on the line) to adopt a more entrepreneurial orientation toward their work. Meanwhile, administrators are hard at work rewriting conflict-of-interest guidelines to allow (and encourage) faculty to be ever more enterprising. What then happens to all of those medical students who accompany these physicians on their patient care rounds and examinations? What happens when students identify these doctors as role models and flock to catch their "clinical pearls"—which are accompanied by not-so-subtle messages that the only *real* career in medicine is to exploit/maximize their access to patients and push for new medical discoveries? Will these students be able to discern what differentiates genuine conflicts of interest from those patient contacts where the primary of the patient truly is the guiding value? My own surmise is that there is a substantial and positive (statistical) relationship between the willingness of faculty to identify genuine conflicts of interest and the ability of students to tease out the nuances that are inevitably present in medical work. Conversely, the more routinized conflict-of-interest practices become, the less able students will be to even recognize (yet alone do something about) situations that contain the potential for unprofessional behavior.

A Closing Note

Organized medicine has taken impressive steps under the banner of professionalism. Since the mid 1980s, there has been a stunning and sustained commitment within medicine to advance the principles of professionalism. Considerable resources have been expended (time, energy, and resources) and considerable space has been earmarked for issues of professionalism in medical academic journals. I applaud—and concur—with Jordan Cohen's position in the preface to this volume that the most important task facing medical educators today is having our students "consistently demonstrate the attributes of medical professionalism."

There remains, however, one glaring problem. Medical educators cannot accomplish all of this alone. In fact, none of what organized medical education has accomplished thus far (and it is considerable) will matter a whit if organized medicine remains unwilling to bite that most distasteful of all bullets—namely, the implementation of a meaningful system of peer review—and do so with particular attention to what Cohen and other medical leaders have identified as the nemesis of professionalism: commercialism and self-interest. Metaphorically, all still can appear well within the monastery, but the city lights still beckon our students with the siren call of self-interest and entitlement. These lights also blur the boundaries between self-improvement and self-indulgence. If medical students are to internalize the "true meanings" of professionalism, then organized medicine will need to rid the streets (as best as possible) of these commercial enticements, for this is where our students go (and learn) after classes end and after their teachers have retired for the evening. Furthermore, organized medicine must take this painful and internally unpopular step and do all this in the most public of ways so that students—and the public at large—will know, beyond a shadow of a doubt, that organized medicine means what it says about professionalism being sacred and core. As it stands now, the current picture contains a multitude of conflicting messages. Commercialism is condemned (rhetorically it seems) while it also continues to flourish within the domains of clinical and research medicine.

The problems posed by commercialism are compounded by a particular fantasy. In this fantasy, medical schools will enculturate future students with the ways and mores of professionalism, and over time, these students will take the places of those currently practicing physicians—all of whom were trained in "preprofessional" times.

The fantasy's key chimera is that these raw recruits never come to the medical marketplace in dribs and drabs so that the forces of commercialism, inimitable within the current generation of practitioners, can wreak havoc with those carefully laid messages of service and selflessness. Instead—and somehow—these new physicians (who have schooled within pedagogically sophisticated, competency-oriented, and morally affirming learning environments) will be held in some form of social suspension, awaiting the retirement of all those never properly socialized physicians—so that, in one fell swoop, the new professionally competent physicians can move into place. Nothing distasteful or confrontational will need to happen. The "old" will disappear and the new will flower (professionally speaking). Within this fantasy, all that medical education needs is "a little more time."

Well, it's not going to happen—at least not this way. The reason has to do with the assumptions that underscore this Rip Van Winklesque scenario. To date, medicine has focused its professional attentions and resources almost exclusively on organized medical education—with a corresponding lack of attention to what is happening within clinical practice settings (which not so incidentally are the domains where the informal and the hidden curriculums hold sway). There are, of course, no "germ-free" learning environments within medical training. Actually, with the rise of commercialism, our sites of training are more germ infested than ever. And this is the point. How do we keep the classroom lessons from being undone in the clinic? The answer seems obvious (not easy, just obvious)—yet organized medicine continues to ignore the ever-encroaching marketplace of medicine.

In sum, the basic issue is whether organized medicine is going to take some of the energy it has lavished on medical education and begin to direct its efforts more toward the clinical practice environment—and in doing so make significant statements about what practicing physicians can and cannot do under the banner of professionalism. Moreover, organized medicine needs to infuse these steps with normative "teeth." This is not a matter of what physicians can and cannot do legally. This is an issue of *professionalism*. There is no point in touting professionalism in the classroom if students are left to precept with physicians who extol the legality of selling Amway products, facial creams, or research patients. Unfortunately, organized medicine has been sitting on the legal-professional fence so long that many practicing physicians are honestly confused about just what is and is not "professional." Nonetheless, if organized medicine fails to address issues of professionalism within the domains of clinical practice, then all it has done within its classrooms will be for naught.

As noted at the beginning of this chapter, this volume provides a benchmark for addressing issues of professionalism and its assessment. Within this quintal, I see five fundamental issues that must be taken into account in medicine's continuing march of professionalism. First, organized medicine must make clear its definition of professionalism and, in turn, its conception of commercialism—including specific points about the dynamics of conflict and conflation. Second, medical educators must not only establish formal curricula in practice environments that stress excellence and professionalism but also must harness and marshal the informal and hidden curricula of undergraduate, graduate, and continuing medical education to provide learners with a thematically consistent and seamless learning environments across the trajectory of lifelong medical learning. Third, we need to better attend to our vocabularies of success and failure. Fourth, and referring now to an issue not previously addressed in this chapter, we need to develop multiple learning environments across the continuum of medical education that will promote (and consistently reinforce) the principles of professionalism. Deviance (both positive and negative) is a functional and necessary part of all group dynamics and structure. We may, indeed, consistently stress the positive side of attributes and goals as a critical part of "group health," but nothing is accomplished if the pursuit of affirmation is built on a Lake Wobegon foundation. Whatever the particular focus or stage of training, tools to assess professionalism must be able to identify students and/or practitioners who reflect suspect as well as exemplary behaviors. Fifth, and most fundamental, professionalism is not a "thing." It is a process. Like the quarks of particle physics, professionalism does not function while "at rest." As such, professionalism must remain a topic and focus for debate and discussion. The surest enemy of professionalism is the assertion that we have developed the necessary measurement tools and learning environments—and thus we can call a halt to the arguments, debates, and discussions.

And so, organized medicine must act. This volume provides educators and regulators alike with a framework within which they can develop instruments and collect information for action. At the student and resident level, this action is the responsibility of deans and program directors. At the practicing physician level, the responsibility lies with professional societies and state medical boards.

Nonetheless, and positive affirmations notwithstanding, if organized medicine truly desires professionalism—if it actually (and actively) envisions a medicine that is reenergized by professionalism—then organized medicine is going to have to say "there's a new sheriff in town"—and mean it.

References

AAMC. Report 1. Learning Objectives for Medical Student Education: Guidelines for Medical Schools. Medical School Objectives Project. Washington, DC: Association of American Medical Colleges, 1998.

Allison JJ, Kiefe CI, Weissman N, Person SD, et al. Relationship of hospital teaching status with quality of care and mortality for Medicare patients with acute mi. JAMA. 2000;284:256–262.

American Journal of Bioethics. 2004;4(2):1–72.

Angell M. The doctor as double agent. Kennedy Inst Ethics J. 1993;3:2 79–286.

Angell M. Is academic medicine for sale? N Engl J Med. 2000;342;1516–1518.

Arnold L. Assessing professional behavior: yesterday, today, and tomorrow. Acad Med. 2002;77:502–515.

Baldwin DC Jr., Daugherty SR, Rowley BD. Observations of unethical and unprofessional conduct in residency training. Acad Med. 1998;73:1195–2000.

Beatty S. New wrinkle: hot at the mall: skin-care products from physicians: "cosmeceutical' creams tap antiaging market: questions about claims: Dr. Perricone's TV specials. Wall Street Journal 2003;A1, A8.

Becker H, Geer B, Hughes EC, Strauss AL. Boys in White: Student Culture in Medical School. Chicago, IL: University of Chicago Press, 1961.

Bosk CL. Forgive and Remember. Chicago, IL: University of Chicago Press, 1979.

Branch W, Kroenke K, Levinson W. The clinician-educator—present and future roles. J Gen Int Med. 1997;12(suppl):A1–A14.

Branch WT, Pels RJ, Lawrence RS, Arkey R. Becoming a doctor: critical-incident reports from third-year medical students. N Engl J Med. 1993;329:1130–1132.

Brown-Saltzman KB, Diamant A, Fineberg IC, Gritsch HA, et al. Surrogate consent for living related organ donation. JAMA. 2004;291:728–731.

Bucher R, Stelling JG. Becoming Professional. Beverly Hills, CA: Sage Publications, 1977.

Burack JH, Irby DM, Carline JD, Root RK, Larson EB. Teaching compassion and respect: attending physicians' responses to problematic behaviors. J Gen Int Med. 1999;14:49–55.

Christakis DA, Feudtner C. Ethics in a short white coat: the ethical dilemmas that medical students confront. Acad Med. 1993;68:249–254.

Christakis DA, Feudtner C. Temporary matters: the ethical consequences of transient relationships in medical training. JAMA. 1997;278:739–743.

Clouder L. Becoming professional: exploring the complexities of professional socialization in health and social care. Learn Health Soc Care 2003;2:213–222.

Croasdale M. Professional issues: balance becomes key to specialty pick: family practice and general surgery are taking the biggest hit, but fewer students are choosing medicine overall. Chicago, IL: American Medical News, 2003. Available at: http://www.AMNews.com. Accessed September 22, 2003.

DeAngelis CD, Drazen JM, Frizelle FA. Clinical trial registration: a statement from the international committee of medical journal editors. JAMA. 2004;292:1363–1364.

Doctor X. Intern. New York: Harper and Row, 1965.

Dorsey ER, Jarjoura D, Rutecki GW. Influence of controllable lifestyle on recent trends in specialty choice by US medical students. JAMA. 2003;290:1173–1178.

Eichenwald K, Kolata G. Research for hire: drug trials hide conflicts for doctors. New York Times, 1999a. Available at: http://www.nytimes.com/library/national/science/health/051799drug-trials-industry.html. Accessed May 16, 1999.

Eichenwald K, Kolata G. Research for hire: a doctor's drug studies turn into fraud. New York Times, 1999b. Available at: http://www.nytimes.com/library/national/science/health/051788drug-trials-industry-2.html. Accessed May 17, 1999.

Eichenwald K, Kolata G. Hidden interests—special report: when physicians double as entrepreneurs. New York Times, 1999c. Available at: http://www.nytimes.com/library/financial/113099medical-devices.html. Accessed November 30, 1999.

Eisner EW. The Educational Imagination: On the Design and Evaluation of School Programs. 2nd ed. New York: Macmillan, 1985.

Eron LD. Effect of medical education on medical students. J Med Educ. 1955;30:559–566.

Eron LD. The effect of medical education on attitudes: a follow-up study (pt 2). J Med Educ. 1958;33:25–33.

Gawande A. Complications: A Surgeon's Notes on an Imperfect Science. New York: Metropolitan Books, 2002.

George JH. Moral development during residency training. In: Scherpbier AJJA, Van Der Vleuten CPM, Rethans JJ, Van Der Steeg AFW, eds. Advances in Medical Education. Dordrecht: Kluwer Academic Publishers, 1997;747–748.

George JH. Med students enter the "lion's den." Philadelphia Bus J. 1998. Available at: http://philadelphia.bizjournals.com/philadelphia/stories/1998/06/08/focus1.html. Accessed September 24, 2004.

Ginsburg S, Regehr G, Hatala R, McNaughton N, Frohna A, Hodges B, Lingard L, Stern D. Context, conflict, and resolution: a new conceptual framework for evaluating professionalism. Acad Med. 2000;75(10 suppl):S6–S11.

Ginsburg S, Regehr G, Stern D, Lingard L. The anatomy of the professional lapse: bridging the gap between traditional frameworks and student perceptions. Acad Med. 2002;77:516–522.

Goffman E. The Presentation of Self in Everyday Life. Garden City, NY: Doubleday, 1959.

Goffman E. Interaction Ritual. New York: Pantheon, 1967.

Goldie JGS. The detrimental ethical shift towards cynicism: can medical educators help prevent it? Med Educ. 2004;38:232–538.

Haas J, Shaffir W. The professionalization of medical students: developing competence and a cloak of competence. Symb Interact. 1977;5:71–88.

Haas J, Shaffir W. Taking the role of doctor: a dramaturgical analysis of professionalization. Symb Interact. 1982;5:187–203.

Hafferty FW. Managed medical education. Acad Med. 1999;74:972–979.

Hafferty FW. In search of a lost cord: professionalism and medical education's hidden curriculum. In: Wear D, Bickel J, eds. Educating for Professionalism: Creating a Culture of Humanism in Medical Education. Iowa City, IA: University of Iowa Press, 2000; 11–34.

Hafferty FW. Greetings from the Lake Wobegon school of medicine: competencies, social control, and the future of American medical education. In: Proceedings of the Central Region Group on Educational Affairs, Association of American Medical Colleges, Spring Conference; March 15–18, 2001; Minneapolis, MN. Washington, DC: Association of American Medical Colleges.

Hafferty FW. What medical students know about professionalism. Mt Sinai J Med. 2002;69:385–397.

Hafferty FW. Unpublished class report. September 28, 2004.

Hafferty FW, Franks, R. The hidden curriculum, ethics teaching, and the structure of medical education. Acad Med. 1994;69:861–871.

Henningsen J. Why the numbers are dropping in general surgery: the answer no one wants to hear—lifestyle! Arch Surg. 2002;137:255–256.

Kassirer JP. Academic medical centers under siege. N Engl J Med. 1994;331:1370–1371.

Kassirer JP. Managed care and the morality of the marketplace. N Engl J Med. 1995;333:50–52.

Kassirer JP. Managing managed care's tarnished image. N Engl J Med. 1997a;337:338–339.

Kassirer JP. Our endangered integrity—it can only get worse. N Engl J Med. 1997b;336:1666–1667.

Kassirer JP. Managing care—should we adopt a new ethic? N Engl J Med. 1998;339:397–398.

Kassirer JP, Angell M. The high price of product endorsement. N Engl J Med. 1997;337:750.

Klass PA. Not Entirely Benign Procedure: 4 Years as a Medical Student. New York: G. P. Putnam's Sons, 1987.

Klein SA. Firm Cashes in on Drug Trials; Some Patients Worth Up to $37,000. Chicago: Crains Chicago Business, 2003. Available at: http://www.crainschicagobusiness.com. Accessed December 8, 2003.

Konner M. Becoming a Doctor: A Journey of Initiation in Medical School. New York: Penguin, 1987.

Lingard L, Garwood K, Szauter K, Stern D. The rhetoric of rationalization: how students grapple with professional dilemmas. Acad Med. 2001;76 (suppl):S45–S47.

Linzer M, Beckman H. Honor thy role models. J Gen Int Med. 1997;7:76–78.

Lundberg GD. Medicine—a profession in trouble? JAMA. 1985;253: 2879–2880.

Lundberg GD. Countdown to millennium: balancing the professionalism and business of medicine: medicine's rocking horse. JAMA. 1990;263: 86–87.

Lundberg GD. The business and professionalism of medicine. JAMA. 1997;278:1703.

Lundberg GD. Severed Trust: Why American Medicine Can't Be Fixed. New York: Basic Books, 2001.

Marion R. The Intern Blues: The Private Ordeals of 3 Young Doctors. New York: Ballantine Books, Fawcett-Crest, 1990.

Marion R. Learning to Play God: The Coming of Age of a Young Doctor. New York: Ballantine Books, Fawcett-Crest, 1993.

Marion R. Rotations: The 12 Months of Intern Life. New York: Harper-Collins, 1998.

McArthur JH, Moore FD. The two cultures and the health care revolution. JAMA. 1997;277:985–989.

Members of the Medical Professionalism Project. Medical professionalism in the new millennium: a physician charter. Ann Int Med. 2002:136: 243–246.

Merton RK, Reeder LG, Kendall PL. The Student-Physician: Introductory Studies in the Sociology of Medical Education. Cambridge, MA: Harvard University Press, 1957.

Morris R. Student soapbox: decent into cynicism. Student BMJ. 2000;8:203.

Motulsky H. Intuitive Biostatistics. New York: Oxford University Press, 1995.

New York Times. Patients for hire, doctors for sale. 1999 May 22;A12.

Nolen WA. The Making of a Surgeon. New York: Random House, Mid List Press, 1970.

Paukert JL. From medical student to intern: where are the role models? JAMA. 2001;285:2781.

Pound ET. Report: Rush in human clinical trials can lead to abuse: investigators cite misleading promotions, researchers recruiting their own patients. USA Today. 2000 June 12;A1,A9.

Relman AS. The new medical-industrial complex. N Engl J Med. 1980; 303:963–970.

Relman AS. Practicing medicine in the new business climate. N Engl J Med. 1987;316:1150–1151.

Relman AS. Shattuck lecture: the health care industry: where is it taking us? N Engl J Med. 1991;325:854–859.

Relman AS. What market values are doing to medicine. Natl Forum Atl Mthly. 1993;73:17–21.

Relman AS. Dr. Business. Washington DC: The American Prospect 1997;91–95.

Relman AS, Lundberg GD. Business and professionalism in medicine at the American Medical Association. JAMA. 1998;279:169–170.

Rice B. What's a doctor doing selling Amway? Med Econ. 1997;74:79.

Rosenthal GE, Harper DL, Quinn LM. Cooper GS. Severity-adjusted mortality and length of stay in teaching and nonteaching hospitals. JAMA. 1997;278:485–490.

Rowley BD, Baldwin DC Jr., Bay RC, Karpman RR. Professionalism and professional values in orthopedics. Clin Ortho Rel Res. 2000;387:90–96.

Schwartz RW, Jarecky RK, Strodel WE, Haley JV, Young B, Griffen WOJ. Controllable lifestyle: a new factor in career choice by medical students. Acad Med. 1989;64:606–609.

Schwartz RW, Haley JV, Williams C, Jarecky RK, Young B, Griffen WO Jr. The controllable lifestyle factor and students' attitudes about specialty selection. Acad Med. 1990;65:207–210.

Self DJ, Baldwin DC Jr. Does medical education inhibit the development of moral reasoning in medical students? A cross-sectional study. Acad Med. 1998;73(10 suppl):S91–S93.

Self DJ, Jecker NS, Baldwin DC Jr. The moral orientations of justice and care among young physicians. Camb Q Health Ethics. 2003;12:54–60.

Self DJ, Skeel JD. Facilitating healthcare ethics research: assessment of moral reasoning and moral orientation from a single interview. Camb Q Health Ethics. 1992;4:371–376.

Shem S. The House of God. New York: Dell, 1978.

Skeff KM, Mutha S. Role models: guiding the future of medicine. N Engl J Med. 1998;339:2015–2017.

Stern DT. Practicing what we preach? An analysis of the curriculum of values in medical education. Am J Med. 1998;104:569–575.

Testerman JK, Morton KR, Loo LK, Worthley JS, Lamberton HH. The natural history of cynicism in physicians. Acad Med. 1996;71(10 suppl): S43–S45.

Uhari M, Koddonen J, Nuutinen M, Rantala H, Lautala P, Vayrynen M. Medical student abuse: an international phenomenon. JAMA. 1994;271: 1049–1051.

Whitcomb ME. Fostering and evaluating professionalism in medical education. Acad Med. 2002;77:473–474.

Winslow R, Carrns A. Harris, MediciGroup join to recruit test patients. Wall Street Journal February 2000;10:B21.

Wright SM, Kern DE, Dolodner K, Howard DM, Brancati FL. Attributes of excellent attending-physician role models. N Engl J Med. 1998;339: 9186–9193.

Index